NURSING STUDENT
to
NURSING LEADER:
THE CRITICAL PATH TO
LEADERSHIP DEVELOPMENT

To Carolyn —
Thank you so
much for your
support of nursing
students! I hope
you enjoy the book.
  Carol A. Fetters Andersen,
          BSN, RN

NURSING STUDENT
to
NURSING LEADER:
THE CRITICAL PATH TO
LEADERSHIP DEVELOPMENT

Carol A. Fetters Andersen, BSN, RN

Dementia Care Specialist

1991/1992 President National Student Nurses' Association

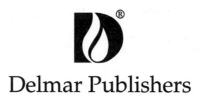

Delmar Publishers

an International Thomson Publishing company I(T)P®

Albany • Bonn • Boston • Cincinnati • Detroit • London • Madrid
Melbourne • Mexico City • New York • Pacific Grove • Paris • San Francisco
Singapore • Tokyo • Toronto • Washington

NOTICE TO THE READER

Publisher does not warrant or guarantee any of the products described herein or perform any independent analysis in connection with any of the product information contained herein. Publisher does not assume, and expressly disclaims, any obligation to obtain and include information other than that provided to it by the manufacturer.

The reader is expressly warned to consider and adopt all safety precautions that might be indicated by the activities herein and to avoid all potential hazards. By following the instructions contained herein, the reader willingly assumes all risks in connection with such instructions.

The publisher makes no representation or warranties of any kind, including but not limited to, the warranties of fitness for particular purpose or merchantability, nor are any such representations implied with respect to the material set forth herein, and the publisher takes no responsibility with respect to such material. The publisher shall not be liable for any special, consequential, or exemplary damages resulting, in whole or part, from the readers' use of, or reliance upon, this material.

Cover design: Scott Keidong

Delmar Staff

Publisher: William Brottmiller
Acquisitions Editor: Cathy L. Esperti
Project Editor: Patricia Gillivan

Production Coordinator: Barbara A. Bullock
Art and Design Coordinator: Timothy J. Conners
Editorial Assistant: Darcy Scelsi

Copyright © 1999
By Delmar Publishers
a division of International Thomson Publishing Inc.

I(T)P The ITP logo is a registered trademark under license.

Printed in the United States of America

For more information, contact:

Delmar Publishers
3 Columbia Circle, Box 15015
Albany, New York 12212-5015

International Thomson Publishing—Europe
Berkshire House
168-173 High Holborn
London, WC1V 7AA
England

Thomas Nelson Australia
102 Dodds Street
South Melbourne, 3205
Victoria, Australia

Nelson Canada
1120 Birchmount Road
Scarborough, Ontario
Canada, M1K 5G4

International Thomson Editores
Campos Eliseos 385, Piso 7
Col Polanco
11560 Mexico D F Mexico

International Thomson Publishing GmbH
Konigswinterer Strasse 418
53227 Bonn
Germany

International Thomson Publishing—Asia
60 Albert Street
#15-01 Albert Complex
Singapore 189969

International Thomson Publishing—Japan
Hirakawacho Kyowa Building, 3F
2-2-1 Hirakawacho
Chiyoda-ku, Tokyo 102
Japan

Dedication

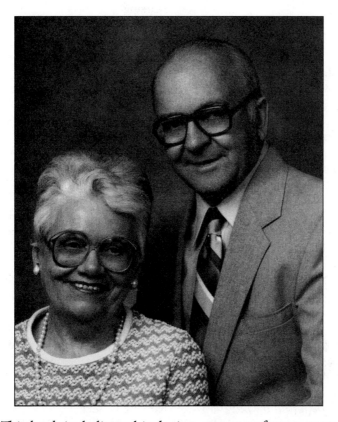

This book is dedicated in loving memory of my parents,
Ed Wandling (1918–1995) and June Wandling (1918–1996),
who helped me believe I could accomplish any dream,
and gave me a strong foundation of both faith in God and
humanity towards my fellow man, which has empowered
me to keep trying—even when I stumble or fall.
So thank you. For by your gift,
I'm a better nurse and a better leader.

I miss you both,
Carol

Contributors

RADM Carolyn Beth Mazzella, RN
Chief Nurse Officer, United States Public
Health Service
Rockville, MD
Biography can be found on page: xxii

Lucille A. Joel, RN, EdD, FAAN
First Vice-President International Council
of Nurses
Professor
Rutgers, The State University of
New Jersey
College of Nursing
Newark, NJ
Biography can be found on page: 16

Mary P. Tarbox, EdD, RN
Professor and Chair
Mount Mercy College
Department of Nursing
Cedar Rapids, IA
Biography can be found on page: 34

M. Louise Fitzpatrick, EdD, RN, FAAN
Dean and Professor
College of Nursing, Villanova University
Villanova, PA
Biography can be found on page: 46

Geraldene Felton, EdD, RN, FAAN
Executive Director, the National League
for Nursing Accrediting Commission
Past Dean University of Iowa–
College of Nursing
Iowa City, IA
Biography can be found on page: 64

Ellen M. Strachota, RN, PhD
Professor and Head of the Division of
Nursing
Grand View College
Des Moines, IA
Biography can be found on page: 76

Carol Toussie Weingarten, PhD, RN
Associate Professor
College of Nursing, Villanova University
Villanova, PA
Biography can be found on page: 86

Mary E. Foley, RN, MS
Director of Nursing
Saint Francis Memorial Hospital
San Francisco, CA
Biography can be found on page: 108

Michael L. Evans, PhD, RN, FACHE
Vice-President for Nursing Services
Presbyterian Hospital of Dallas
Dallas, TX
Biography can be found on page: 120

Pamela F. Cipriano, PhD, FAAN
Chief Operating Officer and Chief
Nursing Officer
Medical University of South Carolina
Charleston, SC
Biography can be found on page: 128

Tim Porter-O'Grady, EdD, PhD, FAAN
Senior Partner Tim Porter-O'Grady
Associates, Inc.
Assistant Professor—Emory University
Atlanta, GA
Biography can be found on page: 138

Diane J. Mancino, EdD, RN, CAE
Executive Director
National Student Nurses' Association
New York, NY
Biography can be found on page: 172

Virginia Trotter Betts, MSN, JD, RN, FAAN
Senior Advisor on Nursing and Policy to the Secretary and Assistant Secretary of Health
Washington, DC
Biography can be found on page: 182

Connie Vance, EdD, RN, FAAN
Dean and Professor of Nursing
College of New Rochelle School of Nursing
New Rochelle, NY
Biography can be found on page: 200

Mary Mallison, BSN, RN
Nursing Leader, Consultant, Journalist
Atlanta, GA
Biography can be found on page: 212

Carole A. Anderson, PhD, RN, FAAN
President of American Association of Colleges of Nursing
Dean-Ohio State University College of Nursing and Assistant Vice President for Health Sciences
Columbus, OH
Biography can be found on page: 228

Geraldine Polly Bednash, PhD, RN, FAAN
Executive Director
American Association of Colleges of Nursing
Washington, DC
Biography can be found on page: 229

Connie White Delaney, PhD, RN
Vice-Chair ANA Nursing Information & Data Set Evaluation Center Advisory Committee
Associate Professor
University of Iowa, College of Nursing
Iowa City, IA
Biography can be found on page: 240

Florence L. Huey, RN, MA
Managing Editor
Medscape Women's Health
New York, NY
Biography can be found on page: 256

Sharon A. Brigner, BSN, RN
Neurology Unit
National Institutes of Health Clinical Center
Bethesda, MD
Biography can be found on page: 272

Beverly L. Malone, PhD, RN, FAAN
President
American Nurses Association
Washington, DC
Biography can be found on page: 290

Sr. Rosemary Donley, RN, PhD, FAAN
Vice-President, Office of Advancement, Sisters of Charity of Seton Hill
Ordinary Professor of Nursing
The Catholic University of America
Washington, DC
Biography can be found on page: 316

Contents

Preface

This book is a collection of essays on a variety of experiences and issues that either consciously or unconsciously provide continuity and wholeness to your nursing career. Each of these processes impact your critical path to leadership development in nursing. They reflect milestones that ease transition from the role of nursing student to full-fledged member of the discipline. In this volume, you will find essay perspectives from two recent nursing student leaders who are transitioning into active nursing leadership roles, as well as perspectives from some of today's most influential nursing leaders.

This collection is an important supplement to your nursing leadership and nursing issues classes. It is intended for the use of students preparing for entry into nursing, as well as for those preparing for active nursing leadership roles. Each topic is treated in a provocative, sometimes tongue-in-cheek, fashion with the intent of stimulating opinion, critical thinking, and controversy. Use of these essays, critical-thinking questions, and suggested additional readings or activities as a focus for individual thought and group discussion is proposed as a learning experience to shape the attitudes and values necessary for a successful career adjustment.

We are very excited to bring you this book and provide you with an opportunity to learn from nursing leaders' experiences and visions about the critical path to leadership development. Remember, the nursing leader of tomorrow is YOU!

Carol A. Andersen, BSN, RN

Acknowledgments

As author and editor of *Nursing Student to Nursing Leader: The Critical Path to Leadership Development,* I would like to take this opportunity to thank the people who helped and supported me in my efforts to make the vision of this book a reality.

First, let me thank the four people who have encouraged me since the idea for this book began—Dr. Lucille Joel, Dr. Robert Piemonte, Dr. Diane Mancino, and Dr. Ellen Strachota. Your encouragement and mentorship over the past few years as the book developed helped me to stay focused on the value and integrity of this project.

Second, I'd also like to thank the contributing authors who joined me in my dedication to providing nursing students and nurses with a new unique text to use in their leadership development. A text that not only tells the history and details of nursing over the years, but through the sharing of nurse leader's personal paths and perspectives, transmits the passion and life of nursing as well. The contributing authors are each listed with their chapters in the Table of Contents, and I know you will find value and enjoyment in each one's valuable work. Thank you each for your contributions and faith in me. It means more to me than I can ever express.

Third, many thanks to the members of the team at Delmar Publishers. You have supported my work as we brought together a group of diverse authors and subjects into one book centered around a leadership model that I developed. The following people have been a valuable asset to me both in support and technical advice:

William Brotmiller—Publisher

Cathy L. Esperti—Acquisitions Editor

Darcy Scelsi—Editorial Assistant

Barbara A. Bullock—Production Coordinator

Patricia Gillivan—Project Editor

Timothy J. Conners—Art and Design Coordinator

Thank you for your hard work and dedication to me as an author, and to the book.

Fourth, my thanks go to the reviewers for their suggestions and ideas as the project developed. Reviewer's work is the part that can often be distasteful to authors, at first glance. But, you have challenged me and all of us to look deeply into the meaning behind our words and have assisted us to achieve what I believe will be a valuable contribution to nursing literature. You have also taught me the necessity to stand up for the words and issues that are paramount to the integrity of the work and to let go of those that are not needed. I've learned a great deal. So, thank you. In many ways, you've made me a better author and editor.

Next, I offer my thanks to my colleagues who have supported my work. First, to the registered nurses at Olsten Health Services who serve on the RN Team that I led as Case Manager during the book's production. You are all professionals, and adjusted schedules as needed so that I could meet the demands placed on me by this project. Second, to my professors and fellow students at the University of Iowa for supporting me and approving of my flexible schedule as I balanced my various roles. The graduate program at the University of Iowa College of Nursing is exceptional, and the graduate advisor Lori Anderson, MA, and my thesis Chair, Dr. Kathleen Buckwalter, RN, have helped me stay on track. I'm pleased to say I expect to graduate with my MSN, CNS in Gerontology in 1998. Thank you all.

And last, but never least I owe my deepest gratitude to my family:

To my husband Harvey who brings joy, faith, love, and peace to every day of my life and has been my best editorial advisor and friend throughout the project. I owe a lifetime of smiles and cackling laughter.

To my son John (J. R.) and my daughter Jamie. Thank you for sharing me and being my best cheerleaders. Both you and nursing are the passions of my life. The opportunity to make the world a better place for you both and to leave nursing better than I've found it are my constant goals. I hope you'll use this book as your example that you too can accomplish any dream.

I have been blessed with skills and am grateful. But mostly, I have been blessed with wonderful mentors, supporters, a loving family including my brother Don Wandling, and good friends—many who are part of this project. Thank you all for placing your faith in my talents and abilities, and for encouraging me to hang on to my dream.

Foreword

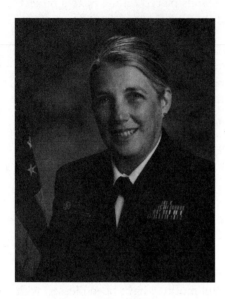

RADM Carolyn Beth Mazzella,
RN

It is a privilege to introduce Carol Andersen's work *Nursing Student to Nursing Leader*. She has thoughtfully explored and mapped out the critical path to leadership development that for many of us began with NSNA and culminated in a career position.

NSNA was indeed a "leadership practicum" during my years as NSNA President, 1970–1971. It was a pivotal organization in student activism in health and health care—a crucible testing professional and national interests, and a proving ground for personal convictions and practice. What I learned and gained from that experience, from work with the Nursing Students Association of South Dakota (NSASD) the previous year, and as the NSNA elected consultant the following year, has been unrivaled in my career. Those lessons were singular contributors to the development of a nursing leader—if the Chief Nursing position can be so characterized.

NSNA taught me to hear and seek to understand divergent viewpoints, and then to analyze and synthesize the positive elements into a coherent and cohesive consensus and plan of action. It taught me how to move from thought and desire to activism, and gave me the opportunity to dare to implement those ideas. And, it provided me the opportunity to work "long term" on the "big picture." NSNA gave me opportunities to see beyond the province of localities or profession into the broader world of health and health care for a Nation. My commitment to public health, to health as a right for all peoples, and to nursing's responsibility to advocate and agitate for health are directly attributable to those experiences.

Andersen identifies key "stones" in the path to leadership—courage, commitment, direction or purpose, and unity buttressed by education and professionalism. These stones are truly diamonds under cover. Leaders cannot lead without standing firmly upon them. My courage to face the frontier of the unknown and the unfamiliar is proportional to my commitment to health for all. My purpose to assure access to basic health care for all people, especially the most vulnerable and underserved is only achieved by bringing others to the work—in unity. One cannot achieve lasting success without working for the societal acceptance of the goal and the investment of the necessary resources.

This brings us to the current challenge of nursing's leaders—mentorship. Andersen carefully and correctly states that mentorship is not cloning our own image. It is the regeneration of enthusiasm and altruism with a new perspective, fostered by shared experience, strength, and hope. I have not accomplished all I dreamed—but I have begun. In order to carry-on and achieve what I may not have even dared to dream, I must imbue another with those aspirations and dedication. Mentorship begins as a nursing student and must continue throughout our professional life. Mentorship is not a generational passing of the baton, but a daily revitalization of spirit.

Carl Sandburg believed that "nothing happens, unless first a dream." When I went to nursing school, that was a dream. Working with NSASD was a dream that took me to a national office with NSNA. NSNA was the dream that opened new doors, introduced new people, and created new frontiers far beyond my imaginings or deepest hopes. As a candy striper in South Dakota in the 60s, I never knew or dared to dream that one day I would be the Chief Nurse of the U.S. Public Health Service. The fulfillment of those dreams leaves one with a tremendous sense of humility and responsibility. A responsibility to assure that the critical path to nursing leadership is sustained and illuminated so that another can accomplish the journey from *Nursing Student to Nursing Leader.*

RADM Carolyn Beth Mazzella,

RN

RADM Carolyn "Beth" Mazzella is the Chief Nurse Officer (CNO) for the U.S. Public Health Service (PHS). As the PHS Chief Nurse Officer, she serves as nursing's voice to the Surgeon General on nursing issues related to professional practice, personnel activities, and advocacy to and for nurses of both the Civil Service and the Commissioned Corps within the PHS. She represents more than 6,000 nurses, of whom more than 1,000 are commissioned officers. The Chief Nurse's functions include direct response to events and issues, policy and position development, advice and guidance to the Surgeon General and the eight PHS agencies. RADM Mazzella also serves as liaison and spokesperson between national and international professional associations and public groups. This entails broad oversight of nursing programs, research, and practice.

RADM Mazzella received her Bachelor of Arts in Nursing in 1971 from Augustana College in Sioux Falls, South Dakota; her Masters of Science from Northern State University in Aberdeen, South Dakota in guidance and counseling; and her Master's in Public Administration from the University of South Dakota in Vermillion. She began her career in 1971 as a Public Health Nursing Intern and went on to spend nearly 16 years with the Indian Health Service as a community health nurse, nurse educator, and Aberdeen Area Hospital Nursing Consultant.

In 1988, RADM Mazzella joined the National Health Services Corps and was instrumental in the development and implementation of PHS recruiting initiatives. From 1990–1996, she served as Deputy Director of the Division of Scholarships and Loan Repayment and administered and managed more than $80 million (FY1995) in seven scholarship and loan repayment programs. RADM Mazzella credits her leadership roles and skills to the many leadership development opportunities she experienced as a nursing student in South Dakota, and while she served as President of the National Student Nurses Association in 1970–1971.

A Note from
the Author:
The Stepping Stones—
From Nursing Student
to Nursing Leader

A s we explore the path to leadership development in nursing, we begin by under-standing why a *Critical Path to Leadership Development in Nursing* is so needed today. In Part 1, we will look at the student's perspective to the path and start to define the path itself. In Part 2, we will explore the path of a seasoned nurse leader who is known nationally and internationally as she shares her Life Review as an ANA President. This review allows you a personal glimpse into a nurse leader's views on the path of leadership. Our journey begins.

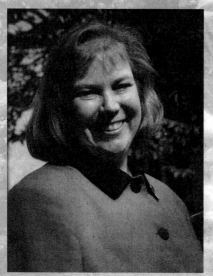

Photo courtesy of Bob Dunphy

Carol A. Andersen,

BSN, RN

Carol Andersen (formerly Carol A. Fetters, BSN, RN) served as President of the National Student Nurses' Association in 1991–1992. She was remarried on Christmas Eve 1996, and lives with her husband Harvey, son John, and daughter Jamie in Urbandale, IA. Carol is an experienced nursing professional and strong patient advocate. Her specialty is dementia care, and she is committed to optimal quality of life and optimal independence for dementia patients and their families from onset through the disease process, including death. In April 1995, Carol was co-presenter of a concurrent session on dementia care at the Mid-American Congress on Aging Convention.

Carol graduated in 1992 with her Bachelor of Science in Nursing from Grand View College in Des Moines, IA. Following graduation, she worked for two and a half years at the Veteran's Administration Medical Center (KVAMC) in Knoxville, IA, on their long-term care dementia unit as a staff nurse, RN Case Manager, and Unit Coordinator. Carol was the author of the *KVAMC Standard of Care on Wandering,* Co-Chair of the Nursing Research Committee, Co-Chair of the KVAMC Assault Task Force, and the KVAMC Unit CQI Coordinator for the long-term care dementia unit. Carol began work during this time at the University of Iowa, on her degree of Masters of Science in Nursing, as a Clinical Nurse Specialist in Gerontology with an additional focus in Informatics. She plans to complete her degree and her thesis work in 1998. From 1995–1998, Carol has worked in home care for Olsten Health Services in Des Moines. Her role with Olsten has been as an RN Case Manager.

More biographical information about the author can be found on page 304.

INTRODUCTION: PART 1

The Critical Path to Leadership Development–The Student's Perspective

INTRODUCTION

The topic of health care in the United States has been a revolving centerpiece of our political debates over the years. More recently, we observed and participated in debates involving national reform of our health care system. The newspapers, television broadcasts, and the internet kept us informed of the current hot issues about providing adequate health care to our citizens.

As Americans, we were exposed to various ideas of how to solve our health care and budgetary problems. Or, if not solutions, at least impassioned pleas for the need to find answers. And yet, as a country, we still struggle for ways to find consensus on how to meet even basic health care needs for many of our citizens. Nursing leaders of the past have challenged us to become change agents and leaders in our society. Leaders who will bring about the needed health reforms of our day.

In 1986, Jessie Scott, then Director of the Division of Nursing of the U.S. Public Health Service asked Mary Ann Garrigan, a faculty member at the Boston University (BU) School of Nursing (who established the Nursing Archive at Mugar Library at BU), to identify some common characteristics of leaders in nursing. Ms. Garrigan replied, ". . . Courage. To work toward a goal when support is not forthcoming; to be willing to start again in a new direction; to believe in yourself and the worth of the work you are doing" (Garrigan, 1986, p. 4).

Martha E. Rogers, one of nursing's theorists, in the text titled, *Changing Patterns of Nursing Education,* commented on a quote from Hafdan Mahler, the former Director General of the World Health Organization (WHO). Mr. Mahler stated "that if nurses all over the globe who shared a common conviction about primary health care would come together as one force they would be the powerhouse behind achieving health for all." Martha Rogers went on to say that the change Mr. Mahler described is coming, and that nurses around the world would help bring it about (Rogers, 1987, p. 130). Nursing's leaders have challenged us to see the needs, have the courage to bring about change, and work toward health for all. These are extensive and exciting goals that will continue to challenge the profession as well as nursing's future leaders.

During 1991–1992, I had the privilege of serving as President of the National Student Nurses' Association. I became increasingly aware of the need for a clearly defined critical path to leadership development for nursing students if our profession intends for us to be both empowered and qualified to become the future leaders in health care reform.

To accomplish those goals, you will need to be actively involved in your own leadership development. You will need a leadership text that: shares the path to leadership as well as the outcome; combines not only the history and facts about nursing but also nursing's passion, its voice, and its vision; prepares and empowers you while still a student to also become one of *Nursing's leaders*—rather than a text that focuses on preparing you to become a nursing leader in one specific setting. And finally, you will need a text that illuminates for all of nursing's future leaders a framework for the critical path to leadership development.

That is how the concept, passion, commitment, and outcome of this book became a reality. Through the various nurse leader's stories and visions found within this text, it is our collective hope that you will scrutinize our paths and ideas, glean the most valuable stepping stones for your own path, and depart from your experiences with us empowered, visionary, and committed to walking beside us towards nursing's vision.

OUR JOURNEY BEGINS

I invite you to review with me the need for both health care reform and an effective way to train leaders for that reform. We will explore some of the current leadership development opportunities that are available to you as nursing students. We will define the framework for your own path to leadership development. And finally, we will be challenged to establish our future vision for nursing—one that emphasizes commitment, direction, and a spirit of unity.

HEALTH CARE REFORM

The health care system in the United States could more appropriately be called an illness care system. Frequently, because of lack of funding and inequities in access to affordable preventative/health promotion and community based treatments, health care dollars have been spent on costly acute care. The result has been that too many Americans delay care until they are too sick to go without it. This focus on costly acute care has impacted our economy and is now demanding our collective attention to find solutions.

In spite of the levels of technology we have attained in acute care, when we look at our country's health statistics, we find some surprising health outcomes. In 1991, I wrote an article for *The American Nurse* and talked about those health statistics. "More than 60 million Americans are either uninsured or underinsured. The nation's infant mortality rate is often equated with that of third world nations. Homelessness, inadequate immunizations, lack of prenatal care, the needs of an expanding geriatric population, the need for excellence in treatment options—including compassionate care for AIDS patients and their families—are some of the challenges facing our society" (Fetters, 1991, p. 2). These challenges and the related problems of geographical and financial access to care often lead some of our citizens to avoid treatment. Although we have seen federal legislative efforts to improve and maintain access to health insurance (such as the Insurance Portability Law resulting from the Kennedy-Kassebaum Bill), and some collaborative efforts between the public and private sectors of health care funding, we still have millions of Americans falling through the cracks without access to even basic health care. In our nation's health care debates and decisions those citizens' voices often go unheard. Nursing must remain committed to advocating for those patients who have no voice.

Today, we see federal legislative efforts to shift fiscal responsibilities and moral responsibilities for programs that address injustices in access to health care back to the states. The good news is that this can lead to some important community level decisions about hospitals and clinics sharing services when possible, rather than having each facility buy every piece of diagnostic equipment available. These will be tough changes for us to accomplish when we have been accustomed to thinking more was better. It will also require that we give attention to providing care to patients in rural settings close to their homes. As a result, there will be a need for primary care providers in those rural settings, including Advanced Practice Nurses. And finally, the development and access to telemedicine will be encouraged. The bad news is that this shift of responsibilities could be devastating to states that are unprepared to meet the financial burden of funding and administering such programs. Do you know the status of your community? As state legislatures address these health care access issues, it is essential that nurses are there. Now is a critical time for nurse leaders to consider running for state legislature positions and seek appointment to state legislative committees.

Since we will not have a blank check for health care in each state, we will be faced with rationing care in some way to meet the determined critical needs of our state's citizens. Although critical care or acute care has taken a large portion of the health care dollars in the past, that may not be where each state decides to allocate the majority of their funds. Determining who will receive coverage for what services will pull at our collective conscience. As we ration care, are we really ready in the states to accept the moral responsibilities for our citizens when their assistance options run out? Officials report that in some states over half the homeless population is made up of children and families. We also find in both the uninsured and underinsured population that people are forced to choose between medicine and food. It is indeed much easier to discuss budgetary cuts impersonally as a number on a page. But in the states and communities where those numbers have a face, are we still prepared to deny basic services? How will you react?

It is imperative that we clearly understand the financial impact of our current health care system. Health care costs are consuming an increasing share of our gross national product (GNP). In 1991, the United States spent $756 billion on health care (National Leadership Coalition for Health Care Reform, 1991, p. 2). If our health care system continues to grow at the same rate, we are projected to spend between $2.1 and $2.7 trillion on health care as a nation by the year 2000 (U.S. Department of Commerce, 1991, pp. 1–6). As nursing's future leaders, we will need to keep a current picture of both the financial impact of our current health care system and our nation's health care statistics. These are the facts that we must bring to the decision table with us as we help determine where we go from here with health care in the United States.

In the area of health care and many other areas of public concern, the nation is looking towards leaders who will be change agents on their behalf. In recent presidential races, as well as in congressional elections, we have witnessed increasing demands by the public to find leaders who will speak out for the public's needs regardless of political party affiliation. The public desires leaders who can effectively work together to bring about needed changes. I hope this is striking some familiar chords as it becomes clear that the public deserves and demands that the various parties involved in health care also work together for change. Indeed, our country's current and future leaders in legislative roles, insurance, and both in medicine and in nursing would be well served to understand the importance of developing effective skills in collaboration.

THE CRITICAL PATH TO LEADERSHIP DEVELOPMENT

In a research study conducted as part of the National Ad Council's project called NCNIP (National Commission on Nursing Implementation Project) that promoted the image of nursing to the public in 1990, results showed that the public overwhelmingly viewed nurses as the most qualified to help reform the health care system. They viewed nurses as their strongest patient advocates (McCarty, 1991, p. 1). As nurses, we see the need for change and have the public's vote of confidence to bring that change about. But will you, I, and tomorrow's nursing leaders rise to the challenge? Or will we merely sit back and only react to changes orchestrated by someone else?

The nursing leaders of the future will not just appear. It is our professional responsibility to help develop our own leadership and the leadership of those nursing students who will follow after us by clearly defining the path that will help create tomorrow's leaders. There are stepping stones within that path that nursing students currently utilize to varying degrees. They are the stepping stones that involve the areas of education, practice, professional nursing involvement, mentoring, and networking. By emphasizing the completeness of the path, and increasing the efficacy of its use, we can help future leaders rise to meet the challenges they will face. So, the critical path to leadership development in nursing begins to take shape.

Education

One of the first stepping stones that you will experience as a nursing student is *education*. Starting now you need to be exposed to the various theories of leadership that you can utilize in your future profession. Today, curriculums in nursing must reflect the need for primary health care, the movement towards community based care, nursing practice that meets cultural diversity needs, and nursing research that validates appropriate interventions that lead to definable positive outcomes for patients in both improved quality of life and improved wellness. We must learn to articulate what nursing does and the impact that quality nursing care has on outcomes. We must understand and be actively involved in the ever changing environment of health care.

There are many leadership models that can be used by nurses in their roles as leaders and change agents. You'll find numerous buzz words in leadership theories today: connective leadership; transformational leadership; team leadership; situational leadership, and many others that will be valuable for you to understand. One specific leadership theory that can be especially helpful to newer nursing leaders was developed by Paul Hersey and Kenneth Blanchard. The situational leadership model that they published, in its 1988 form, was based on the "interplay among (1) the amount of guidance and direction (task behavior) a leader gives, (2) the amount of socioeconomic support (relational behavior) a leader provides, and (3) the readiness level that the followers exhibit in performing a specific task, function, or objective" (Hersey & Blanchard, 1988, pp. 169–201). This model can help nursing's future leaders develop the skills to assess a situation and, with the parties involved, choose the most appropriate leadership style to accomplish the goal at hand. It encourages us to learn that good leaders also know how to follow. We have only touched the surface in this area, and I recommend further exploration by you or your class in leadership theories and areas such as conflict resolution. As a suggestion, these may be good areas for you and some fellow students to cover in a seminar presentation. Also, through formal and informal educational offerings sponsored by nursing student or nursing groups you can be exposed to a wide variety of leadership theories that can help you function as an effective leader when new and challenging situations arise. Begin today internalizing a commitment to lifelong learning. The dedication, passion, commitment, and drive that this philosophy requires will provide you with the energy and rigor needed to become one of nursing's leaders in the twenty-first century.

Supportive Involvement in Practice

The second stepping stone you'll begin to experience as you enter clinical rotations in your courses involves the *practice* of nursing. Through supportive involvement in practice you can begin to flourish as a leader. As a student, you bring new and fresh ideas and commitment to your clinical practice.

Our society as a whole, including health care, is changing at a more significant rate than ever before. We know that change can cause stress as people react to it differently, especially unplanned change. Often this leads people to cling to the familiar and resist new ideas. As a future leader, it is important that you are sensitive to this very real concern for individuals. As a result of reacting to unplanned change in health care settings, there is more of a tendency for some practicing nurses to avoid straying from their established routines and ideas. Unfortunately it still happens in some settings that new grads are viewed as idealistic. I try to point out to nursing students when I speak on this status quo philosophy that experiencing practice can help us *all* see both the strengths and shortcomings of our knowledge, ideas, and practice. Carl Sandburg once wrote, "Nothing happens, unless first a dream" (from the poem, "Washington Monument by Night," 1922). In nursing, the shortcomings of knowledge and ideas (theory) must be weighed and explored to see if problems that arise are with current practice (application of theory), or with a theory in its present form. The challenge of overcoming resistance should not dissuade you as a student or new nurse from dreaming and discovering new and better ways for us to practice.

I am absolutely convinced that if we, in nursing, squelch student's and new graduate's critical thinking and creative problem solving by insisting on cloning them in our image, we will single-handedly destroy the nursing leaders of tomorrow. Instead, as nurses, we must all continue to apply new ideas, and clinical and outcome nursing research utilization to our daily practice.

Nursing leaders and nursing students together will need to explore effective internship, externship, and preceptor programs as practice moves more and more towards community based care. While working for Olsten Health Services for the past two and a half years, I have encouraged them as an innovator and advocate of quality patient care, to explore the development of a national preceptor/internship program in the company for new nursing graduates. In the past, the rule of thumb has been that a new nurse needs at least one year of medical-surgical nursing experience before entering home health care. The problem for new nurses now is that those jobs are not available in many settings. With growing technology and the market need for more community based care, dynamic home care companies are well poised to be proactive by working with nursing leaders and nursing students to develop the transitional path for the home health nurses of tomorrow. You must, as one of nursing's future leaders, become an active participant in decisions that will affect both our profession and the patients/clients that we will serve.

Professional Involvement

Third, another vital stepping stone in the critical path to leadership development is *involvement in professional nursing organizations*. For you as a nursing student, that involvement begins by joining the National Student Nurses Association (NSNA). In 1991, Diane J. Mancino, executive director of NSNA stated, "Over four decades, thousands of nursing students have experienced first hand leadership development and organizational analysis through participation in all three levels (national, state, and school) of NSNA. This exposure provides students with important new skills in dealing with the vast complexities of a large association. When graduation arrives, NSNA alumni comfortably make the transition to state nurses associations and to complex work situations. Without question, NSNA is the leadership practicum that broadens the boundary of a nursing student's formal education and reaches far beyond the classroom setting by providing opportunities for interaction on state and national levels" (Mancino, 1991, p. 5).

The American Nurses Association uses a federation model for membership, which means that as a new nurse you will join your state nurse's association and the state is the member of ANA. In many states, graduates who join their state nurse's associations within six months of graduation and licensure, receive a 50 percent discount on their first year's membership dues. In some states in 1996, free first year memberships were offered to graduates who were NSNA members, and met that same criteria. This financial incentive sends a clear message to you as a nursing student that professional involvement is an important step in becoming a future nurse leader. The health care environment is changing daily—and along with it, the future of nursing. As nurses, we no longer have the luxury of delaying professional and political involvement. As a future nurse leader, you must quickly become articulate in the discussion regarding nursing and patient care.

Will you be involved and proactive to change? Or will nursing and health care change without your input? We have all spent countless hours preparing to be the nurses of tomorrow. What will *you* do to positively impact nursing's future and to advocate for quality patient care?

Mentoring

Fourth, it is important that you understand the value of nursing leaders mentoring students and new graduates into leadership roles. Your next step in the path should be onto the stepping stone of *mentoring*. The state nurse's associations who offer discounted or free first year memberships to graduates are now following up with those new members by offering mentoring programs on the district and state level to encourage active involvement.

It is absolutely critical that as you have been mentored, you strive to mentor other future nurse leaders. In an editorial which appeared in the October, 1991, issue of the *American Nurse,* Deborah Smith, MN, RN wrote about the importance of mentoring and socialization of nursing students. She writes, "Each of us has an opportunity to influence the future by helping to create the right kind of twenty-first century nurse. Support autonomy, not dependence. Recognize sound performance and good judgment. Build self-esteem, not sacrifice. Encourage creativity, not conformity. Reward thinking, not obedience. Foster professionalism and commitment. Stimulate participation in NSNA and ANA. Promote accountability. Nurture excellence" (Smith, 1991, p. 4). I cannot find a more articulate description of the mentoring role that will be required of us as we help develop the nursing leaders of tomorrow.

Networking

Fifth, and finally, the critical path to leadership development in nursing includes the valuable stepping stone of *networking*. I would define networking as the process of developing and utilizing a web of contacts or connections that one can access for education, influence, opportunities, and support. In nursing, you will want to develop your own network of contacts or connections. These may include some or all of the following groups: teachers, fellow students, NSNA leaders, clinical nurse leaders, nursing leaders, business and political leaders, insurance leaders, health care leaders, community leaders, and others that can help you as you work to obtain goals. Later in the book (Chapter 13), I have included some exercises for you to do involving networking. These exercises are designed to help you begin developing your own networking potential. Networking is a process that is best understood by practicing it. I have a creativity exercise that I like to share with nursing students when I am invited to speak to them. It involves solving some word puzzles, and requires a great deal of creativity and abstract thought. Independently, very few students can solve over half the problems. But when they are allowed to network with their peers to find answers, almost all the answers are soon discovered. I enjoy the exercise as much as they do, because it provides a fun method for me to share the value of working with others to solve problems. This is a valuable lesson for nursing's future leaders who will be active in health care reform.

ESTABLISHING NURSING'S VISION

As we move along the stepping stones in our path which involve education, practice, professional nursing involvement, mentoring, and networking, we are led to look ahead to nursing's future vision of health for our nation, and our profession's role in that health.

That vision is still taking shape. The future participants in the vision are being trained, and with the shape of that training, our path solidifies and our vision receives direction. Our predecessors in nursing still call out to us to proceed in a spirit of unity with the welfare of our patients driving our movement forward. Nurses have been the advocates for patient rights, for quality care, and for preventative care for generations. If ever there was a time that you as a nurse or future nurse should be actively involved at the decision table for health care in the United States, I am convinced that it is today.

UTILIZING THE CRITICAL PATH

We have reviewed together the critical path to leadership development for tomorrow's nursing leaders, and have looked at some alarming health statistics that currently exist in the United States. I hope you found it refreshing to realize that the public views nurses as their advocates and the change agents who can successfully help them obtain primary health care—which most view as each person's right.

The current stepping stones to our critical path include (1) *education:* both formal and informal; (2) *practice* and the clear vision that results when the environment is supportive; (3) *professional nursing involvement* (in NSNA, SNA/ANA, and Specialty Nursing Organizations), which develops strength and depth of leadership; (4) *mentoring* that occurs as nursing leaders challenge, support, involve, and encourage students and new registered nurses; (5) *networking* contacts and connections that nursing students can develop while still in nursing school and later in practice—both within nursing and with other disciplines as well.

What an exciting moment, when nursing students grasp the concept that their peers and the nursing leaders they meet will be their colleagues throughout their professional careers. This glimpse of being one student or one nurse in practice, and yet being a part of a nation-wide and even a world-wide profession is life changing! That life changing event moves us into active roles of collaboratively helping develop nursing's future vision.

As we utilize more areas of the critical path, we will become more and more the leaders and change agents that can make that vision a reality. It will demand leaders with commitment to health for all and a strong knowledge base. A base that through critical thinking and creative problem solving will provide direction to nursing's vision. As we move toward that vision, we must hold fast to our patient advocacy and be leaders in efforts to promote healthy communities and access to affordable quality health care for all of our citizens.

MEETING THE DEMANDS OF CHANGE

Our nation needs to develop leaders who understand that effective health care reform begins when the various parties in health care work to effectively communicate and collaborate together. Nursing took a proactive step towards beginning that communication and collaboration by developing *Nursing's Agenda for Health Care Reform.* The debates on national health care reform have taken a back seat to debate about budgetary demands on social entitlement programs such as Medicare, Social Security, and Medicaid.

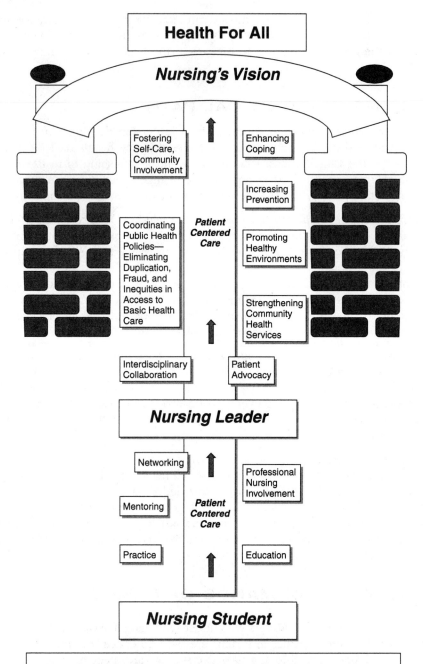

Health For All

Nursing's Vision

Fostering Self-Care, Community Involvement

Enhancing Coping

Increasing Prevention

Patient Centered Care

Coordinating Public Health Policies— Eliminating Duplication, Fraud, and Inequities in Access to Basic Health Care

Promoting Healthy Environments

Strengthening Community Health Services

Interdisciplinary Collaboration

Patient Advocacy

Nursing Leader

Networking

Professional Nursing Involvement

Mentoring

Patient Centered Care

Practice

Education

Nursing Student

The Critical Path To Leadership Development In Nursing

This led nursing to respond to market changes that are occurring in a different forum. A new document is being developed by ANA to address the current area where we are experiencing health care reform. That area involves managed care. While our forum and focus is now different than in *Nursing's Agenda for Health Care Reform,* I believe that the central tenets of the agenda are no less applicable to tomorrow's health care environment. Whether future reform takes place on a state by state level, through managed care, piece-meal, or resurfaces as national reform, nursing's future leaders will find the overall guidance in *Nursing Agenda's* central themes valuable. Those themes call for accessible, affordable, quality health care for all citizens, at least at a minimum basic level. (If you do not have a copy of *Nursing's Agenda for Health Care Reform,* one is located in the back of this book in Appendix A.) This change in direction we have experienced, as nursing remains involved in health care reform gives Mary Ann Garrigan's (1986) words even more meaning. To paraphrase her words, . . . We, as the nursing leaders of tomorrow, must have courage. We must continue to work towards nursing's vision of health for all. Even when support does not come, as occurred in our efforts for national health care reform, we must start together in a new direction, and continue even more committed to the worth of the work we are doing.

Perhaps the most important lesson for us in future health care reform is that nursing must be at the decision table of such reform. That means as nurse leaders you must be active, earn and demand a seat at the table, while still embracing collaborative outcomes. Because, transforming *Nursing's Agenda's* central concepts into laws and policies "will take the combined vision and commitment of many groups—politicians, teachers, corporate leaders, the insurance industry, nurses, physicians, and countless others. The energies of nursing students can play a role in moving this important effort ahead" (Fetters, 1991, p. 2). As we take steps to become the nursing leaders of the future, the skill to communicate and collaborate with professions other than nursing must still be some of the mortar that holds our path together. "Today, perhaps more than at any other time in history, we have the opportunity to communicate with respect for each other's roles and to collaborate in improving the health of our nation" (Fetters, 1992, pp. 18–19).

SUMMARY

As you and I train to become nursing's future leaders, without the skills of communication and collaboration, our path towards nursing's vision will become like quicksand and our efforts on behalf of our patients will be at risk.

I challenge each of you to move along the stepping stones we have discussed and then to place your own unique stones into the mosaic of our path. For some of you, they will be practice stones, for some educational, for some administrative, for some technical as nursing joins the lead in health informatics, and for some—new creative stones that are yet to be named. However, all stones will be important and provide a strong foundation for us as future nurse leaders to walk together side-by-side with our patients towards health.

Just as all stones in the path are part of the greater work, each voice in nursing is a part of the greater whole. I challenge you to not let your missing stone in the path cause a fall nor your missing voice prevent our voice from being heard. The nursing leader of the future is YOU. Develop your leadership skills well and continually add supporting stones to the path that students who follow after you must walk. It is my hope that the conceptual model for the critical path to leadership development in nursing will serve as a first step in our becoming effective leaders. I am proud to work and walk beside you.

CRITICAL THINKING QUESTIONS

1. What are the most valuable things for you to know, be able to discuss, and be actively involved in related to health care reform in our country? In your state? your community?
2. How does your nursing curriculum prepare you for nursing roles including community based care, health promotion and wellness, nursing informatics, and nursing leadership?
3. What is the difference between preparation as a clinical nurse leader and a nursing leader? How can you prepare yourself for both?
4. What will nursing's role be in the twenty-first century? What will the state of health care be in this country? What will access to health care be for citizens working full-time? part-time? the Unemployed? the Retired? the Disabled? nursing students? those who are homeless, including: men, women, families, and children?
5. What goals do you have for your leadership roles in nursing and health care in the twenty-first century?

ACTIVITIES

1. Do an in depth study of one of your favorite nurse's involvement in health care reform. What is their definition of nursing? What has their educational experience been like? What got her or him involved in the bigger picture of nursing and health care?
2. Go to Chapter 13 of this book and complete the mentoring and networking exercises found there.

REFERENCES

Fetters, C. A. (1991, October). Message to nursing students: This is where the change begins. *The American Nurse,* 2.

Fetters, C. A. (1992, May 22). Viewpoints from Colleagues in Training: A Strong Future for Nursing. *The Pharmacy Student, 2,* 18–19.

Garrigan, M. A. (1986, November 2). A tribute to Mary Ann Garrigan. *Journal of Nursing History, 1,* 4.

Hersey, P., & Blanchard, K. (1988). *Management of organizational behavior* (5th ed.). Englewood Cliffs, NJ: Prentice-Hall, Inc.

Mancino, D. (1991, October). Four decades of shaping nursing's future. *The American Nurse,* 5.

McCarty, Patricia. (1991, October). Image campaign boosts student enrollments (NCNIP). *The American Nurse,* 1, 24.

National Leadership Coalition for Health Care Reform, 1991, "A Comprehensive Reform Plan for the Health Care System," p. 2.

Rogers, M. E. (1987). *Changing patterns of nursing education.* New York: National League for Nursing.

Smith, D. (1991, October). Creating the 21st century nurse. *The American Nurse,* 4.

U.S. Department of Commerce (1991). Health and medical services. U.S. *Industrial Outlook 1991* (chapter 44, pp. 1–6).

ADDITIONAL SUGGESTED READINGS

Benner, P. (1984). *From novice to expert: Excellence and power in clinical nursing practice.* Menlo Park CA: Addison-Wesley.

Chenevert, M. (1996). *Pro-nurse handbook: Designed for the nurse who wants to thrive professionally.* (3rd ed.). St. Louis, MO: Mosby.

Chitty, K. K. (1996). *Professional nursing: Concepts and challenges.* (2nd ed.). Philadelphia, PA: W. B. Saunders.

Ellis, J., & Hartley, C. L. (1995). *Nursing in today's world: Challenges, issues, and trends.* (5th ed.). Philadelphia: Lippincott.

Hansen, R., & Washburn, M. (1990). *I Light the Lamp.* Vancouver, WA: Applied Therapeutics Inc.

Hein, E., & Nicholson, M. (1994). *Contemporary leadership behavior: Selected readings.* (4th ed.). Philadelphia: Lippincott.

Kelly, L. Y., & Joel, L. A. (1995). *Dimensions of professional nursing.* (7th ed.). New York: McGraw-Hill.

Leddy, S., & Pepper J. (1993). *Conceptual bases of professional nursing.* (3rd ed.). Philadelphia: Lippincott.

Marquis, B., & Huston, C. (1995). *Leadership roles and management functions in nursing.* (2nd ed.). Philadelphia: Lippincott.

Mitchell, P. R., & Grippando, G. M. (1993). *Nursing perspectives and issues.* (5th ed.). Albany, NY: Delmar.

Porter-O'Grady, T., & Wilson, C. K. (1995). *The leadership revolution in health care: Altering systems, changing behaviors.* Gaithersburg, MD: McGraw-Hill.

Strickland, O., & Fishman, D. J. (1994). *Nursing issues in the 1990s.* Albany NY: Delmar.

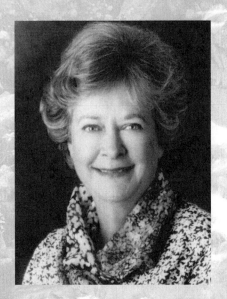

Lucille A. Joel,

RN, EdD, FAAN

Lucille Joel is a Professor at Rutgers—The State University of New Jersey College of Nursing. Dr. Joel is Past President of the American Nurses Association (ANA) and First Vice-President of the International Council of Nurses headquartered in Geneva. Dr. Joel holds official status as the Non-Governmental Organization (NGO) representative to the UN and UNICEF on behalf of the ICN. She is Editor-at-large of the *American Journal of Nursing* and co-author of *Dimensions of Professional Nursing* and *The Nursing Experience,* both published by McGraw-Hill.

Dr. Joel has served as a professional-technical advisor to the Joint Commission on the Accreditation of Health Care Organizations and chaired the Food and Drug Administration's steering committee on nursing and medical devices. She was the ANA representative to the board of the Computer-Based Patient Record Institute and is currently the association's liaison with the Health Care Financing Administration's Multi-State Nursing Home Case Mix and Quality Demonstration Project. She served as a member of the Federal Salary Council of the US Office of Personnel Management and as a member of the Health Care Administration Board of the state of New Jersey.

INTRODUCTION: PART 2

Life Review of an ANA President—The Path of Leadership

INTRODUCTION

The process of a life review sounds ominous and may infer that there is no life after ANA. Actually, the ANA presidency is only one step, and not the last, along a critical path towards the finest service that you can offer your profession. In conceptualizing the critical path of leadership, there is a beginning. And the outcome is largely dependent on the environments we were exposed to, the people who shaped us, and the opportunities that present themselves along the way.

THOSE FIRST HESITANT STEPS TOWARDS LEADING

I am the exception to the assumption that leaders are born. From early on I was quite the extraordinary follower, judged by the standard of parochial and diploma school education of my era. I learned the rules well and followed them exactly. I was always too intimidated to question authority. I knew myself as intellectually gifted, but this was not an asset valued by my peer group. As a consequence, I lacked confidence and most of the qualities that would target me for leadership roles. What set me apart were my brains, a cooperative nature, a good work ethic, and a presentable appearance. A perfect 10 on the follower scale.

I would caution those students who see some of themselves in me to sit up and take pride. There were very valuable lessons learned during this period of my life. I was well socialized to respect the work that nurses do. I knew when I was responsible and what I needed to know and do to be accountable. I learned respect for precision and attention to detail. Contrary to the experience of many of today's new graduates, it was not my clinical practice ability that left me in doubt. In fact, it was my technical proficiency that allowed me to hide all of my other insecurities. I was secure in the belief that I was one more link in the human chain that is nursing. I saw myself as part of a grand tradition with rich support systems of all ages.

There are some lessons to be learned here by both students and your teachers. Attention to socialization to the discipline of nursing is as important as the behavioral and natural sciences, and the liberal arts. It should be the constant theme throughout the educational experience. Socialization should include some forceful lessons about responsibility and accountability, and keep you ever mindful that we are a practice discipline and exist to serve the public in a very essential way. Requirements for dress, grooming, and hygiene should be an integral part of this lesson.

Full clinical days and realistic case loads are also a necessity. The value of a sound work ethic and a cooperative nature should not be understated. Students who work should be encouraged to seek positions that allow them to be involved in the activities of nursing, albeit at a low level. Work as a nurse's aide or physician's office assistant allows exposure to patients and some of the things that nurses do. Work-study programs, summer internships, and even post-graduate residency programs are opportunities to enhance your practice and become comfortable with the conduct of your role. None of these are bad choices given that employers expect a finished product.

Students can also be compromised in their learning by exposure to an unnecessary number of clinical placement sites. Concentrating clinical experiences in a limited number of carefully selected sites promotes more supportive relationships between students and staff and reduces the time invested in adjusting to each new setting. Serious thought should be given to having staff nurses take a more active role in teaching and precepting.

These details are lessons learned by personal experience and later reassessed through the critical eye of an educator. The principle being that there are basic attitudes and values that are synonymous with professionalism. To socialize well to these values, it has been common to create support systems through incumbents in the field and do some active ego building. The student physician's apprenticeship relationship with practicing physicians has served well in this way. And it is no secret that student physicians are indoctrinated into the "captain of the ship" philosophy early in their education. The food for my ego was my intellectual ability and clinical skill. These attributes were very personally mine and not situational. How much did this reinforce an internal locus of control? This poses some interesting questions about nursing, leadership, and personality. Leaders are often alone, opposed in making decisions, and need the courage of their convictions. Personality studies on students who choose nursing deserve to be revisited given the changing demands in health care.

My first position in nursing brought me to the specialty area of psychiatric nursing, although my preference and talent had been for medicine/surgery and the adult patient. Psychiatry offered better economic rewards. My motivation was very shallow as I attempted to establish myself financially after years of student impoverishment. The other benefits of that choice were hidden from my eyes.

In the early 1960s, public sector mental hospitals were crowded and there was little more than a token presence of registered nurses. The learning opportunities were great for the willing and able. No one questioned your right to practice autonomously and that practice included ample occasions to work directly with patients. Work with unlicensed assistive personnel was constant, creating the perfect laboratory to develop both managerial and interpersonal skills. Survival was dependent on being able to work through others, evaluate them correctly, and develop them boldly and cooperatively. What was initially a strange and uncomfortable situation became a daily challenge. I began to thrive on the role, and I was good at it. I acted like a nurse; people treated me like a nurse. They even expected me to have all the answers. If there was a place and a time when I made contact with my talents and recognized them, it was during this period. I began to lead and did so comfortably and confidently. The followers were initially nonprofessionals, with a growing number of professionals during the course of my tenure in that system.

In considering models of leadership, different qualities are necessary to secure the cooperation of assistive personnel as compared with professionals. Whether actual or assumed, in that era nursing assistants saw themselves accountable to registered nurses. In effect, this interpretation put the registered nurse in a position of authority. Your clinical credibility was established by your license. But different qualities, mostly interpersonal, assured cooperation.

Developing a productive working relationship with assistive personnel was a lesson in humility. I came to appreciate the rich information their many years of experience represented and how these individuals could be developed to extend your time and capabilities. They knew the complex bureaucratic system and were experts at working it to their advantage. They introduced me to the political process. I have come to the opinion that my leadership grooming started here. It was quite by accident that I found challenges galore, a situation where whatever you did would profit the system and your patients, plenty of people with history to promote your socialization, and an advocate who dismissed your insecurities as so much rubbish.

These years held my first exposure to mentorship of a sort. I have never really decided what term best describes my relationship with this patron. She was the chief nurse in this highly political and bureaucratic system. She was majestic in conduct and appearance and protected her privacy to the extent that she was surrounded by an aura of mystery. She knew the power of having friends in high places and never hesitated to use those contacts to further her own interests or those of her mentees, staff, or patients. She singled me out for new experiences and responsibilities, but never even indirectly hinted that she saw talents to be developed. I learned beginning lessons about building and using power. I learned that there is more to be gained by collaboration than by flaunting your strength and sources. In the true fashion of mentorship, I was there for her as she slipped from her public role. This is the obligation of the mentee, no matter how distanced in time and space you are from those early favors.

Though there were other noteworthy environments in my career trajectory, my natural talent to lead was unleashed working in a public sector psychiatric facility. My advice to new graduates is to seek out those settings where you will be allowed to experiment and take on new and demanding responsibilities: "You will rise to the occasion." In today's more sophisticated practice environments, I would look for the presence of advanced practice nurses to facilitate this learning.

THE BUILDING YEARS

Early in my nursing education, I became convinced that I owed myself a baccalaureate degree. This was not so much because I recognized the need for higher education in nursing, but rather that I felt denied a college degree. It would have been simple and even somewhat honorable to abandon my baccalaureate aspirations given my full-time employment and growing family responsibilities. But with tenacity and an ego to feed, I persevered towards this new benchmark and was awarded my degree.

Even at this point in my development, I found it difficult to look beyond the horizon. I had few aspirations after the baccalaureate. In retrospect, it is amazing who moves you to establish new benchmarks. In my case, it was an instructor in the inevitable leadership course that is often the capstone of the BSN program. She informed me quite matter-of-factly that I was talented and should go on to graduate study without delay. She touched my life personally for but a fleeting moment, but left an indelible mark. I have always wondered whether I would have moved on to another educational benchmark without that subtle push. I have never forgotten this incident as I deal with students, and my suspicions are verified when former students comment on how one word of encouragement made the difference.

Even as I moved on to graduate school, I was uncomfortable with the magnitude of the commitment facing me. My priority became the search for a program that would leave room for the other facets of my life—home, family, work. This was a tall order in the 1960s.

I was actively discouraged by two programs before finding my way to Teachers College, Columbia University. Here was an educational institution where the corridors radiated history, and students were taught the value of networking. To this day, the TC network remains one of my richest support systems. The TC days were filled with supportive faculty and rich role models. But it is surprising for me that no one person stands out as most prominent. It is the collective community that is responsible for the TC experience, TC the international melting pot, TC which attracted students who were already established nursing personalities.

My passion for organizational work can be traced to a class where Veronica Driscoll was a fellow student. Driscoll, later to become Executive Director of the New York State Nurses Association, decried our ignorance about the business of the profession. She created a discomfort and embarrassment in me that was impossible to ignore. She eloquently described the strategic necessity for collective action.

It is impossible to dismiss Teachers College briefly. These were years of hard work without restrictions on the hours or days devoted to learning, and few regrets. It was an environment frequented by leaders with few lessons about being a good follower. This is not a criticism, but reality. Students may be better served when the leader-follower paradigm is addressed more openly and honestly.

The pressures and frustrations of graduate study will be labeled pain or pleasure depending on the adequacy of your support systems. Support systems can be derived from many places. Mine was my husband—always assuring that family life continued undisturbed, often placing his own career goals secondary to mine, and offering encouragement when academic demands seemed to outpace my ability or resources. There are lessons here; assess the nature of your support systems. Are they a help or a hindrance? The significant people in your life can easily become distanced if you don't actively plan to have them grow with you.

INVISIBILITY TO VISIBILITY AND BACK AGAIN

Achieving the necessary credentials for practice is the first step in most fields. That has not always been the tradition in nursing. We often prepare for the roles we have already assumed. I was no exception. The days of my graduate education paralleled the initiation of my academic career, my first significant involvement in organized nursing, and the beginning of many years of practice as a nurse-psychotherapist.

Entry into the academe was probably the most traumatic event of my life. Orchestrating the activities of psychiatric attendants and the rigors of Teachers College only partially prepared me for teaching. The missing element was strong advanced clinical practice skills. Those were the days when there was little said about nursing theory and advanced clinical content was only slowly making an appearance. TC offered some good advanced practice exposure, but only enough to convince me of all I didn't know. I was forced to be honest about my deficits. I chose to remedy them through peer support systems and private practice.

Those early days of teaching offered my next lesson in humility: never doubt the importance of personal presence. There is an art and science of teaching that is separate from clinical competence. I have no affection for those days, preparing for class until the gong of the bell to satisfy my insecurities, assuming that I had to know everything. I learned you can't necessarily teach it just because you can do it. You grow in your ability over time. Teaching as well as nursing is dependent on experience. Pat Benner's work outlined in her book *From Novice to Expert* provides a paradigm for nursing practice that recognizes the value of experience. It tells us to trust intuition once we are seasoned practitioners (Benner, 1984). The same standard can easily be applied to the role of teacher. Master teachers are those who have worked hard at their art.

There is an art to organizational work, as well. My own long history in organizational work started with membership in my state nurses association upon graduation from diploma school. It was an expected first step into the profession and mandatory in spirit. In those days, many voluntary actions were de facto mandatory and very few questioned the standard. It became a mindless habit to continue paying dues, but my participation was infrequent.

In the late 1960s, I was volunteered to assume a more prominent role in the New Jersey State Nurses Association (NJSNA). My dean, a newcomer to the state, was appointed to the Board of Directors of NJSNA after a major restructuring of the association. Being limited in the number of people she knew, she was quick to volunteer faculty for appointments. And so through this very thoughtful process, I was requested to chair the newly established Psychiatric-Mental Health Nursing Practice Division. I was elected and then reelected to that position for over twelve years. My tenure in that office started with my usual insecurities. I was about to assume leadership for a specialty practice area dominated by Rutgers—The State University of New Jersey. But I wasn't a Rutgers graduate and saw this as threatening my credibility.

The years of providing leadership to this fledgling practice division were an opportunity waiting to happen. The division's accomplishments were significant in moving New Jersey nursing forward and drew national attention. The state insurance laws were modified to include many categories of advanced practice nurses. A state certification for clinical specialists in psychiatric-mental health nursing, which predated ANA's national certification program, was established and recognized by the Board of Nursing as the legal credential for independent practice as a nurse-psychotherapist. After almost thirty years, I am still impressed at what we were able to achieve. The cooperative relationship between specialists and staff nurses in psychiatric nursing flourished. And psychiatric nurses assumed a prominence in interdisciplinary causes that still exists. We established rich liaisons that have allowed us to challenge mental health benefits in managed care programs, oppose licensing of marriage counselors as a separate provider group, and support police intervention in situations of spousal abuse. These are but a few of the consumer advocacy, professional and public policy areas where we were able to leave our mark. The lessons learned are those of respect for collective action and the diversity of the nursing community. Never will I minimize the contribution every nurse can make by sacrificing personal goals in order to support something more critical to the profession.

My first tentative involvement with the association's work expanded rapidly. The state Psychiatric Nursing Practice Division became the national Practice Division (American Nurses Association) that led to the national Congress on Practice, state first vice-president, member of the national resolutions committee, state president, national first vice-president, and ultimately President of the American Nurses Association. Each period and office held its landmark events, significant accomplishments, and memorable personalities.

My tenure as NJSNA president had a rousing start. The annual meeting, during which I assumed the presidency, turned into a major confrontation over the educational requirements for entry into practice. This issue, still unresolved, lies beneath the surface in many testy situations where nurses are pitted against one another. The schism that existed within the association required that the work of healing become the priority, and that we fervently search for a unifying agenda. That agenda was provided by the reimbursement model that was being refined in the state for eventual federal use. New Jersey was the testing ground for Diagnosis Related Groups (DRGs) and nurses were unified in the belief that the intensity of nursing varied significantly from DRG to DRG.

Creating the proof and then the mathematical equations to move the dollars for nursing to the clinical situations where they are justified is consumer advocacy of the highest order. Additionally, this model allowed nursing to surface as a major player in hospital finance. Though this seminal work was the undertaking of the New Jersey Department of Health, the political leverage of NJSNA was essential for protection and to eventually have Relative Intensity Measures of Nursing (RIMs) cast into public policy. The strength of RIMs as a statistical equation is irrelevant. RIMs are a symbol and a landmark event. They are the first recognition in public policy that nursing is a significant financial factor in health care. I not only personally lobbied for RIMs, but began an intense interest in the relationship of public policy to the profession's agenda.

Landmarks during my service as an officer of ANA's Division on Practice and the Congress for Practice included the publication in 1980 of *Nursing: A Social Policy Statement*—the profession's ultimate statement of responsibility to the consumer. It was during this same era that the ANA underwent the transition to a federation model of governance. As part of that reorganization, debate focused on whether the association should continue to address specialty practice interests. This is still a controversial issue, especially given that most nurses identify closely with the specific populations they serve.

A summary of major events during specific periods of my organizational life does not infer that these are my personal accomplishments. Yet in some way, either by my presence, protection, or silence, I did contribute. No one can forget the nursing shortage of the late 1980s. And I was catapulted into this world following my election as ANA President in Louisville, Kentucky in June of 1988. I immediately beat a path to Chicago and the annual meeting of the American Medical Association (AMA). My attendance was not merely social, but a public statement to challenge the right of the AMA to propose the creation of a new health care worker, the Registered Care Technologist (RCT), as a solution to the national nursing shortage. The AMA's proposal was in such bad taste and so insulting to the nursing community that it created a solidarity among nurses never before achieved in our history. Nurses throughout the country, those networked through membership in some nursing organization and others who lacked any apparent linkages, came together to defeat the RCT and hold the medical community accountable for their intrusion into our internal affairs. Not only did nurses agree to speak with one voice, they contributed hard dollars to the work needed to defeat the RCT.

Nurses also moved forward as a unified force to create a better work environment and to recruit more men and women to the profession. The profession's efforts were so successful that a surplus was upon us within a few short years. The details of this period are fascinating, but too lengthy to chronicle here. What is important is the observation that an external threat can create the perfect opportunity to lead. Though the circumstances surrounding the shortage were very painful for a new president, and in some ways testimony that we had not carefully monitored the emerging problems in our own field, it was the perfect opportunity to create internal solidarity. The historic issues that had polarized nursing for generations, especially educational requirements for entry into practice, were put aside in favor of coming together to protect our control over our field of work.

The establishment of the National Center for Nursing Research was a premier event. Where managing the nursing shortage thrived on solidarity, the debate around the Center created dissension at the highest levels of leadership. Many prominent nurses openly opposed creation of the Center. They saw center status as permanent relegation to secondary status at NIH. Those with more political savvy knew that gains are usually incremental and half a cup is better than none at all. The legislative battle for the NCNR was resolved to our advantage with the override of a Presidential veto. And ANA lobbyists were proven right as funding for the Center flourished and the Center became an Institute in 1992.

The work of building unity and common cause among nursing organizations was also labeled as foolish by many nursing leaders. The reality is that most nurses identify strongly with their area of specialty practice and some are also ready to invest in the broader issues of the profession. Together, we would be a force to be reckoned with. Our management of the RCT issue made the point that nurses are more successful together than apart.

The creation of the Agency for Health Care Policy and Research (AHCPR) by the federal government moved nursing's organizations closer. AHCPR was the government's response to the growing consumer demand for medical consensus about the preferred treatment of frequently diagnosed conditions. AHCPR was mandated to produce these guidelines. And through a coalition of ANA and specialty societies, AHCPR was convinced to include a nurse on each of the guideline panels and to expand their agenda to include conditions that are highly nursing-sensitive: incontinence, pain, pressure sores.

The success with AHCPR created a climate where ANA and the specialties could dare to speak with one another about standards of practice. Through the processes of joint authorship and endorsement, standards began to emerge which had the credibility of both the specialty community and the ANA. These organizational coalitions continued to generate practice guidelines, and work on developing databases and classification systems—all intellectual products that would become part of the next generation of public policy.

It was this community of nursing that welcomed *Nursing's Agenda for Health Care Reform* (1991). The *Agenda* represents the first time that nursing presented a comprehensive platform for health care reform to Capitol Hill. It is the final product of serious negotiation among the major national associations and builds on the theme of our stewardship to the public. Lobbying the *Agenda* has been funded by the entirety of nursing, and the principles contained in the document have been publicly commended by many influentials, including the President of the United States. (See *Nursing's Agenda for Health Care Reform,* Appendix A.)

For ANA the years from 1988–1992 were tempestuous and absent stability. The movement to a federation model in the mid-1980s created many questions about who could be in membership and what internal structure would best serve us in these changing times. These questions were studied by the Commission on Organizational Assessment and Renewal (COAR). Their report was disseminated to the states for study, and facilitating by-laws changes were entertained at the 1989 House of Delegates. Setting detail aside, there were some landmark decisions that set the tone for ANA's continuing work. The membership reaffirmed their support for a free-standing credentialing center (The American Nurses Credentialing Center) that would take on the work of certification and an evolving number of other recognition programs. The International Nursing Center was established and gave the message that American nursing was ready to participate as a full partner in the world community. The American Nurses Foundation was empowered with staff and authority to boldly move forward as the tax-exempt and philanthropic arm of ANA.

Simultaneous with this radical internal restructuring, the association prepared to move its national headquarters from Kansas City to Washington, DC by 1992. The association's constantly increasing prominence in politics and public policy has verified the wisdom of that decision. As the president who executed this move, I recall many days of uncertainty. And there is no event in my life that more clearly exemplifies the advice, "Stay focused and never look back." But there were many sleepless nights. You were not only gambling with the future of the association, but the working lives of hundreds of employees.

Here are some of the lessons I learned and relearned during my presidency. Success is dependent on being surrounded by those who can be trusted and know their business, anticipating change before it is upon you, the ability to focus and follow things through to conclusion, a healthy ego which can absorb failure and move on, the sensitivity to know when others need to be credited with successes, and the optimism to see damage control as part of larger process and not label it as failure. Issues management and damage control are an on-going part of the organizational modus operandi.

Your victories will be in direct proportion to the quality of the relationship between staff and elected officials. The interaction between the president and chief executive officer is of necessity unique. One holds responsibility and authority for implementation of policy, and the other provides leadership for policy development. Be aware that the line between these roles is not always so clear, and that is when the trust and respect between these two individuals comes into play. An association is properly driven by the elected and appointed officials, and the staff exist to make those who have assumed these offices look good. Staff are the figurative "power behind the throne," providing continuity and stability. And given the complexity of today's health care issues, staff must possess a sophistication about specialized issues that outpaces most officers of the association. Staff are carefully selected; officers are the products of an often fickle political process. The lesson learned here for aspirants to any presidency is to work on the relationship with your chief of staff, though titles may vary. Personality clashes have no place here and will ultimately compromise the work of the association.

Organizational work has provided satisfaction and prominence, but has not been the mainstay of my professional life. Teaching and the mission of unifying education and practice have provided continuity to my work. After my initial tentative and tremulous venture into the academe, I grew in confidence and pride over the students I had touched. Sometimes I left an indelible imprint on their persona, and other times they taught me bigger lessons. In honesty, an academic life with its inherent flexibility allowed me to invest heavily in the politics of the profession. I would have been forced to assume much more modest roles without that freedom. I do not want to leave the impression that teaching requires any less than full effort and more, but often academic obligations can be honored in a time and place suited to your convenience. Appreciating these unique circumstances, I am in awe of the organizational investment of those who have the least flexibility and sometimes no freedom—the staff nurse.

The students who have moved through my life these many years are an endless source of satisfaction. It is through them that I will leave legacy. So many of those students have become my peers, colleagues, and even intimates. I have to periodically remind myself that I was younger than many of those first students. Though many like to claim me as a mentor, I have an aversion to the liberal use of that term. Mentorship is a bonding of two people in a relationship which frequently spans an entire career. There is a mutual commitment and a definite chemistry. But there are many varieties of patron relationships that can be just as fruitful and useful as mentorship. For many I have been a role model, given my ability to combine career and family. For others, though falling short of the distinction of mentorship, I have been the source of opportunities. And to a few, I have been a true mentor, but those have been very few and carefully selected. In my own mentor-protégé relationships, I have tried to emulate my personal experience with mentorship. Mentorship is never trivial, it is attention given freely with no expectation of any return, but an opportunity to leave legacy. But at its best, it is also a savings account, the banking of favors and opportunities given for courtesies returned at some later date as your own vitality and prominence decline.

I was only able to make a home in the academe because I could create situations that allowed me to maintain and nurture my roots in practice, even if indirectly. Due to a rich psychiatric nursing network in my own state and our success in dealing with obstacles to advanced practice, I have been able to maintain a private practice, albeit shrinking. In retrospect, my association work made it impossible to retreat to an "ivory tower," dismissing the needs of the nurse at the bedside. Neither did I want to lose contact with the thrill of seeing the basic decency and value of the work we do firsthand. My passion for the work of nursing became even more intense as I began to teach for the advanced practice role.

In 1979, I found the "dream" position for an academic with my practice and political inclinations. As Associate Dean for Clinical Affairs in the Rutgers College of Nursing, I had the opportunity to develop a joint appointment system between the College and its clinical affiliates. This created the vehicle to involve the best practitioners of nursing in the education of our students and for faculty to get seriously involved in the work of our affiliate agencies. It also provided an environment for the establishment of the Rutgers Teaching Nursing Home Program, one of eleven Teaching Nursing Homes originally funded by the Robert Wood Johnson Foundation. Contractual agreements were negotiated giving the college authority and responsibility for the standard of care in a 600 bed public sector home. Interdisciplinary respect and the innovative use of nursing personnel, including nurses in advanced practice, produced significant positive clinical outcomes. Among the adventures in my professional life, the Teaching Nursing Home ranks high in excitement and fulfillment. The camaraderie among the staff was unprecedented in my experience. We thrived on change and proved that what we were doing made a difference.

NEW AND DIFFERENT WAYS TO SERVE

The ANA presidency provided occasional exposure to the global nursing community. These opportunities were not so frequent, but they were memorable. Most were connected in some manner with the International Council of Nurses (ICN). The scheduled liaisons with the Canadian Nurses Association, attendance at biennial meetings of the Council of Nurse Representatives (CNR), and quadrennial Congresses of ICN all demonstrate the common cause of the nursing community. Communication has made distance a minor obstacle to the international exchange of ideas and resources. The best lessons were learned from international colleagues who did not allow themselves the luxury of seeing distance and culture as barriers. Need forced them to be venturesome.

My international appetite was satisfied in 1993 when I was elected as the North American representative to the Board of the International Council of Nurses, and in 1997 I became First Vice-President. The international world of nursing revives all sorts of feelings of inadequacy. It helps to focus on the consistencies first. Nurses are consistently humanitarian and prisoner to their feelings of moral compromise. They are also undervalued and subject to many of the human rights violations that their patients suffer.

The philosophy of ICN is to network nurses in every country into the world of organized nursing. ICN serves as the conduit for nations to help one another, always remaining sensitive to the reality that help must lead to self-help or the outcome is crippling. With 114 countries in membership and emerging associations in the remainder of the world, ICN's constituency is so large that progress will only come from outreach and partnering. This strategy parallels my own philosophy for living. Dependence is not only crippling but denigrating.

There have been exciting opportunities associated with ICN. I assumed the role of ICN's official representative in forums associated with the United Nations in a variety of ways: The Committee on the Status of Women, UNICEF, the NGO forum (nongovernmental organizations). Additionally, I have represented ICN with the World Hospital Federation and the Commonwealth Medical Association.

Moving beyond what may appear to be an impressive list of experiences, what are the lessons learned? First, another lesson in humility. The contributions of American nursing are well respected, but they are more often not the answers for the rest of the world. The content, tempo, and pace of international politics is at first a strange fit with the American way. There are so many who do so much more with so much less. I have learned not to judge others by the standard which exists in this country. But I fear that others will aspire to our standard and inherit our dilemmas and frustrations.

But where does one go after the bells and whistles of the most prominent and visible association service? The greatest opportunities to serve lie beyond the status of the office, which by its nature and constituency is highly political. Liberated from the competitiveness of politics, there is the obligation to continue to serve in other ways, often less visible but critical for the profession's stability. A very wise and seasoned executive director once offered the advice that the perfect work for past presidents is fund raising. Words offered as humor often ring true. By simple reasoning, one would have to assume a deep affection for any association where they had labored so tirelessly over the course of their professional life. It is unnatural to walk away from those commitments and never look back. Just as I think it is impossible to have the same intensity of identification with several associations. In one of her brilliant editorials, Lucie Kelly pokes fun at nursing's recyclable leadership (Kelly, 1988).

The end of my ANA presidency did not represent closure on my work with the association. I became Editor-at-Large of *The American Journal of Nursing*. My willingness to serve was clearly based on the fact that AJN was an ANA property, and I was there to safeguard the interests of the association from the editorial perspective and to emphasize the bond between ANA and AJN by my presence. I am a constant source of information and opinion to ANA staff, who I may now deal with more freely and openly. I continue a long relationship with the Health Care Finance Administration on ANA's behalf.

My allegiance to my state association is similar. I continue to work behind the scenes and up front where it can help. I am cautious to stay as apolitical as possible. I have no need to set policy or to sit on decision-making bodies. My power is subtle and deserved by my history of service. I resist any temptation to criticize current leadership, appreciating that I cannot know all the facts and that it is an imposition and politically naive to expect leaders to justify every action. I offer support, chair fund raising campaigns, and make myself physically present as much as possible. In a manner of speaking, you can best serve by assuming the role of statesperson.

A RETROSPECTIVE ON LEADERSHIP

It is easy to be analytic about leadership. The secret is to offer practical and timely advice. Given human nature, you may have already assigned yourself a leadership quotient. Be careful of preconceptions. They limit you in developing your natural talent and send a message to others. Maintain an open mind. We all have the capacity to become either leaders or followers and both are necessary. There are no leaders without followers, and no matter how high you climb the leadership ladder, there is always the requirement to follow some of the time. Neither is the follower at one end of the leadership continuum and the leader at the other, with intermediate points where these qualities are blended in different proportions. Both leader and follower have a continuum. There are those who are more accomplished as leaders or followers. They realize these roles are not in competition, but rather natural compliments to one another's success.

The best advice for successful leadership is to realize there must be a good fit between the circumstances, the qualities of the leader, and the traits of the followers. Many combinations are possible and some examples may help to both place yourself and groom yourself. Some believe that we are born with leadership qualities. A better interpretation is that we are exposed to experiences and role models that demonstrate leadership qualities—and some choose to pay attention.

Charisma is a valuable attribute when followers are asked to make sacrifices that could only be expected based on personal loyalties. Most revolutionary leaders were charismatic. Literature verifies that there are certain traits commonly associated with leadership talent: intelligence, emotional maturity, creativity and ability to see novel solutions for problems, initiative, careful and sensitive listening, ability to cut through a confusing situation and derive meaning, persuasiveness, sociability, good judgment about people, and adaptability (Kelly & Joel, 1996).

Traditional theories of leadership have emphasized control, the power of one person over another, and have inferred a hierarchy of some sort. They have assumed that the major point of analysis is the relationship between the leader and followers, and that the environment is relatively stable. Instead today, we see a tumultuous environment and the need to create a bond between the leader and follower. The goal is for the leader and follower to fuse and move together towards a common goal. This is a comparison between the transactional paradigm of another generation and the transformational leadership more suited to today and to the needs of professionals. Transformational leaders work to create a shared vision with their followers. They focus on process not content and unify followers by a goal. Roles are not predetermined but emerge over time and in response to the work needed to accomplish the goal, and hopefully the personal talents of participants. Feelings are recognized, accepted, and worked through. When complexity and ambiguity make progress difficult, these transformational leaders seek novel solutions to problems using creativity and intuition. They facilitate the work of followers, protect them, and empower them. The leader becomes much more dependent on the follower in a transformational model (Kelly & Joel, 1996).

These principles can easily be applied to my own leadership trajectory. First, don't prejudge yourself. Although I had no design to seek out leadership challenges, they came and went, and I was all the better off for the experience. If you find yourself in a bad situation, make it your laboratory for leadership development—don't run away too quickly. Instead, seek the counsel of someone wiser and more seasoned. Seek the counsel of a faculty member—they do not cease to serve you at graduation. Or reach out to the state or district nurses association—ANA and the state associations have established a mentorship program for new graduates. Again, the word mentor may be used indiscriminately, but the program is well intentioned and useful.

A principle as old as leadership, and for the most part absolutely correct, is that you must "pay your dues" before assuming more leadership prominence. Simply put, most people start at the bottom or somewhere near it. My entry into organizational leadership at the state level was atypical, but suited the immediate need of the organization. However, from that point on I moved forward rung after rung. A good place to start is the district nurses association, or whatever the smallest unit of the state nurses association is called in your situation. You will have the opportunity to observe the operations of the association and volunteer for smaller projects while you become known and get to know others.

Hard work is not always the ingredient that makes for success. Instead, you have to cultivate that uncanny ability to be in the right place at the right time and take advantage of opportunities waiting to happen. To identify those opportunities takes vision, and vision is often linked to the extent of your networks and the degree to which you monitor trends. Reading broadly and voraciously helps, even skim reading. My major area of scholarship has become public policy, more specifically case mix and reimbursement models. My interest was first piqued by the New Jersey State Nurses Association's work on DRGs and the relative intensity measures of nursing. The association was not motivated to latch onto this area as a legislative or regulatory priority, but the economic messages in health care supported the prediction that this would eventually be a "hot" item.

SUMMARY

Cultivation of leadership ability requires patrons, whether they are role models, preceptors, mentors, or a peer support system. Choose wisely or place yourself in situations where you will be chosen. Remember that mentorship is a very weighty relationship. It assumes a long-term obligation and probably a decent attempt to pass on the privilege. Mentorship is not adulation at a distance, but a two-way street. I have had one true mentor, and another personality in my life who accessed me to favors and singled me out for leadership, but I am reticent to call that relationship mentoring.

Over time peer networks become increasingly valuable. They will be as rich as your experience, and you will be judged by your associations. Remember, if you want to fly with the eagles, don't hang out with the crows.

Nursing has richly endowed my life. I can only wish you as much as you travel the critical path ofi leadership development in nursing.

CRITICAL THINKING QUESTIONS

1. Which of your qualities predict success in leading or following? What are your most problematic attributes related to these areas? Back each statement with an example to illustrate your point.

2. What are some likenesses and differences among the qualities of two prominent nursing leaders, either historical or contemporary.

3. What is your style in relating to authority figures or leadership personalities in your life? Be as descriptive as possible.

4. What leadership experiences have you had? How successful were they?

5. What leaders have you known in your life? How do you judge their effectiveness? Establish criteria for your opinion.

ACTIVITIES

1. Share your answer to Critical Thinking Question #1 with a classmate, preferably someone who does not know you well. Supply additional information as needed to allow her or him to understand your opinion. Reflect on and consider their feedback.

2. Select two historical nursing leaders. Read widely to allow understanding of their formative years and experiences. Offer an opinion on why they developed leadership ability and style as they did.

REFERENCES

American Nurses Association. (1980). *Nursing: A Social Policy Statement*. Kansas City: The Association.

American Nurses Association. (1991). *Nursing's Agenda for Health Care Reform*. Washington, DC: American Nurses Publishing.

Benner, P. (1984). *From Novice to Expert*. Menlo Park, CA: Addison-Wesley Publishing Company.

Kelly, L. (1988, September–October). Nursing, nothing but nursing, *Nursing Outlook 36,* 227.

Kelly, L. Y., & Joel, L. A. (1996). *The Nursing Experience*. New York: McGraw-Hill.

ADDITIONAL SUGGESTED READINGS

Joel, L. A. (1996, April). An American nurse returns from abroad, *AJN 96,* 4, 7.

Joel, L. A. (1997, July). The leader-follower connection, *AJN 97,* 7, 7.

Joel, L. A., & Wade, J. W. (1988). Rutgers—The State University of New Jersey and Bergen Pines County Hospital. In Small, N., & Walsh, N. (eds.), *Teaching nursing homes: The nursing perspective* (pp. 211–237). Rockville, Maryland: National Health Publishing.

The Stepping Stone of Education

Unit One begins solidifying the nursing student's path to leadership development by going back to nursing's roots and laying some valuable groundwork. Chapter 1 looks at *the history and nature of nursing itself.* Chapter 2 explores the *history, milestones, and vision of nursing education*—an area that currently consumes a large part of your time, energy, and talent. Chapter 3 discusses *nursing research and its impact on both education and practice.* Finally, Chapters 4 and 5 finish the unit with content from two strong advocates of leadership development in nursing students. Chapter 4 reviews the need for *developing accountability in future nurse leaders.* Chapter 5 provides an overview of *faculty's role in the leadership development of nursing students.*

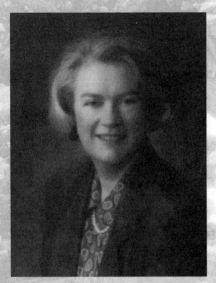

Photo courtesy of Lasswell's Studio.

Mary P. Tarbox,

EdD, RN

Mary P. Tarbox, EdD, RN, is the Professor and Chair of the Department of Nursing at Mount Mercy College in Cedar Rapids, IA. Dr. Tarbox graduated from Mount Mercy and the University of Minnesota with a clinical specialty in community health nursing. In addition to inpatient experience in pediatrics, Dr. Tarbox has worked with children with severe and profound disabilities and with families in the community setting. Following several years as a faculty member at Mount Mercy, Dr. Tarbox pursued a doctorate in nursing education administration with a research emphasis in nursing history. As a stu-

dent at Teachers College, Columbia University, she was a member of the Society for Nursing History and one of the early members of the American Association for the History of Nursing in the Sisters of Mercy in the United States. Dr. Tarbox continues to research the influence of religious women on nursing and has presented papers on the topic locally, regionally, and internationally. In addition to an interest in nursing history, Dr. Tarbox also serves on the research team for the Iowa Nursing Interventions Classification project with faculty and staff members of the College of Nursing at the University of Iowa.

Dr. Tarbox has supported nursing student organizations since joining NSNA as a student and serving as a state officer. As an advisor for the nursing student association at Mount Mercy, she has worked with students to encourage their participation in NSNA and their attendance at state, regional, and national conventions. One Mount Mercy student served as a member of the NSNA board of directors (1989–1990), and several students attend the annual convention each year.

Dr. Tarbox is an active member of the Iowa Nurses Association, the American Association for Colleges of Nursing, and the National League for Nursing. Her work in nursing history and nursing education received recognition from the Iowa Nurses Association through the Teresa Christy Award in 1993.

CHAPTER 1

The Nature of Nursing—Yesterday, Today, and Tomorrow

INTRODUCTION

Why are nurses so reluctant to belong to collective bargaining units? Why is the nursing profession still predominantly a female profession? Why are nursing students so adamant about learning technical skills in spite of efforts by faculty to incorporate more skills in critical thinking and analysis? Why is public opinion consistently favorable toward nursing and nurses? Questions like these are common among the members of the nursing profession, and usually they are answered by a shrug of the shoulders and a renewed effort to combat the identified "problem." Such questions are not new, nor is it necessary to shrug off attempts to answer them. The answers can be found in the critical review of the history of nursing from its beginning to current times.

Although it is well understood by most nurses that they should be familiar with the general history of their profession, some may believe that details of that history are not very interesting. They may find it difficult to read, and they may feel that it is not necessary if one is truly interested in being a good "clinical practitioner." Lavinia L. Dock (1858–1956), one of nursing's great leaders and a strong advocate for women's rights, believed that nurses needed to understand the importance of nursing history.

She believed that any nurse who knew only her own time and surroundings would be unprepared to correctly estimate and judge the current events that were likely to affect her own career (Dock & Stewart, 1937).

The study of chronological events that describe the historical development of nursing may be of considerable interest to nurses who are fascinated by the course of human events as they shape the present world. To others, the chronology is not as important, nor as interesting, as the study of a specific event within the context of the society and time in which it occurs. However, nursing leaders have long acknowledged that an understanding of the past can bring additional clarity to decisions that will shape the future (Kelly & Joel,1995). Although nurses may not be aware of the historical events that have shaped their own practice, they may still be able to provide care. However, their acceptance of nursing as a profession, rather than an occupation, will require their long-term commitment to nursing and a willingness to work toward its future development. Nurses' efforts to fulfill the obligations associated with the nursing profession, without an understanding of its history, may lead to the repetition of errors of the past (Kelly & Joel, 1995).

This chapter focuses on nursing history as one element in your development of a professional identity. It emphasizes learning from those who have gone before, who are here now, and who will continue to shape the profession in the future. Chronological listings of events and characters in nursing history are available in a variety of texts and have been effective in bringing nursing history to the attention of not only nurses but also members of the public (Donahue,1996, Kalish & Kalish, 1995).

This chapter asks potential nurse leaders to consider the context of those events and individuals in history, as well as in the succeeding developments of the nursing profession. Only a few events and individuals are noted in this chapter as examples of ways to use history to appreciate the present.

A SENSE OF PLACE AND TIME

"An understanding of the past" is a phrase often used to suggest what is essential to one's comprehension of the present. How one obtains this understanding is an individual effort that takes many forms. To play on a phrase from physics, history abhors a vacuum, meaning that one must acknowledge the context within which history occurs. Nursing history, in particular, must be studied within the context of time and place, and with a recognition of the many factors that have directed its progression.

Events in nursing history are influenced by and do indeed influence events around them. It is readily apparent in accounts of the Civil War in the United States, for example, that disease and poor sanitary conditions were more to blame for battlefield deaths than the battles themselves. It may not be as readily apparent that the "nursing care, provided by women volunteers and women of religious orders, was recognized as an important step in the development of organized hospital nursing and as a call for formal education of nurses throughout the country" (Kalish & Kalish, 1986, p. 53). The Civil War, studied by every child in American schools, is viewed by nurse historians as a complex, vivid setting for the beginning of the development of modern nursing in the United States. The nurse who studies the places, times, and events of the Civil War with an eye toward the women and men who were instrumental in the care of the sick and wounded will find an intricate view of the conflict. That nurse will also find a new understanding of the circumstances that shaped the future development of nursing. Neither nursing nor the war is viewed the same way when one is cognizant of the complexity of the events and individuals involved (Maher, 1989).

As historical events have influenced nursing, so too has nursing influenced historical events. The work of nurses in the Civil War is directly responsible for changes in the operation of general hospitals and in furthering the call for formal training for nurses. Nursing education programs offered opportunities to women that were not available in previous times. Women now had another option to provide them with the skills and confidence necessary to face the complexity of the society in which they lived.

Consider the young woman who chose to pursue nursing as an option. The nursing school of the late nineteenth century offered a protective environment compared to homes or factories, which may have been her only other options. She could fulfill a desire to help others and herself with the independence that a position in nursing would offer. There were many pitfalls, however, in the form of long hours, hazardous conditions, and no guarantees of employment. There were few long-term benefits for those in this dangerous occupation. But, these perils were far outweighed by the provision of an altruistic service and the potential for independence, advancement, and social standing as a professional and potential leader in nursing. These are many of the same motivators identified by nurses today.

THE PATTERNS OF NURSING HISTORY

As one explores the context and events of nursing history, it is evident that certain patterns occur. These patterns help one recognize the historical basis for current situations, both positive and negative, that occur in health care. Appreciating these patterns will assist nursing's future leaders in directing the profession into the next century.

Gender

One identifiable pattern is the influence of gender on the course of nursing history. The association of women and nursing has been influential in both the constructive development of the profession and the detrimental events that caused a regression or backlash within the profession. As sociologists and historians study women and society, nurses are the focus of many of those studies (Lewenson, 1993).

Since the beginning of families, and the recognition of structured roles within those families, women have been the predominant providers of care for the sick. This led to the characterization that women have a predisposition to be nurses, and that nurses do what comes naturally as women. Histories of nursing that chronicle the events of earliest times identify women as caregivers in every society, and at all times in history as an expectation of their roles.

Men are identified as caregivers only when they are exceptions to their gender, are a part of an organized movement such as the Knight Hospitalers, or are monks in a monastery. Although physicians are consistently portrayed as men, caregiving is not seen as their established role. Until the most recent history of the twentieth century, women identified as physicians were viewed as exceptions to historical patterns.

In history, there were both positive and negative consequences to identifying nurses as women. Positive results occurred when women functioned in roles that otherwise would not have been open to them in their societies. These occurred in military conflicts where women were involved as caregivers to the sick and wounded and also in religious movements where women could offer services to others in the name of their god, in spite of restrictions placed on them by the male leaders of the movement. Just as frequently, however, identifying nurses as women led to negative consequences when nurses wished to be in command of those providing care, to be property holders of the institutions in which nursing took place, or to be recognized for their education and expertise in a world that did not value skills "naturally" associated with one's gender.

Religion

The association of nursing with religion is another pattern to consider. Early historical accounts of nurses often affiliate their services with those of priests and priestesses, nuns, and even witches. These earlier accounts of caregiving are likely to be in the context of ridding one's patient of evil spirits or mollifying the displeasure of the gods. But organized nursing in Western civilizations was clearly founded on the principles of Christianity. At that time, efforts to live in the image and likeness of Christ led women and men to be motivated and sanctioned to organize services that provided care to individuals other than family members. Those women and men who wished to be of service to others found that Christianity gave them "permission" to practice their desired work in societies that had not allowed, or even seen, such services offered. When posed in the context of service, nursing received approval from both secular and religious bodies to provide the care certainly needed, but so difficult to procure through less altruistic means.

On the other hand, providing care for those in need out of a religious motivation has often served as a barrier to recognition and compensation for nurses. In other words, why recognize nurses for the care they provide when they are doing it out of dedication to religious beliefs and their own needs to be of service to others?

The question of religion and altruism in the development of nursing as a profession continues to motivate researchers and historians in their efforts to grasp the influence of both on nurses, even in the context of current health care. It is not unheard of to find opposition to nurses bargaining for contracts or threatening to strike based solely on the notion that nurses are working out of dedication to the betterment of all humans and in service to their god. This underlying philosophy can also impact some nurses' decisions about belonging to bargaining units.

Military Action

A third pattern that emerges throughout nursing history is the influence of military action on the development of the profession. Wars, as they changed the course of human events, were just as influential on the course of nursing as a profession. Along with the patterns of gender and religious influence, war and military actions served both to enhance and to impede the progressive movement of nursing.

Chronicles of nursing history account for the impact of such events as the Fall of the Roman Empire, the Crusades, the Crimean War, the Civil War, and the two major world wars as being pivotal in the development of nursing. Such events not only called for the assistance of those with caregiving skills but also provided the context for the exercise of authority, expertise, and evaluation that was seldom offered through any other event in society. When nurses are perceived as persons who can truly improve the situation, whether through either their presence as guardians of the sick and wounded or their expertise as skilled providers of health care, the roles of both women and nurses are enhanced.

The military influence on the development of nursing obviously had positive repercussions, as women received recognition for their services and expertise beyond their "natural calling." The first women to receive rank in the military in the United States were nurses in service to their country. When the country needed nurses, support was granted to assure that nurses were available for both military and civilian duty through such programs as the Cadet Nurse Corps in World War II. It is thought by some researchers that the uniforms and caps of nurses and the early reference to rank, such as head nurse or chief nurse, have military derivations. These were helpful in their origins to assure respect and compensation for nurses but have become less appropriate in recent times in an environment where function and safety are the deciding factors in uniform style.

One of the most significant chapters in the history of men in nursing begins during the Crusades with the establishment of nursing orders to assist the European pilgrims going to the Holy Land. The Crusades offered the context for the work of the Knight Hospitalers. The military order and rule provided the structure for the organization that would eventually grow to include thousands of recruits and multiple facilities. The Knights, originally known for their care of the sick and wounded, eventually became soldiers themselves, in defense of the Holy Lands (Kalish & Kalish, 1978).

As one considers the influence of the military on nursing, one can see pivotal milestones in the development of the profession. The Crimean War certainly propelled Florence Nightingale into the public eye and gave her access and resources for her future work, which may not otherwise have been available. The Civil War launched nursing in the United States into modern times with formal nursing education, progressive work in hospitals and communities, and recognition of the role of women in military service. World War I saw nurses enlisted in the military and serving overseas in treacherous conditions, as did World War II, when nurses were recruited, enlisted, and expected to serve under dangerous uncharted conditions for women. The Cadet Nurse Corps brought thousands of nurses into service who may not otherwise have been involved and launched nursing education into the university setting.

Wars forced nurses to rethink their roles, their education, and their service. From war emerged nursing specialties such as psychiatric and intensive care nursing. War also left little time to debate or impede some of the most significant changes in nursing education and services. As nurses considered the positive effects of such changes, they also considered the threats toward future progress of the profession.

Out of their war experiences have come nurses who fight for the rights of veterans (including themselves), nurses who seek to improve the conditions of all women in the military, as well as nurses who oppose further military action of any kind, including the use of nuclear weapons.

Other Patterns

Other patterns in nursing history help one to understand past incidents and to analyze current events. Each pattern encompasses the context within which events occurred and urges the nurse to consider any number of other variables that may influence the outcome. While researching the history of a women's religious order and its early influence on nursing in the United States, I was compelled to also consider the history of women, religion, immigration, industrialization, and urbanization. No event exists in a vacuum, and every event deserves full examination to be of use to nurses in their understanding and initiative toward professional development. Further exploration of these patterns is encouraged by nursing's future leaders.

FOUNDATIONS OF CURRENT THEORY AND RESEARCH IN NURSING

Modern students of nursing are introduced to the phenomenon of theory building in nursing. Since the 1960s, nursing has seen a concerted effort on the part of nurse educators and practitioners to define nursing as an entity separate from medicine and to further explain what it is that nurses do. Serving as a chart or map for the course of action taken by nurses in defining and conducting nursing practice, a theory makes it possible to provide rationale for those actions based on definable phenomenon (Bullough & Bullough, 1984).

Florence Nightingale is often identified as the first nurse theorist because of the emphasis she placed on assessing and manipulating the patient environment to enhance recovery by facilitating the natural course of healing. This knowledge of Nightingale's writing is an example of using the past to better understand the present and further advance the development of nursing. Although one may not depend only on Nightingale's theory to direct modern practice, it is helpful to know that rationale, developed to explain nursing actions, has been a part of the profession since its modern beginnings.

More recently, theory development has become important to professional nurses who wish to have a foundation for their practice. Although theories vary, they offer nurses direction and sound rationale for the complex practice of nursing. Knowing a variety of nursing theories allows the nurse a number of options for guided practice, as well as a variety of perspectives on caring for diverse client populations. Historically, knowing that practice may guide theory or that theory may guide practice allows the nurse to function in either direction with some foundation for decisions that are made. As with other efforts to understand what has gone before and to be able to better comprehend what is happening now, nurses who are familiar with the dynamics of nursing theories will be better able to use them in their current practice. And most important, this understanding can provide nursing's future leaders with the knowledge of theory development that will be needed for the twenty-first century.

Nurses have learned that the early practice of nursing was founded on the tradition, rather than the theory, of providing care to those who needed assistance that they or their family members could not provide. Such care was first dispensed outside the home by religious men and women who offered their services in very small institutions or in designated areas of their monasteries. These were the hostels or hospitals of the medieval period. As these care institutions changed throughout history, they continued to serve the poor and infirm who were away from home and alone. Almshouses, prisons, and asylums came to be known as last resorts for those who were ill. Their caregivers were often fellow inmates or those sentenced to service in those institutions. Actions on the part of caregivers in these situations could hardly be defined as nursing practice. Care was inconsistent, because there were few, if any, models of nursing until the nineteenth century. Even then, models were based on trial and error. Caregiving included what might be seen as one's "natural tendency" and "keenness" toward care of the sick (Dock & Stewart, 1937, p. 95). Those who provided care learned from each other. Then what worked was taught to the next generation.

Formal education would lead nursing care into the modern era as nurses learned from those who had practiced and documented the results of their work. Florence Nightingale's *Notes on Nursing; What It Is and What It Is Not* (1860) (Harrison, 1989) continues to be considered one of the first written instructions to nurses. Although not based on formal research, Nightingale's skills in observation and deduction were most effective in providing rationale for the practice of nursing, which she proposed.

Empirical, clinical research, as a basis for nursing practice, was not seriously considered until the second half of the twentieth century (Abdellah & Levine, 1979). By that time, nurses had established curricula for schools of nursing and hospitals had become the primary location for nursing practice. Even at this time, however, research inclined toward studies of who nurses were, where they worked, and how they were educated. It would be many years before the first research studies that focused on patient care and the rationale and effectiveness for specific interventions would evolve. The 1950s saw both changes in nursing research due to support from nurse leaders and increased numbers of masters prepared nurses with knowledge of research techniques and funding. Most nursing research funding at this time was available through research grants from the federal government.

The journal *Nursing Research* was established in 1952 and gave nurses the opportunity to disseminate their research findings and concerns (Burns & Grove, 1993). Clinical nursing research had an early start in military nursing, and additional studies in the outcomes of nursing interventions continued during the 1960s. As funding became more available through the federal government, more nurses earned doctoral degrees. Clinical nursing research became the focus of most nursing research in the 1970s and 1980s and continues to be emphasized through federal funding and identified needs expressed by nurses in practice today. Research conferences held at the local, regional, and national levels did, and continue to, provide nurses with access to giving and gaining new insights into practice and lead to an empirical base for the practice of nursing.

An appreciation of the historical course of nursing theory and research provides future nurse leaders with an understanding of the past that is so important in the comprehension of current issues and concerns. Recognizing that theory and research are fairly new in the course of events gives one pause to think of the tremendous progress nursing has made in so short a time. It should also bring nurses together to know that those who have gone before had struggles and triumphs many of which were solved and are directly reflected in current nursing practice. Such knowledge can give strength to those who lead. For those who understand what has gone before may be able to avoid the errors of the past and to progress with more confidence and success.

SUMMARY

Learning about nursing's past can be an optimistic experience as one discovers individuals, groups, and organizations that have succeeded in the face of adversity. History will also enlighten us to the setbacks and difficulties that influenced the progress of the nursing profession. What history will not tell nurses is how to chart their future.

What lies ahead for the profession of nursing is a question very much on the minds of nursing leaders, educators, and practitioners as the new millennium approaches.

More answers will be posed for the question of nursing's future in the next few years than at any time in the history of the world. In answer to those who ask if there is a future for nursing, those who have studied its history know that nurses of the past would answer "yes" and would be first in line to carry us on into that future. Among those who have already suggested answers are those concerned about the tension of a century ago that still exists between the "scientific base of nursing and its moral base of care." Will nurses be the forerunners in health promotion instead of illness care? Will nurses be able to access and acknowledge the value and cost of caring at a time when costs count for more than concern and contentment? Nursing must be seen as an essential solution in the current health care system rather than a contributor to the problems (Kitson, 1997).

While some authors may suggest very specific changes for nursing to advance successfully into the future (Korniewicz & Palmer, 1997; Bartels, 1997), others will be more general and contemplative in charting a direction for the profession. As future nurse leaders, nursing students must study what has gone before, examine what is currently transpiring, and listen carefully to what is being suggested for the future. The challenge is upon nursing, and there is every indication that such an eminent profession will continue to be successful and influential in the future.

CRITICAL THINKING QUESTIONS

1. The year is 1910, and you are a young adult wishing to enter a school of nursing. What will you tell your parents about this opportunity? What is your motivation for selecting nursing, and how do you anticipate they will respond?

2. In 1935, the hospital in which you are employed as the head of the surgical nursing services decides that students are no longer cost effective and graduate nurses must be hired in the operating room. What are your concerns? What changes do you anticipate because of this decision?

3. The year is 1950. You have been hired as the new director of nursing of a small community hospital in the midwest. You recognize that the community holds this hospital as "sacred" in the history and current operation of the community. What measures would you take to learn more about the hospital and the community so that you can better understand its place in the community?

4. As an experienced staff nurse on the neurology unit of a large university hospital, you are asked to serve on the nursing research committee. Discuss some of the ways you can contribute to that committee.

5. The members of your staff in a home health agency approach you with a proposal to begin a service for mothers of newborn infants who are discharged after twenty-four hours in the hospital. As you work with the staff nurses to further develop this idea, what would you identify as (a) the historical basis for such service, (b) the current challenges and opportunities available for such services, and (c) projections for future opportunities related to such services?

ACTIVITIES

1. Look for the references that describes the beginnings of the nursing education program in which you are currently enrolled. If you are in a baccalaureate program in a college or university, find out if a hospital school of nursing preceded the current program.

2. As nursing history becomes more recognized as essential to understanding the current issues and trends in nursing, more nursing journals are publishing nursing history articles. Review CINAHL for current listings of articles associated with nursing history. Often anniversary issues of nursing journals feature history articles.

3. Consider joining the American Association for the History of Nursing. This organization meets annually in September for a conference on nursing history. The membership collaborates with local nursing history groups and international history of nursing associations. Publications of the association are the *Bulletin* and the *Nursing History Review*. For additional information contact the association at: AAHN, PO Box 90803, Washington, DC 20090-0803.

REFERENCES

Abdellah, F., & Levine, E. (1979). *Better patient care through nursing research.* (2nd ed., p. 3) New York: Macmillan Publishing Co.

Bartels, J. (1997). Creating meaningful accreditation practices for the next millennium. *Journal of Professional Nursing, 13,* (3), 140.

Bullough V. & Bullough, B. (1984). *History, trends and politics of nursing.* Norwalk, CT: Appleton-Century Crofts.

Burns, N., & Grove, S. (1993). *The practice of nursing research: conduct, critique, and utilization.* (2nd ed., p. 21) Philadelphia: W. B. Saunders Co.

Dock, L., & Stewart, I. (1937). *A short history of nursing.* (3rd ed.). New York: Putnam's Sons.

Donahue, M. (1996). *Nursing: The finest art: An illustrated history,* (2nd ed.). St. Louis, MO: Mosby.

Kalish, P., & Kalish, B. (1995). *The advance of american nursing,* (3rd ed.). Philadelphia: J. B. Lippincott Co.

Kalish, P., & Kalish, B. (1978). *The advance of american nursing,* (p. 5–6) Philadelphia: J. B. Lippincott Co.

Kalish, P., & Kalish, B. (1986). *The advance of american nursing,* (2nd ed., p. 53) Philadelphia: J. B. Lippincott Co.

Kelly, L., & Joel L. (1995). *Dimensions of professional nursing* (7th ed.). New York: McGraw-Hill, Inc.

Kitson, A. (1997). Johns Hopkins Address: Does nursing have a future? *Image, 29,* (2), p. 111–115.

Korniewicz, D., & Palmer, M. (1997). The preferable future for nursing, *Nursing Outlook, 45,* (3), 108–113.

Lewenson, S. (1993). *Taking charge: Nursing, suffrage, and feminism in America: 1873–1920,* New York: Garland Publishing.

Maher, M.D. (1989). *To bind up the wounds: Catholic sister nurses in the U.S. civil war.* New York: Greenwood Press.

Nightingale, F. (1989). *Notes on nursing: What it is and what it is not.* London: Harrison. (Original work published 1860)

ADDITIONAL SUGGESTED READINGS

Alcott, L. (1885) *Hospital Sketches.* Boston: Roberts Brothers.

American Association for the History of Nursing. (1992–1997). *Nursing history review.*

Ashley, J. (1996). *Hospitals, paternalism, and the role of the nurse.* New York: Teachers College Press.

Bullough, V. & Bullough, B. (1978). *Care of the sick: The emergence of modern nursing,* (p. 38–41) New York: Prodist.

Bullough, V., Church, O., Stein, A., & Sentz, L. (1988–1992). *American nursing: A biographical dictionary.* New York: Garland Press.

Lageman, E.C. (Ed.) (1983). *Nursing history: New perspectives, new possibilities,* New York: Teachers College Press.

Melosh, B., (1982). *The physician's hand: Work culture and conflict in american nursing,* Philadelphia: Temple University Press.

Reverby, S. (1987). *Ordered to care: The dilemma of American nursing* 1850–1945. New York: Cambridge Press.

Woodham-Smith, C. (1951). *Florence Nightingale.* New York: McGraw-Hill.

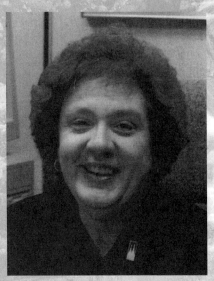

Photo courtesy of Carol Toussie
Weingarten, PhD, RN.

M. Louise Fitzpatrick,

EdD, RN, FAAN

M. Louise Fitzpatrick is Dean and Professor of the College of Nursing, Villanova University—a position she has held since 1978. Prior to that time, she was a faculty member in the Department of Nursing at Teachers College, Columbia University, where she served as major advisor for master's degree students in community health nursing and guided doctoral study in nursing history and historiography.

Dr. Fitzpatrick is a graduate of the Johns Hopkins School of Nursing and received her bachelors degree in nursing from Catholic University. She earned two masters degrees—one in the Administration of Community Health and one in the Teaching of Public Health Nursing, and her doctorate in Curriculum and Teaching in Nursing Education from Teachers College, Columbia University. She also holds a certificate from the Institute for Educational Management, Harvard University.

Dean Fitzpatrick is active in community and professional affairs and has held many elected and appointed nursing leadership positions. She has served as Chairperson of the ANA Cabinet on Nursing Education, and Chair of the NLN Accreditation Committee. Her research, scholarly interest, and publications are in the area of nursing history and nursing education.

Dr. Fitzpatrick has extensive experience in international activities including the former Soviet Union, Spain, Morocco, Egypt, Jordan, the West Bank, the Persian Gulf, and the People's Republic of China.

Dr. Louise Fitzpatrick is a strong supporter of leadership development in nursing students and is an individual sustaining member of the National Student Nurses' Association (NSNA).

CHAPTER 2

Nursing Education– The Vision and Milestones

INTRODUCTION

As the next millennium approaches, nursing emerges a mature, respected profession and a progressive force within American health care. The genesis of professional nursing is rooted in responses to the many political, economic, demographic, and scientific changes that the country experienced at the last turn of the century.

THE EMERGENCE OF NURSING AS A PROFESSION

The result of nursing's progress over the years is amazing. Today, nurses in clinical practice act both independently and collaboratively with physicians and other kinds of practitioners. They are full partners with their patients in making critical judgments about what will best meet their health goals at individual, family, and community levels. Nurses provide leadership in the administration of health services by conducting research that improves patient care and results in measurable outcomes. They serve in both the civilian and military sectors at home and abroad and participate in political activities, including holding elective office, and assuming key positions in shaping health policy for an ever-changing diverse population. Nurses are found in nontraditional roles more frequently. Some are nurse attorneys, others are employed by insurance companies and the pharmaceutical industry, and others are found within the growing health-related business community.

Nurses are providing leadership in the managed care environment as case managers and entrepreneurs. Some are experts in informatics using their experience and expertise in nursing as a rich database for designing health-related information systems. Many are faculty members and deans of educational programs preparing nurses for the future. Not unlike the early public health nurses of the 1800s who brought care and health education to disenfranchised immigrants, the community health nurses and primary care nurse practitioners of today deliver care to all ages and all socioeconomic groups—at home and in ambulatory settings. The achievements of American nursing in little more than 100 years are enormous.

Reflecting on this remarkable progress, we can raise questions about what has stimulated this growth and development during what is actually a very short period of time. Certainly our history can identify the numerous leaders, significant landmark studies about nursing, and the chronological events and contextual circumstances (such as scientific discoveries and military conflicts) that had a profound effect on nursing and influenced its development.

EDUCATION: THE KEY TO PROGRESS IN NURSING

The most important, single factor in the development of American nursing, and the reason that contemporary nursing clearly meets the established criteria of a true profession, is the role that education has played in catalyzing nursing's opportunities for progress. Nursing education, and the education of nurses throughout many decades, has provided the framework, the foundation, and the developments in the areas of theory, clinical practice, and research. The profession's commitment to education has formed its vision and its future, and has brought American nursing in post-modern America to maturity.

THE ROOTS OF NURSING EDUCATION IN AMERICA

At the end of the 1800s and continuing into the early 1900s, the country witnessed the proliferation of hospitals that served as laboratories for the training of physicians. Nurses were needed to manage these facilities and care for patients. As a way to meet this need, nursing schools were opened by the hundreds—even the smallest hospitals had a nursing school. There was no prepared faculty—the small amount of instruction given was provided by local physicians. In most situations, the pupil nurses worked long hours in the wards and were exploited. Few graduate "trained" nurses were employed by the hospitals. Instead, students provided the hospitals with cheap labor, and graduates were employed in private homes as private duty nurses.

THE VISION OF EARLY LEADERS

The few nurse leaders who began to reform this situation typically were women in their thirties. They had previous education as teachers and had adopted the fledgling field of nursing as their life's work and as a second career. They received their nursing educations in the schools of nursing at Bellevue, Massachusetts General Hospital, Johns Hopkins Hospital, and the Illinois Training School, to name a few of the larger and more prestigious schools producing the leaders of the day. In these schools, the resources and the approaches to teaching, as well as the quality of the clinical experiences for learning, far surpassed the average programs. Early leaders such as Isabel Hampton Robb, S. Lillian Clayton, and Adelaide Nutting believed that preparation for nursing required education, not just training in tasks that nurses performed. The idea of these visionaries centered on independent nursing schools that would be separate from the hospital, economically stable, and autonomous. This concept for educational programs was an adaptation of the Nightingale model used at St. Thomas Hospital in London. However, in practice this concept had a short life in America. The economics of the hospital and inadequate financial resources to endow and operate separate nursing schools prevented the vision of the leaders from becoming reality. From the beginning, nursing education was plagued by financial constraints, which continue in different but no less significant forms today.

CONCERNS FOR QUALITY IN NURSING EDUCATION

A major concern of these early leaders was the absence of educational standards, criteria for admission, and a paucity of nurse faculty to teach. Related to these issues were the problems resulting from the hospital environment where these nursing schools operated. The subservient role of women, difficult working conditions that made a good level of care for a large number of patients difficult, and the dominance of medicine, all contributed to the problems of quality in nursing education and nursing practice. The early leaders had intelligence, vision, and tenacity giving them the ability to elevate nursing through the vehicle of education.

THE EMERGENCE OF NURSING ORGANIZATIONS: CATALYST FOR REFORM

The founding of the American Society of Superintendents of Training Schools for Nurses (1893), in 1912 called the National League of Nursing Education (NLNE) and changed again in 1952 to the National League for Nursing (NLN), represented a concerted effort to set standards for schools of nursing as a first step in improving nursing education and practice. Shortly after, in 1896, an offspring of the Society called the Nurses' Associated Alumnae of the United States and Canada was formed. (Its name was changed to the American Nurses Association [ANA] in 1911.) In 1912, the National Organization for Public Health Nursing was formed and was later followed by the National Association of Colored Graduate Nurses in 1908. Clearly, the agenda for improving nursing through education was supported by the establishment of organizational structures such as these, that could deal with the myriad of issues confronting the profession.

The campaign for individual licensure for nurses that began with the passage of the North Carolina Nurse Practice Act in 1903 ushered in several decades of important activities undertaken by nursing organizations to safeguard the public, standardize curriculum, develop standards of practice, and organize nurses relative to the economic and general welfare issues affecting them. Issues such as the eight hour workday and adequate financial remuneration became the concerns of these associations. Only graduates of approved schools meeting the Superintendents' Society standards were admitted into membership in the Associated Alumnae. By successfully improving reasonable standards, peer review, and controls, nursing education—despite its location in hospitals—was regarded as a more respectable and forward moving occupation than it had been. Although the vision of the leaders continued to be college-based education, early efforts were concentrated and focused on improvement of nursing programs that had developed rapidly within hospitals.

DEVELOPMENTAL MILESTONES IN NURSING EDUCATION

The period before and following World War I was significant in the development of contemporary nursing education. The world was changing rapidly, and nursing education was responding to the forces impinging upon it, while laying a foundation for the future.

Waves of immigrants had created a need for community-based nursing services, and as public health nursing developed in both urban centers and rural areas, there was a clear recognition that public health nurses required knowledge and skills well beyond the traditional hospital training. In 1917, the National League of Nursing Education (NLNE) produced a *Standard Curriculum Guide for Schools of Nursing*. It encouraged a higher standard of curriculum development and implementation in the hospital-based schools. However, the rapid increase in the numbers of visiting nurse agencies, the demonstration and "model" community health projects flourishing in the 1920s, as well as the needs of patients and families for health teaching and health promotion underscored the need for advanced education for public health/community nurses. Principles of teaching and learning were viewed as integral to community nursing practice. In addition, these nurses needed knowledge of community organization, politics, hygiene and environmental health, and childhood growth and development. They also needed the ability to adapt practice to the home environment, and to practice independently and innovatively in these nonhospital settings. Most of all, they required an understanding of various cultures and the impact of cultural differences on health practices and beliefs about illness and wellness.

Simultaneously, there was growing recognition that preparation of superintendents of training schools, as well as faculty and those primarily concerned with the administration of nursing services, required education at an advanced level. Visionaries of the day set their goals high in order to move nursing education to a higher level and to respond to the obvious needs of those involved in public health nursing and those preparing for leadership positions in nursing education and administration. The vision of individuals like Isabel Hampton Robb, Lillian Wald, Adelaide Nutting, and their acumen to influence those who could help them develop the resources needed to accomplish their objectives resulted in the initiation of university-based courses to prepare nurses for these new and challenging roles following graduation from the three year hospital school programs that had awarded them diplomas in nursing.

COLLEGIATE EDUCATION FOR NURSING

A major accomplishment in the history of American nursing education was the founding of the nursing program in 1899 at Teachers College, Columbia University, which became a department in 1910. There, graduate nurses received education that led to the award of a bachelor's degree and prepared them for leadership positions in teaching and administration, as well as positions in public health. At other institutions, such as the University of Minnesota (1909), a model of basic undergraduate nursing education under the auspices of the university began to develop. However, for many years, programs like the one at Minnesota were not truly collegiate programs in the contemporary sense. Rather, they combined the three-year hospital education with some college courses.

The concerns about educational standards were great. Equally critical was the belief on the part of nursing's leadership that education was the key to elevating the status of the profession, the quality of practice, and ultimately the improvement of patient care. Through the intervention of nursing leaders, the Rockefeller Foundation financed a major study in 1918 that marked a milestone in American nursing education. The study led to revolutionary outcomes including support for university education of nurses and the strengthening of programs designed to prepare nurses for leadership roles.

This landmark study, called *Nursing and Nursing Education in the United States* was directed by a sociologist, Josephine Goldmark, and is frequently referred to as *The Goldmark Report*. Initially, the study was designed to examine education for public health nursing practice. But it was later expanded to address preparation for nursing in general. The report, published in 1921, provided direction and leverage for preparing nurses within colleges and universities to respond to the changing needs of the American public.

Experiences of American nurses who served with the Red Cross in Europe during World War I reinforced the belief that more education and a different kind of education for nurses was required. The ideas for two levels of nurses began to emerge. The vision was to educate professional nurses in a college or university environment in order to prepare them to assume leadership roles.

A MODEL FOR BASIC COLLEGIATE NURSING EDUCATION

In 1923, the Yale University School of Nursing was established with Annie Warburton Goodrich as its first dean. Teachers College had established a milestone by offering collegiate preparation for graduate nurses, and Yale's generic program was an innovative model that enrolled basic students who wished to become nurses. Endowed in 1929 with one million dollars by the Rockefeller Foundation, the Yale program reflected the vision that early nurse educators had hoped to achieve for the profession. Similarly, some other schools of significance were also endowed and provided additional models of nursing education that were futuristic. Examples were the Frances Payne Bolton School of Nursing at Western Reserve University that was endowed in 1923 (now called Case Western Reserve University) and the School of Nursing at Vanderbilt University. Despite the establishment of these and similar innovative models of collegiate nursing education, hospital schools continued to predominate, and as a result of the revised NLNE Curriculum Guides of 1927 and 1937, many of the hospital schools improved greatly. In addition, other major studies that examined the work situations and economic status of schools of nursing and practicing nurses themselves assisted in elevating standards in the schools and encouraged increased financial support for schools of nursing.

Some of these studies were included in the *Report of the Committee on the Grading of Nursing included in the Schools* (1928 and 1934). They had three distinct and important subsections:

1. **Nurses, Patients, and Pocketbooks,** a study of supply and demand.
2. **An Analysis of Nursing,** a study of what nurses did and how they should be prepared.
3. **Nursing Schools Today and Tomorrow,** a study which attempted to grade nursing schools. However, the results were never implemented due to lack of financial support at the end of the study.

By the late 1920s, the zenith in the growth of hospital training schools occurred with approximately 2,300 operating at the time of the Great Depression. That historical economic event halted the growth. Many hospitals went bankrupt, and their nursing schools were closed and many nurses were unemployed. Weak schools closed as well, and by 1936 the number of state approved schools for nursing had declined to 1,472. With the reduction in the number of schools, a discernable increase in quality was experienced. In general, curricula were strengthened and classroom and clinical instruction improved. However, there was still relatively little attention given to providing nurses with a well rounded education in the liberal arts and sciences.

A MATURING PROFESSION

A hallmark of the 1930s was a developing maturity on the part of the nursing profession. Strong hospital schools emerged as models for other programs, and the curricula reflected the growing sophistication of the health care system. College graduates who were drawn into nursing careers during World War I began to assert their leadership. With the collaboration of social scientists and funding from a variety of private foundations, studies continued to be undertaken that had as their goal, the improvement of nursing and nursing education for the future.

As a result of the Federal Relief Program and the passage of the Social Security Act (1935), new kinds of nursing positions developed. Of significance was the development of community-based services under public auspices, as municipal and state health departments were established. Frequently, these were developed as relief projects. Through legislation designed for the national recovery, federal monies became available to prepare nurses for advanced study in public health nursing. Increasingly, public sector support replaced the private philanthropy of the earlier era. Many of the private sources had suffered greatly during the stock market crash of 1929 and the economic depression that followed. New positions that developed as a result of the Federal Relief Program greatly assisted nurses who had experienced significant unemployment during the depression.

The Consequences of World War II

As reprehensible as wars are, nursing education and the profession as a whole have been stimulated by military conflicts. The need to care for the wounded led to major breakthroughs in the development of drugs, such as antibiotics, as well as psychotropic agents. Mechanical equipment and prostheses designed to meet the needs of individuals who sustained disabling injuries ushered in an era that witnessed the development of the speciality of rehabilitation. The influences of these innovations and methods of care brought changes to the roles of practicing nurses.

The declaration of war on Japan, which resulted from the bombing of Pearl Harbor on December 7, 1941, required both an immediate and dramatic increase in the nursing workforce to serve the country both at home and in military efforts abroad.

A partnership was developed between the federal government and the major national nursing organizations, forming the National Nursing Council for War Services. Through this cooperative effort in conjunction with the United States government, massive recruitment campaigns were undertaken to admit large numbers of students to nursing education programs at several times during the year. The campaigns glamorized nursing and were evidenced through posters, movies, books, radio shows, and face-to-face recruitment. In 1942, 42,000 nurses resided in the country. The government estimated that it needed 125,000 more nurses to meet the national emergency. Many college graduates enrolled in the accelerated programs that developed, and the patriotic spirit in combination with an unprecedented public relations effort to encourage a career in nursing, drew an overwhelming response. Then, as an added incentive to educate more nurses for the war effort, Congress passed the first federal legislation specifically designed to assist nursing students and educational programs.

Nursing Education and the National Agenda

Through the sponsorship of Representative Frances Payne Bolton, the Republican congresswoman from Cleveland, the Bolton Act created the United States Cadet Nurse Corps in 1943. Clearly, this was a significant milestone in the history of nursing education—not only because it made a significant investment in the war effort, but also because it was precedent-setting by designating specific funds in the federal line item budget for nursing education. In addition to the immediate result of preparing large numbers of nurses rapidly for the war effort, the $176 million program administered by Lucile Petry Leone set the stage for federal support of nursing education, which has continued in various degrees for fifty years.

Strategic planning to meet the war effort demonstrated that nursing education could be organized and delivered to students in new ways. In 1944, as part of the veterans' benefit package called the GI Bill of Rights, funding was available for nurses who served during the war which allowed them to continue their educations. Approximately fifty percent of nurses returning from the military took advantage of this opportunity and prepared themselves for advanced roles in administration, education, public health nursing, and the newly developing roles called clinical specialties.

ASSOCIATE DEGREE EDUCATION: A CONSEQUENCE OF WORLD WAR II

A major milestone and consequence of the war was the development of the two-year community college which offered associate degrees. Primarily and initially developed for adult students who wished to learn an occupation, the programs prepared people in technical fields as well as those students who planned to transfer to a senior college or university program upon completion of two years of liberal arts and sciences.

In 1949, an experiment funded by the Kellogg Foundation was conducted by Dr. Mildred L. Montag of Teachers College, Columbia University. A model of nursing education that was a new paradigm was created and implemented in two-year community colleges. Montag's vision was reinforced by an important study conducted by

Eli Ginsburg of Columbia University entitled *A Program for the Nursing Profession*. It recommended that nursing functions be divided among two groups: professional and practical.

NURSING FOR THE FUTURE: THE BROWN REPORT

Another landmark study of nursing and nursing education resulted from the activities of this post-World War II period. Supported by the Carnegie Foundation and sponsored by the National Council on War Services, a major study of nursing education was conducted by Esther Lucille Brown. The war had demonstrated that nurses could be prepared in accelerated programs. There were 28 recommendations made in the 1948 publication of the study report called *Nursing for the Future*. One recommendation was for the development of baccalaureate nursing programs in colleges and universities as the preferred model of basic nursing education. In addition, a system of accreditation of schools was recommended, and the inclusion of psychiatric nursing and public health nursing in all nursing programs was encouraged. The most significant thrust of this study was its recommendation that all nursing education be conducted under educational auspices rather than inpatient care environments.

The Brown and the Ginsburg Reports set the stage for serious consideration of Montag's 1951 treatise: *The Education of Nurse Technicians*. Montag posited that nursing information and practice could be classified into those areas circumscribed and predictable, requiring independent judgment, and having a broader nursing and scientific knowledge base. The former would be prepared in community colleges and awarded the associate degree. The programs would include general education and an integrated nursing major. The baccalaureate graduate would be the independent practitioner who would receive a four year college education with a nursing major that was built upon a strong foundation in the liberal arts and sciences.

Originally, the associate degree programs were called "terminal" and were not conceived as the first step of a nursing education career ladder. Over the years, the associate degree programs grew rapidly. In 1980, there were 707 associate degree programs in nursing. In 1996, there were 850. They continue to be the largest in number and produce the largest number of graduate nurses. Most of their graduates now continue their educations for the BSN. It was originally thought that associate degree programs would replace Licensed Practical Nurses and hospital diploma schools, thereby reinforcing the idea that there be two levels of nursing, both prepared under educational auspices rather than in hospital-based schools. At the time, the challenge was great enough to get individual state licensing boards to permit associate degree graduates to sit for the state board licensing examinations for registered nurses. Because of this, differentiation between and among those prepared in different kinds of programs through the development of different licensing mechanisms was not attempted. Therefore, even today, one licensing exam, now called the NCLEX, is used to test all students irrespective of whether they have been educated in hospital, community college, or senior college and university programs.

FOCUS ON STUDENTS: NATIONAL STUDENT NURSES' ASSOCIATION

Another major historical event within the development of nursing education that occurred in post-World War II America was the founding of the National Student Nurses' Association (NSNA) in 1952. This occurred after the reorganization of the national nursing organizations that same year. Over the years, the NSNA has contributed greatly to the development of nursing students and to the educational process. More discussion of the benefits of NSNA involvement can be found later in this book in **Unit Three: The Stepping Stone of Professional Involvement.**

PROLIFERATION OF COLLEGIATE PROGRAMS FOR NURSING

Simultaneous with the post-World War II developments, and encouraged by the Brown Report, was the development of numerous basic nursing education programs under senior college and university auspices. Unlike earlier college programs, a relatively standard model was developed in both private and public institutions. Students met the same admission criteria as all college freshmen. And like their counterparts in engineering, business, and a variety of liberal arts and science majors, they enrolled in curricula that included courses in the liberal arts, sciences, and the social sciences designed to educate the whole person while laying a foundation for professional preparation in a specific field or major, such as nursing. Although different schools often included a different array of courses in the arts and sciences consistent with their institutional missions, and the nursing curricula were organized in different ways, the outcomes were to be the same. The programs qualified students for award of bachelor's degree in nursing and eligibility to take the licensing examination for professional registered nurses in the various jurisdictions of the country. Unlike the hospital-based programs, baccalaureate programs utilized hospitals and a variety of other health care agencies such as nursing homes, clinics, public health agencies, and industry to provide clinical experiences that were taught by nursing faculty from the college or university.

THE DIVISION OF NURSING: NURSE TRAINING ACT

The federal commitment to nursing education engendered by the war, continued well into the 1970s and exists, to a lesser degree, today. Through the passage of the Nurse Training Act of 1964 and its subsequent renewals, schools of nursing benefited enormously. Jessie Scott, the Director of the Division of Nursing, United States Public Health Service, presided over the disbursement of funds that would provide the resources needed for nursing education to take its next giant step. The nursing influentials of the day had a vision passed along to them from former generations of nursing leaders. Congress and the White House provided the resources, while Ms. Scott and her staff facilitated the shift in support of nursing education from hospital-based to college- and university-based education through the allocation of federal funds.

Between 1960 and 1975, the number of BSN programs rose significantly. Government funding provided financial resources for curriculum development and revision, special projects, pre- and post-doctoral study, and traineeships awarded to applicant schools and then dispensed to students by them so that full-time study was possible for advanced degrees. In addition, federal grants from the Division of Nursing funded buildings, labs, and equipment for schools of nursing. Did your school of nursing benefit from funding during these times? If there was a golden age of nursing education in America, it was surely then. The positive outlook and belief that moving up was the only direction nursing education could go stimulated and excited the nursing leadership and socialized hundreds of students into believing that all things were possible for nursing and nursing education. It was an exciting time to be a nursing student. There was no talk of financial constraints or obstacles to progress, and the strong traditional beliefs about nursing's contributions to the improvement of society were considered limitless. It was a wonderful time to be in nursing education, which was moving forward at a very fast pace.

The proliferation of collegiate programs in the 1950s underscored the pressing need for increasing the numbers of nurse educators with graduate degrees. Faculty were needed to teach in these programs. Although it would be many, many years before nursing faculty had academic degrees commensurate with other professors in the university, the goal was set, and there was intense activity directed toward realization of that vision.

ADVANCED EDUCATION

Graduate programs in nursing had been limited in number and kind before the 1960s. As master's degree programs in nursing developed, the emphasis was on role preparation, especially in the fields of administration and teaching. Hospitals and public health agencies were becoming more sophisticated and required strong nursing leadership that was conversant with business techniques and the workings of complex organizations. Schools of nursing in colleges and universities required faculty who were familiar with the system of higher education, with curriculum development, with measurement and evaluation, and with teaching techniques. Most nurses who sought graduate education were already established in their careers and often incumbents in positions for which they needed academic credentials. Gradually, there was a beginning interest in preparing nurses at the master's level who would have advanced preparation in clinical nursing practice, rather than preparation only in areas concentrated on role development related to their current positions or the positions they would assume after graduate education. As more graduate programs were developed, this growing emphasis on developing clinical experts or clinical specialists, as they were called, created a controversy within nursing education circles. Frances Reiter, Hildegard Peplau, Virginia Henderson, Faye Abdellah, Dorothy Mereness, and others all supported the trend to advanced clinical practice at the master's level. In time, programs began to develop that prepared nurses for specialized practice areas. The programs also included opportunities for graduate students to elect minors in subjects related to teaching or administration of nursing services in order to also prepare them for their employment roles.

The passage of the Nurse Training Act of 1964 further stimulated the growth of master's education. From 1964 to 1971, over $334 million was appropriated by Congress for nursing education. Guiding the development of graduate education were nursing sections within regional education planning and accreditation groups such as the Southern Regional Educational Board and the Western Interstate Commission on Higher Education in Nursing. In addition, leadership within the accrediting body, National League for Nursing, and leaders involved in the development of the American Association of Colleges of Nursing (1969) encouraged this emphasis on graduate education. Simultaneously, hospitals began experimenting with new models of care delivery. These changes included primary nursing models and the development of new positions for these newly created clinical specialists who served as expert practitioners.

THE NURSE PRACTITIONER MOVEMENT

In 1965, Dr. Henry Silver (a Denver pediatrician) and Dr. Loretta Ford (a nurse) developed an innovative model of clinical practice that slowly, over a period of 25 years, began to take route as a track within graduate programs. Today it dominates the scene in master's programs of nursing. The development of the nurse practitioner movement and preparation for this role at the master's level met with about the same reaction as clinical emphasis had years previously. Nursing had existed within the shadow of hospitals and medicine for so long that the educative leadership, having emancipated nursing education from the hospital and moving it into academic settings of colleges and universities, then had serious concern about preparing nurse practitioners. They feared that they would become "junior doctors or physicians' assistants."

Today, curricula of nurse practitioner and clinical specialist programs prepare large numbers of advanced practice nurses for the care of children and adults in community-based primary and tertiary care settings. The preparation of nurse anesthetists and nurse midwives, whose roles developed outside the formal structure of advanced nursing education, have also moved these roles into alignment and the mainstream with other forms of advanced practice preparation leading to award of a master's degree in nursing. In response to the needs of a changing field and the managed care environment of the 1990s, master's programs in case management and joint MSN-MBA programs were developed to prepare nurses to manage care delivery in new ways. These new graduate programs drew upon students' clinical knowledge and also equipped them with contemporary management skills for the administration of services.

FORGING THE FUTURE

As advanced practice and clinical specialization have developed, a system of specialty credentialing has also emerged. In addition to the basic license for professional nursing, some governmental jurisdictions issue a second credential that legally enables practitioners to engage in advanced practice as prescribed by law. Specialty organizations and the ANA offer certification examinations to nurses prepared in specialties who meet specified criteria to sit for the certification examinations. Specialty certification identifies nurses with advanced education and clinical experience whose expertise goes beyond basic preparation.

THE ANA POSITION PAPER OF 1965: REVOLUTION AND EVOLUTION

The nurse practitioner movement that began in the mid-1960s was indeed significant to advanced practice nursing. But in basic nursing education, the most significant event of the 1960s was the development of the *American Nurses Association Position Paper on Education for Nursing*. The goal of the position paper was to facilitate support for the development of collegiate nursing education at all levels.

After many years of study and controversy, the ANA's Committee on Current and Long Term Goals proposed in 1960 that the baccalaureate degree be the basic level of preparation for professional nursing. Issued in 1965, the official statement, known as the *ANA Position Paper,* was adopted for study at the historic 1964 biennial convention of the ANA. It was approved by the ANA House of Delegates in 1966. It stated that preparation for those employed in nursing should take place in institutions of learning within the general system of education.

Studying the significance of this position paper and its consequences will provide you, as a future nurse leader, with a historical framework to better understand the current nursing education environment. It will empower you to help shape nursing education's future. The "entry issue," as it was called, was bitterly contested by hospital schools that had not been affected by financial retrenchment and graduate nurses from those schools who believed that completion of the bachelor's degree by already licensed nurses was merely a repetition of the education they had already received. A scission within the profession emerged and emotions ran high. However, there were countervailing forces, as well. In addition to the growing strength of collegiate programs (both BSN and associate degrees) and the financial resources of the Nurse Practice Act, our American society had adopted a philosophy of educational goals and attitudes that encouraged some form of college education for young people. A college education and a career for every American had been the vision of post-World War II American society. It was being realized, and this climate supported nursing in its quest to advance academically.

DOCTORAL EDUCATION AND RESEARCH DEVELOPMENT

Doctoral education in nursing experienced relatively slow growth until the 1980s. Before the 1960s, the pool of candidates was limited, and many nurses who chose to earn the doctorate studied in a related field. Before 1961, there were only three doctoral programs in nursing in the United States: Teachers College, Columbia University awarded a doctorate in nursing education, Boston University offered a doctorate in nursing science, and New York University initially offered a degree in education. But soon Boston University became the first school to award the PhD in nursing.

In 1981 there were 23 programs offering doctorates in nursing in the United States. A continuing concern has been the proliferation of programs that now number 65 in 1997, and the ability of those programs to employ well-qualified faculty to teach in them. A related concern continues to be the allocation of resources required for doctoral programs that during times of financial exigency can negatively affect undergraduate and master's education and drain resources from them.

Research development and the increase in the number of doctoral programs have gone on simultaneously and are strongly linked to one another. Nursing research and theory development have made enormous progress in a few short decades, but despite improvement in the quality of doctoral programs, there is still much to be attained in terms of research preparation and the research production of nurses. Like preparation for leadership positions, research has moved from studies about nurses, health care delivery systems, and student learning to a more in-depth focus on clinical practice problems and outcomes. This can positively influence direct patient care. The influence of nursing organizations such as the ANA, and Sigma Theta Tau with its emphasis on scholarship, and the influence of funds from the Nurse Training Act that made an increase in the number of doctorally prepared nurses possible, all converged to stimulate the interest and understanding of the importance of nursing research. Establishing nursing education within colleges and universities further stimulated and encouraged the need for such activity as part of the academic pursuit of faculty.

Evidence of educational progress in nursing and the results of advanced education and research can be demonstrated in several ways. For example, several research journals, research courses at all levels of nursing education, and the application of research findings in patient care reflect the advancement of the field in attaining its goals and realizing its vision. Perhaps the most conspicuous example of nursing's progress in this area was the establishment of the Center for Nursing Research in 1986. It had as its ultimate goal the establishment of an Institute for Nursing Research on the campus of the National Institutes of Health in Bethesda. This dream was realized in 1993 when the National Institute for Nursing Research (NINR) was formally established. Its 50-year-old counterpart, the Division of Nursing, Division of Health and Human Resources, has nurtured all the developments in American nursing education since World War II. It is identified as a single most influential initiative of the second half of the century that has affected the course of nursing education. Federal support and leadership provided the framework and resources for nursing to mature and develop, move permanently into American institutions of higher education, and it enabled nursing to develop its own body of knowledge through academic programs and the support of students and research. It gave birth to the NINR and was the lens through which the vision of American nursing education and its leadership was sharpened and constantly refocused throughout the decades.

In addition to the established forms of nursing education, there are examples of innovative models that emerged to prepare college graduates with a first professional degree of nursing at the post baccalaureate level. Like social work, law, and medical education, these programs were limited in number, but have made a creative contribution to the history of nursing education in the United States. Some examples are, the program at Yale that admits college graduates with an MN degree, and the Frances Payne Bolton School of Nursing at Case Western Reserve University, which under the leadership of Rozella Scholtfeldt instituted an ND for the same clientele. These degrees were not to be confused with advanced master's of science degrees in nursing and the PhD, DNSc, and EdD programs in nursing, but were modeled after the first professional degree programs in other fields. They represent an important vision of what could be. But, for reasons related to traditional professional issues in the field, the cost of nursing education, the influence of the health care system on nursing education, and a lack of sound economic foundation for nursing education, they have never taken hold, nor had the impact that the visionaries who created and developed them had anticipated.

SUMMARY

As we approach the new millennium, American nursing and nurses worldwide are taking stock of their heritage and are contemplating their vision of the future. Clearly, our progress as a profession over the last century has been inextricably linked to advances we have made in the education of nurses. Education will continue to set the pace and direction for the profession as it responds to societal influences and new demands for care. Our ability to advance in the future will depend, as it always has, on the quality of our education and our commitment to advancing nursing as an intellectual and scholarly pursuit, as well as a compassionate human service. Clearly, the vision that American nursing has had for itself has made possible the achievement of significant milestones and events that have advanced the field. Every profession in every decade has its visionaries. American nursing has been no exception. The ability of nursing's leaders to forge ahead and to accomplish goals that have moved the profession forward is an important part of the history of nursing and, equally, it is an important part of the history of American higher education.

CRITICAL THINKING QUESTIONS

1. Nurse leaders have consistently concerned themselves with the quality of nursing education. What were some of their concerns? What are some actions they took to elevate the educational standards in the field?

2. What influences and effects did military conflicts have on nursing education? World War I, World War II, Korean conflict, Vietnam?

3. The movement of nursing education from hospitals to colleges and universities was stimulated by several factors and officially articulated in the 1965 *ANA Position Paper.* What did the paper propose? What historical antecedents contributed to advancing collegiate nursing education?

4. Private foundations and federal funding have both figured significantly in advancing nursing education. What are some examples of each and how did they influence nursing education and the nursing profession?

5. How did national nursing organizations advance nursing education? What roles did these organizations play?

6. How did graduate education in nursing evolve? What factors influenced its direction and redirection?

ACTIVITIES

1. Continue your education. Nursing is a profession of lifelong learning and holds vast opportunities for nurse leaders. Invite your state's colleges of nursing to submit information about their graduate nursing programs. Compare and contrast them in your nursing leadership class.

2. Select a historical nursing education leader and complete an indepth study of her/his life, nursing practice and leadership roles.

3. Invite your Dean or Director to share the history of the development of your nursing program with your class.

ADDITIONAL SUGGESTED READINGS

American Nurses Association. (1965). *A Position Paper.* New York: ANA.

Ashley, J. (1976). *Hospitals, Paternalism and the Role of the Nurse.* New York: Teachers' College Press.

Brown, E. (1948). *Nursing for the Future.* New York: The Russell Sage Foundation.

Burgess, M. (1928). *Nurse, patients and pocketbooks, report of a study on the economics of nursing.* New York: Committee on the Grading of Nursing Schools.

Goldmark, J. (1923). *Nursing and Nursing Education in the United States.* New York: Macmillan.

Lysaught, J. (1970). *An Abstract for Action, Report of the National Commission for the Study of Nursing and Nursing Education.* New York: McGraw-Hill.

Montag, M. (1951). *The Education of Nurse Technicians.* New York: G. P. Putnam's Sons.

Rines, A. (1977). Associate degree education: History, development and rationale. *Nursing Outlook,* 25(8):496–501.

Scott, J. (1972). Federal support for nursing education, 1964–1971. *American Journal of Nursing,* 72(10):1855–61.

Stewart, I. (1943). *The Education of Nurses.* New York: Macmillan.

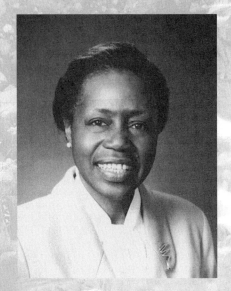

Geraldene Felton,

EdD, RN, FAAN

Geraldene Felton, EdD, RN, FAAN came to The University of Iowa in March, 1981, as Dean of the College of Nursing. She earned her BSN and her MSN in medical surgical nursing from Wayne State University and her Doctorate in Nursing at New York University. Felton is a retired Army Nurse Corps officer, having served as staff nurse, nursing supervisor, nurse anesthetist, and Deputy Director of the Walter Reed Institute of Research, Department of Nursing. While a member of the Army Nurse Corps, she held faculty positions at the University of Hawaii and Georgetown University. Upon retirement from the Army Nurse Corps, Felton was Professor and Dean of nursing at Oakland University School of Nursing in Rochester, MI, until she came to Iowa.

Dr. Felton is a charter Fellow of the American Academy of Nursing and a member of Sigma Xi. Past positions include Chair of the National Institutes of Health (NIH) Nursing Research Study Section and member of the Nursing Science Study Section; member of the DHHS Secretary's Commission on Nursing; President of the American Association of Colleges of Nursing; and chair of various NIH advisory groups and *ad-hoc* Special Study Sections for the Division of Research Grants.

She has just completed membership on the Pew/Robert Wood Johnson National Advisory Committee on Strengthening Hospital Nursing; and the National Academy of Sciences, Institute of Medicine, Committee on Enhancing Environmental Health in the Practice of Nursing. Dr. Felton's program of research is in the area of biologic rhythm phenomena. She teaches PhD students studying nursing influence on health policy.

Dr. Felton was named Kelting Family Professor of Nursing in July, 1996 and left the Deanship at the University of Iowa in January, 1997. She is currently serving as Executive Director, National League for Nursing Accrediting Commission.

CHAPTER 3

Nursing Research– Impact on Education and Practice: The Challenges and the Potential

INTRODUCTION

Much of what has happened to nursing is based upon acceptance of the assumption attributed to Thomas Jefferson that continues to be sound, "An educated citizenry contributes to the common good." Education is viewed as an investment in human potential.

Nursing is a dynamic *process* of human interaction whereby nurses use specialized knowledge, skills, and values to promote, maintain, and restore the health of individuals, families, and communities. The *practice* of nursing is the application of scientifically derived knowledge about human growth and development, the process of nursing intervention, and the evaluation of the outcomes of nursing service—all used in helping human beings preserve and/or achieve the maximum health state of which they are capable. The *artistry* in nursing is being confident in what one has to contribute, what one knows, how one uses knowledge, and the bringing together of knowledge and skills imaginatively in increasingly creative ways. It is this artistry in nursing that empowers one to accomplish the gamut of nursing's professional work. That said, nurses are successful when they believe that what nurses do is an essential, beneficially consequential, and valuable service to all human beings at some time during their lives. Nurses must embrace their education with a view toward making nursing practice reliable, effective, skillful, humane, just, and ethical, as well as cost-effective.

Standards of education and practice are key elements in how a profession defines itself and presents itself to the public. In order to gain public respect and the right of self-determination, nursing must adhere to the norms of professionals and the key elements of professional education: communication, creative thinking, and quantitative reasoning. Recruitment to professional programs is enhanced only when the credentials and entitlements of the professional are made clear to prospective recruits and to the public, along with delineation of roles, relationships with other health professionals, and lifelong learning.

In brief, higher standards of care; clear public recognition; and specificity in authority, accountability, roles, responsibilities, and rewards for the professional nurse are essential goals.

AMERICAN HIGHER EDUCATION

American higher education draws its distinctive character from an attempt to fulfill its three missions, in which knowledge is propagated, created, and applied. Thus, nursing research grows out of the success of the American higher education enterprise and adheres to the same basic assumptions.

The first assumption is the importance of mentors and networks, since science progresses through networks. Nurses who aspire to be scholars must learn how to enter networks. After they know what "nursing science" *is* and what a good education *is* for preparing the nurse scientist, they shift from exploratory studies and surveys to experimental and explanatory studies to determine *why* change occurs, and what, if any, other aspects effect change.

Another assumption is that person-oriented research focuses on critical health problems and has the potential to inform clinical care. Scientists must be aware of the increased need to clearly articulate the value of any program of research bidding for taxpayer support and be accountable for its progress. They need to share with the American public the value and promise of science and technology demonstrating how science adds value to our day-to-day life—improving and advancing our quality of life.

A third assumption is that research and education go together. Research contributes to the knowledge base of the discipline, and the outcomes of research activity in nursing seek to change practice, extend life, improve longevity, improve health-related quality of life, reduce the burden of illness and disability and the impact on health care costs, develop new products and new services, establish better approaches to promote health and prevent disease, and all-in-all contribute to the national welfare by helping to solve societal problems.

A fourth assumption is that focused research efforts are defined by priorities as nurses develop a body of work and programs of research, make a determination to identify and build on strengths and uniqueness, and collaborate in inter- and multi-disciplinary relationships and interactions. Discovery is pluralistic. It springs from the dynamic interplay between one's own interests, intuition, and reason and that of other persons. The more diversity there is among these elements, the more unique the resulting creative product. That means we have to stay receptive to opportunity.

Faculty Productivity

Faculty who are teachers and scholars provide the range of opportunities for educational, professional, and self-development. What they provide to students is founded on faculty scholarship. This presumes that knowledge creation is the most fundamental type of capital formation in a higher education institution.

Giving students a depth of knowledge. Depth is something a research university is particularly effective at providing students. Faculty actively involved in the creation of knowledge develop a deep and extensive understanding of existing knowledge. Many believe it is not possible to be good teachers without this.

Disseminating up-to-date knowledge. Faculty actively involved in scholarship must also be up-to-date on cutting-edge developments in their field. Research universities recruit and promote faculty who are committed to remaining up-to-date, disseminating such knowledge to students, and organizing modern curricula. If a faculty member is not keeping up, it shows in his or her teaching.

Involvement in knowledge creation. Whether we create knowledge in a science laboratory, an artist's studio, a political scientist's survey, or use computer or documentary materials, communicating the essential nuances of the process of knowledge creation requires intimate and thorough involvement in it.

Out-of-the-classroom environment. An environment that stimulates the intellectual development of students and gives them contact with a lively, cosmopolitan environment is an underrated contribution of a research university, albeit a diffuse one.

SCHOLARSHIP IN NURSING

To further develop the discipline of nursing, we need scientists and scholars. The *scientist* deliberately and systematically pursues development or testing of knowledge and finds answers for significant research questions in the discipline. The *scholar* conceptualizes the question as well as pursues the answers; is able to see the questions as parts of the body of the discipline; has a sense of history, a vision of the whole, a commitment to the discipline, and an understanding of how scientific work is related to the discipline's mission and humanity; has a lifelong commitment to the development of knowledge in the discipline and is always engaged in a systemic program for knowledge development; is flexible; has a well-developed theoretical orientation; seeks and engages in pertinent philosophical debates; and has a passion for excellence and a sense of integrity about the science.

Career-minded scientists and scholars properly trained in nursing science as their primary field have programs of research and scholarship. Programs of research and scholarship add to the knowledge (that in the aggregate might have clinical value). They address issues at the core of professional practice—the acceptance and internalization of the concept of high quality; cost-effective nursing care practices; the definition of nursing conduct; and the situational contexts that promote safe and effective health care, and lending support to the concept of scholarly and reflective practice.

Ideally, strong groups of nurse researchers and their colleagues are encouraged to band together and, with other disciplines, provide training opportunities for undergraduate students as well as pre- and post-doctoral students and fellows. They are urged to encourage sharing of resources among and between nurse researchers and clinical agencies under organizational conditions that will endure regardless of the comings and goings of individuals.

Research and Public Policy

Disciplinary research that has—or has had, or may have—policy implications helps policymakers make choices that guide social action and contribute in one or more ways to policy development. Specifically, these include monitoring the course of events that might be relevant to policy, forecasting emergent problems prior to their recognition, identifying and analyzing problem-raising situations, critiquing current policies where they are based on a poor understanding of the problem, redefining the problem, and analyzing the policy-making process itself—including initiation, development, implementation, outcome, and feedback.

Nurse leaders know why they become involved in public policy. It is because decisions on support for nursing science, nursing education, nursing research, and nursing practice generally, and on other policy issues involving scientific and technical considerations, will be made *regardless* of whether scientists and nurses choose to become involved—to ignore legislators is to disregard one's obligation to the nursing and scientific community and to the nation.

Nursing Research Funding

In 1993, the National Center for Nursing Research (NCNR) was funded at $48.51 million (up from $44.9 million in 1992) and language was inserted renaming NCNR the National Institute of Nursing Research (NINR), a part of NIH. Each NIH Institute and Center has its own public, scientific constituency, and research priorities recommended by expert panels. Research awards and contracts for studies help promote existing priorities by generating research on specific topics and prompting further studies in these areas. 1997–1998 funding is expected to be $55 million.

Nursing research addresses biological and behavioral aspects of critical health problems that confront the nation. Nursing research seeks to:

- reduce the burden of illness and disability by understanding and easing the effects of acute and chronic disease
- improve health-related quality of life by preventing or delaying the onset of disease or slowing its progression
- establish better approaches to promoting health and preventing illness
- improve environments in which patients and families seek assistance by testing interventions that influence patient health outcomes and reduce costs and demand for care

NINR research priorities (to date), 1988–1998:

- low birth weight infants: mothers and infants
- HIV infection: prevention and care; caregivers
- long-term care for older adults
- symptom management: pain
- nursing informatics: enhancing patient care
- health promotion for older children and adolescents
- technology dependency across the life span
- community-based nursing models for rural populations/Access and utilization for special populations
- biological/behavioral/environmental approaches to remediating cognitive impairment
- behavioral factors related to immunocompetence
- strengthening patients' personal resources for dealing with chronic illness
- changing health-risk behavior: HIV prevention for women/Biobehavioral markers and nursing effectiveness in HIV/AIDS
- symptom management
- intervention strategies
- quality of life
- older adults

The National Institute of Nursing Research is committed to promoting the development of a career trajectory for research training of nurse investigators through a series of award mechanisms that facilitate research training and career development. Such a trajectory allows the researchers to remain updated and in the forefront of the content and methodologies of their scientific field. The intent of the career trajectory is the development of the body of knowledge that can be used to accurately and predictively guide nursing practice. The purpose of the trajectory is to operationalize the philosophical stance that research training is a career commitment. The steps in the trajectory are not meant to be rigid but to provide guidelines for development and continual preparedness in the nurse scientist role. The nursing research trajectory indicates the mechanisms that are available for support of research training and career development at various stages.

NURSING SCIENCE

Nursing science is a process and a product for making inquiries about health care and health provider performance and evaluating the hypotheses that these inquiries generate.

Theory

It is generally held that there are three major stages in scientific research and that each is meritorious in its own right. First, there is perception of the problem and the search for new phenomena. Second, there is systematic analysis to understand cause and effect. Third, theories and models are developed and tested. Nursing science is a process for making inquiries about the world and evaluating the hypotheses that these inquiries generate.

In support of studies to gain understanding of people, events, interventions, and such things as the ethics or the appropriateness of nursing care and the context and environments in which nurses diagnose and treat patients, one ideally builds a theoretical formulation based upon clinical observations; thoughtful reflection on the nature of human beings; the nature of nursing practice and what others have said, done, and reported on the phenomena and the processes that give rise to them; as well as the constructs and variables within the constructs. Then a model is developed to refine and clarify the conceptual theory. The theory is tested and either discarded or refined until its validity is established, ideally by its ability to predict effective nursing interventions linked to patient outcomes. Models make specific predictions about propositional relationships in theories. A model is evaluated on the basis of usefulness in depicting theory and how closely it matches reality. A requirement is that there are surplus elements in the model that do not emanate from the theory. A basic problem in constructing a model is the failure to identify the theory clearly enough to develop and explain the nursing implications.

For instance, knowledge of rhythmic variations (my program of research) has potential for theory building and theory testing in nursing. Indeed, the construct of biologic rhythmicity turns out to be rather good for model building—demonstrating use of known facts and relationships to build theory. Relatedly, evidence in support of the model requires many and varied investigations. The importance of human time structure and the introduction of chronobiologic principles into our practice and our research requires knowledge of the observed rhythms of specified variables, knowledge of biologic rhythm research, knowledge of measurement issues, and clarification of clinical experiences.

Development of Measures and Models

The essence of science is a search for verifiable truths. Progress in nursing science, as in other disciplines, proceeds in an uneven fashion with periods of rapid growth spurred sometimes by new ideas, but more often by new methods and the data they generate. Nursing research is based upon investigator experiences in collecting data with instruments ranging from the classical and simple (e.g., thermometers, sphygmomanometers, syringes, stop watches, questionnaires, activity monitors, scales, etc.) to solid state data collectors that provide continuous monitoring of numerous physiological parameters (e.g., computerized monitoring of heart rate, blood pressure, temperature, etc.) and self-measures that can be analyzed by electronic aids to calculation. The availability of such "neat" instruments is invaluable. The data obtained provides information about the characteristics of the variable of interest—its range of values, its temporal associations, its effect upon the individual, and its application in nursing. Instruments used by nurses are selected based upon reports in the literature, their noninvasive properties, and their potential for usefulness for evaluation of patient care interventions and outcomes simultaneously. Obviously, those instruments must be applied in multiple, well designed, methodologically rigorous studies, having appropriate samples and large enough sample size to examine effect size. Ideally there will be built-in cost analyses and other contextual variables.

Instrumentation has a major effect upon nursing scientific research in important ways. It makes new experiments possible by providing new information. It makes work much more efficient. It increases the rate at which new things can be learned, because data can be accumulated and analyzed at a much faster rate. Thus, new technology invariably begets new science. Thus, also, the instrumentation revolution in which we currently find ourselves must be among the most exciting things ever to have happened in science. It is a pleasure to marvel at it, to enjoy it, and to benefit from it. Its impact upon our scientific lives is incalculable.

Just as the development of measures is a refinement and clarification of clinical experience, the development of models is a refinement and clarification (when successful) of conceptual theories. Models make specific, quantitative predictions about propositional relations in theories. The basic problem in constructing a model is to identify theories to the point where they clearly have model implications. Then, a quantitative model is constructed with the requirement that there are no surplus elements in the model that do not emanate from the theory. This is a standard caveat of scientific philosophers; however, few such models are used to direct or interpret nursing research. Yet, if the proposition of nursing theories is specifically interpretable, it is clear many nursing phenomena can be cast in this form. Our problem is to describe what is general in the scientific logic of research, and what methodologies are specific to the context of variables and outcomes that are unique concerns to nurse researchers and practitioners.

Limitations of Theory

The limitations of theory must be recognized. A theory is fundamentally an exploration of conceptual relationships couched in hypothetical terms and necessarily abstracts from many features of the real world. Without abstraction and simplification it would not be possible to begin thinking about a research problem. Since different investigators tend to see or at least to focus on different sets of phenomena, there is no option but to leave out what may seem to some people highly important. It is not to be expected that theory should attach significance to the features of the real world according to their prominence in the eyes of the layman, since it is not the purpose of science to describe the obvious in elaborate terms. But abstraction can be carried too far. The theorist may follow paths that lead one further and further from the real world and expose one to the danger of what has been called "theoretic blight." One may be tempted to select problems that lend themselves to sophisticated technical analysis rather than on the grounds of practical importance. One may become lost in admiration of the conceptual schemes one has developed without regard to the unrealistic premises on which they are constructed. One may also make the common mistake of getting things the wrong way round, or leave out what really does matter or that can only be left out provisionally. One may then be deceived into thinking that one understands how things work when in fact the model is misconceived. Theory, as someone once put it, can be "an organized way of going wrong with confidence." To be a useful guide, theory has to separate correctly what is adventitious from what is truly significant.

Theory may suffer from a distortion of emphasis or a quirk of intellectual fashion that throws into prominence the wrong variables, the wrong problems, or the wrong formulations of them; attention may then be diverted from the things with which the theory should be occupying itself. When that happens, the theory must be accounted not just irrelevant, but bad. The primary purpose of theory is to assist us in posing questions, and if we are moved to ask the wrong questions, theory has failed us.

Policy, derived from theory, has to deal with practicality and specific situations. It consists of a set of logically consistent propositions and abstracts from many of the circumstances that may in practice govern the policy pursued. What is to be done is never a simple corollary of theoretical conclusion.

In the application of theory to practical problems, insight needs to be reinforced by imagination and accurate observation. Imagination is kindled by good theory but is powerless or mischievous if fed with inadequate or inaccurate information. Further, theoreticians may tend to treat far too lightly the difficulty of obtaining and presenting the information necessary to a sound decision. If one desires to understand how something works, one needs to have an eye for the information that matters, the relevance of important relationships, and (since the unexpected keeps happening) for up-to-date information and imagination to conceive alternatives.

There is another aspect to consider beyond the development, the application, and the limitations of theory. If, after many years, we find that a theory has held up under experimental scrutiny, then the question arises, why bother to continue to test it? The reason is that fundamental interactions of nature and humans require the most solid empirical underpinning we can provide. Thus, this "testing the consequences" continues to drive model building in nursing. Every test of any theory strengthens that theory or does not. Verified discrepancies between observation and prediction will eventually kill a theory, and another will have to be substituted in its place. That is the circularity of science. It follows that the better we understand the implications for nursing, the better we may be able to extend and refine predictions about the consequences for nursing services.

Integrity and Trust

Simply put, the whole edifice of science, including nursing research, is built on faith in the honesty of other researchers and the veracity of their accumulated insights and accomplishments. Indeed, we are dependent upon each other's integrity. Few things are more damaging to the research enterprise than falsehood—be it the result of error, self-deception, sloppiness, haste, or dishonesty. It is the paradox of research that the presumption of veracity is the source of modern science's resilience and of its intrinsic fragility because there are many gray areas in the progress from planning to data collection, data analysis and interpretation, and then to reporting. A significant part of the problem is that scientists may not adequately explain how they acquire, interpret, and refine data or use the data to test hypotheses, modify hypotheses, and (most often) reject hypotheses. The simple truth is that over our lifetime there has been an increase in the total number of scientists, the expansion of science, an immense competition for scarce research funding, an erosion of honesty and ethical behavior among scientists, and an increase in the total number of visible transgressions.

SUMMARY

The norms of science are not a set of special ethical maxims. The means of science are the intellectual and technical tools with which scientific training equips members of various research communities and the deployment of which allows members to assess work as competent or incompetent, significant or trivial. It will scarcely come as a surprise that there are exciting opportunities for nurse scientists to contribute to the solution of current worrisome problems related to clinical manifestations. Thus, the circularity—research in the aggregate is meant to build on past knowledge to produce new knowledge to be stored in verifiable form for later use by science and by society. If you desire to become one of nursing's future leaders, I encourage you to read, critique, discuss, experience, utilize, and someday be involved in the development of nursing research. Continue your education both formally and informally. It will be essential in the twenty-first century that nursing's leaders clearly articulate what nursing is and the research-based outcomes that quality nursing care provides.

CRITICAL THINKING QUESTIONS

1. Only with a fairly large body of evidence are we really able to evaluate risk, for instance in such areas as diet and life-style. What can nurse scientists and clinicians do to increase the body of evidence to evaluate risks?

2. How can the undergraduate student's learning about nursing research be improved?

3. What techniques could be used to provide graduating seniors who have an interest in doctoral education with better information on the academic job market, potential job prospects, and nursing research priorities for the years in which they are likely to get their doctorates?

4. Inconsistency teaches scientists to be cautious; how can scientists help the public to learn the same lesson?

5. What should the NINR program research inclinations be for the year 2000?

ACTIVITIES

1. Meet and talk with a nurse researcher in your state, either employed in a hospital, at a university, or in a research clinic. Find out if there is a Nurse Research Committee at the hospital where you do clinicals.

2. Attend a nursing research conference. They often give student registration rates.

3. Find a topic that interests you and research the literature to see what has been studied about the subject.

4. As a class, watch the Ida Grove video on Nursing Research Utilization that was done by Horn Productions and Coleen Goode. How could you become involved in a nursing research utilization project?

ADDITIONAL SUGGESTED READINGS

Burns, N., & Grove, S. (1993). *The Practice of Nursing Research: Conduct, Critique, & Utilization* (2nd ed.). Philadelphia: W. B. Saunders.

Goode, C. J., et al. (1991). *Research Utilization: A Study Guide*. Ida Grove, IA: Horn Video Productions.

Horsley, J., et al. (1982). *Using Research to Improve Nursing Practice: A guide*. C.U.R.N. Project. New York: Grune & Stratton.

Iowa Intervention Project. (1996). Nursing Interventions Classification (2nd ed.). St. Louis, MO: Mosby Year Book.

Stetler, C.B. (1989, May–June). A strategy for teaching research use. *Nurse Educator, 13*(3), 17–20.

Titler, M.G. (1994). Infusing research into practice to promote quality care. *Nursing Research, 43* (5), 307–313.

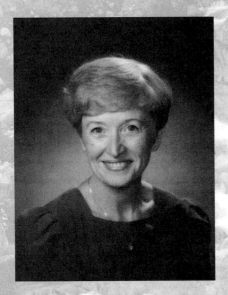

Ellen M. Strachota

RN, PhD

Dr. Ellen Strachota, RN has been a nurse educator for the past 20 years, teaching baccalaureate students at Grand View College in Des Moines, Iowa. She has been administrator of the Nursing Division at Grand View since 1985. Dr. Strachota worked on an on-call basis at Mercy Hospital Medical Center in Des Moines, until May 1992, in order to keep in touch with the hospitalized, critically ill patient and the nurses who served them.

Dr. Strachota values education and has a commitment to lifelong learning. She received her Bachelor of Science in Nursing from Marquette University in 1967, her Masters of Art in Nursing from the University of Iowa in 1979, and her Doctor of Philosophy, major in Education, from Iowa State University in 1989.

Dr. Strachota is an active member of the Iowa Nurses Association (Past President 1989–1993), the Iowa League for Nursing (currently serves as President), Sigma Theta Tau (Gamma and Zeta Chi Chapters), the Iowa Tri Council of Nursing, the Iowa Academy of Science, and the Iowa Association of Colleges of Nursing. Dr. Strachota served on the Council of Baccalaureate and Higher Degree Programs' Accreditation Committee of the National League for Nursing from August 1989–August 1991, and has served as a program evaluator and consultant of baccalaureate programs. Dr. Strachota and the Grand View faculty have implemented a new and innovative *Caring* nursing curriculum at Grand View as a result of her diverse experience and vision. That vision also established the Grand View Model of membership in NSNA. This model emphasizes and encourages membership through grants and work assistance programs with faculty.

Recognizing that nurse leaders of today must be politically active, Dr. Strachota serves as a member of Senator Tom Harkin's Nurse Advisory Committee and has testified on various occasions before national congressional committees/subcommittees as they addressed health care and nursing education issues.

Dr. Strachota is a visionary nurse leader and mentor, and has received many awards and recognitions from nursing student groups, nursing groups, and civic groups throughout her nursing career.

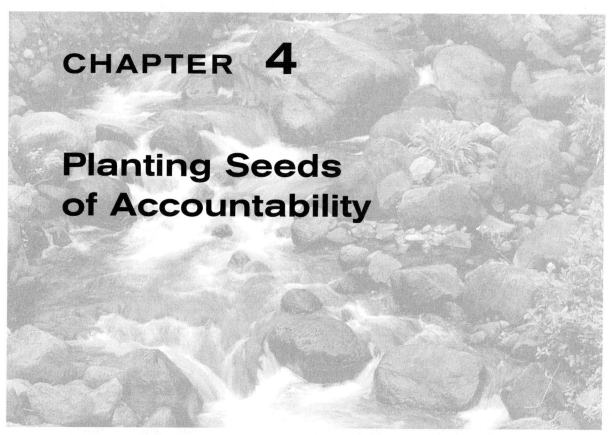

CHAPTER 4

Planting Seeds of Accountability

INTRODUCTION

In this rapidly changing health care environment, very little will remain the same. Students, as they develop into professional nurses, must understand and practice responsible, accountable nursing. Responsibility denotes an obligation to accomplish a task, whereas accountability is accepting ownership for the results or lack there of (Sullivan & Decker, 1997). Accountability is a complex concept with many definitions. It implies that one has both the authority and autonomy in the areas of responsibility (Batey & Lewis, 1982). Hyde (1985) describes accountability as the professional nurse's requirement of ability and willingness to anticipate the results of one's actions, act accordingly, and be held accountable by one's peers. To be accountable denotes an acceptance both of the obligation to disclose and of dealing with the consequence of the disclosure; it means being answerable for ones activities and to stand behind both decisions and actions (Snowdon & Rajacich, 1993).

Accountability is a process that needs to be nurtured throughout the nursing education experience. Because of the health care climate, it is critical to prepare nurses who can practice in a tomorrow full of unknowns. Nurses today and in the twenty-first century must be autonomous, assertive, accountable practitioners who communicate effectively and accept roles in new practice arenas.

Creating a milieu where students develop these needed skills in a time of transition in health care, requires a change in paradigm for faculty. The days of eight to ten students in one hospital clinical rotation with faculty rotating between patient-care rooms are rapidly becoming a teaching modality of the past. Students are learning one to one with preceptors; they are in communities, homes, clinics where there are one to two students with specific learning objectives. Professional education needs to provide opportunities for students to learn, think, and act as professional nurses.

In order for students to be professional nurses who are fully accountable, educational programs must provide students with a high level of skill in management, teaching, professional development, and research (Hancock, 1983). The fully accountable nurse must be comprehensively educated for the role. Students must learn to be accountable to themselves, the public, nursing colleagues, and other health care professions.

LEARNING ACCOUNTABILITY

When the student decides to pursue a nursing educational program, he or she assumes the responsibilities associated with the practice of nursing and develops a set of professional commitments and values. These responsibilities are based on minimum standards of nursing care where nurses justify their actions according to a sound knowledge and theoretical base. A portion of the role of faculty is to stimulate the students to critically think and understand the rationale for nursing care. Students need to be exposed to a variety of clinical and didactic experiences that will help develop these skills.

Resources that faculty can use to cultivate sound clinical judgments include: multiple textbooks and articles, judicious questioning of students, shared information seeking, clinical nurse experts, standards of practice and clinical pathways or protocols, and role modeling. Students should be held accountable for preparatory work for both class and clinical and should suffer the consequences if expectations are not met. For instance, students quickly learn to prioritize their student time to include formulating a plan of care for their clinical client if they are sent home when they arrive at the clinical sites unprepared. The faculty has a responsibility to the profession to instill these values in the developing professional.

THEORETICAL BASE

Sound knowledge and theoretical base for nursing care creates accountability by expecting students to build on standards of care. There are acceptable treatments for specific diseases, and students are individually accountable to know what they are and the expected outcomes. Students also need to be aware when the situation does not conform to the expected and to have an array of other possible nursing interventions. This is an ongoing process because of the rapid changes in technology, pharmaceuticals, and treatment protocols. Research, especially nursing research, is critical to explore new knowledge and skill demands for competent nursing care. Students need to understand how and when findings from nursing research should influence their practice and when it should not.

Faculty role modeling is essential for student development. Faculty cannot always have the "right" answer. The methods of inquiry used by nursing faculty help students understand that they do not have to know everything, but they do need to know how to discover a variety of potential answers. By working with students and valuing their input, faculty empower students to take risks, and share information. The faculty member who has an open and accepting attitude about learning from everyone instills a similar attitude in the learner.

ETHICAL PRACTICE

Embedded in accountable clinical practice is the concept of ethics. Nurses have a moral obligation to provide competent nursing care based on an honest relationship with their patients. That relationship is based on trust; trust that the professional nurse has the knowledge, skills, and abilities of a professional; trust that all that can be done, will be done, or that an explanation will be given.

Ethics has become a problem as nursing faculty have been experiencing a change in students' moral behavior. In a recent study, May and Loyd (1993) reported between forty to ninety percent of all college students cheat. Nursing students' cheating is of great concern for faculty as they mold moral values that will guide the future practice of the nurse.

In a study by Roberts (1997) where she surveyed nursing faculty about unethical student behavior, she found the most frequently identified problems to be lying, cheating, plagiarizing, falsifying information in patients' charts, and fabricating home visits. Examples included incidents from both clinical and classroom settings. The faculty interviewed believed that there was a positive correlation between classroom behavior and clinical behavior. They felt that dishonesty was a reflection of a student's value system and therefore behaviors would be similar in both classroom and clinical environments (Roberts, 1997).

Some specific exemplars included: reported situations where students turned in made-up home visits, indicated correct dosage of medication was given when evidence was contrary, copied newborn infant assessment, fabricated authors and journals in required papers, used articles verbatim in papers without acknowledging the author, and obtained test bank questions from the textbook and did not report it when test questions were the same (Roberts, 1997). Faculty from all types of nursing education programs can give similar examples. A great concern is that students sometimes do not realize that their actions are unethical and only regret the fact that they were caught.

It follows that if students have cheated, lied, been unethical, and falsified their way through their educational program, their knowledge, skills, abilities, and actions as professionals may also be questioned. Pellegrino, a physician, stated that when cheating has occurred in medical school, not only may there be immediate harm to a patient but the gravest harm is to the character of the cheater. Cheating in any manner is reprehensible because it misleads, deceives, and jeopardizes the trust that others have placed in the physician, a trust that is essential to a healing relationship (Pellegrino, 1991). This is also true for nursing, where nurses have a moral obligation to maintain an honest trusting relationship with those they serve (Roberts, 1997).

Nursing faculty can integrate and apply ethical principles throughout the students academic experience. Bosek and Savage (1997) discussed the need for clinical instructors to find teachable moments in the clinical arena. Opportunities to learn can occur through role modeling by staff nurses and the nursing instructor, attending patient care conferences, rounds, ethics grand rounds, and critical incident discussions either real or hypothetical. The students may also attend ethics committee meetings, read classic literature on bioethics, and take required or elective courses on ethics. Bosek and Savage (1997) encouraged faculty to help students separate legal from ethical issues. They also suggested role-playing situations such as questioning a physician's order, whistleblowing, advocating for a patient's refusal of treatment, or renegotiating an assignment to assist students to experience real-life concerns.

Faculty role-modeling ethical ideals in both classroom and clinical settings sends a very loud and clear message to students. It is vital for faculty to treat students ethically such as maintaining confidentiality, advocating for students' rights by seeking fair and just solutions, and demanding ethical treatment from each student.

The American Nurses Association has a Code of Ethics for Nurses, first published in 1950 and updated in 1985, which is frequently used in guiding nursing practice (Gillies, 1994). The Code is being updated again in 1997, and the changes were discussed at the ANA's House of Delegates meeting in June, 1997. Members of the House of Delegates passionately spoke about the importance of this code of ethics in their everyday practice of nursing. As nursing faculty challenge students to become ethical nurses, the Code of Ethics for Nurses will serve as a set of stated principles that all nurses can apply to actual clinical situations.

STANDARDS

When empowering students to be accountable practitioners, nursing faculty must discuss with them established standards of practice and standards of care. Standards of practice focus on the provider and define the activities and behaviors needed to achieve patient outcomes, while standards of care focus on the patient and describe the outcomes that patients can expect (Montgomery, 1997). Several sources for nursing standards include: American Nurses Association, Joint Commission on Accreditation of Health Care Organizations, Speciality Nursing Organizations, U.S. Department of Health, State Department of Health, and graduate nursing programs (Gillies, 1994). The standards range from general to specific depending on the organization and the purpose of the standards. Nurses representing all hierarchial levels and speciality groups in health care agencies should develop specific nursing practice and care standards (Gillies, 1994).

The National Institute for Health has outlined five general areas that standards of care should address. These include:

1. protection from harm: safety infection and environmental issues
2. provision of comfort: emphasis is on decreasing pain and anxiety
3. promotion and maintenance of equilibrium: both psychological and physiological equilibrium or balance
4. fostering autonomy and dignity: respect for cultural and spiritual uniqueness along with establishing a caring relationship with open communication
5. maximizing knowledge and understanding: patient education about illness, protocols, medications, treatments and resources throughout the course of the disease process (Montgomery, 1997).

Standards of practice describe the minimum activities a nurse must do on an ongoing basis for a specific patient. These standards describe assessment factors, interventions, and evaluation criteria that will be considered and utilized by the nurse in caring for patients and moving them toward expected outcomes (Montgomery, 1997). These standards need frequent updating because of changes in health care.

Nursing faculty can integrate these two types of standards into the nursing curriculum by having students read different standards and develop hypoethical standards of practice and care. By having students develop hypoethical standards for both, students can appreciate the similarities and differences. Students need to abide by the standards when they are functioning in the clinical areas. If they do not, it is imperative that the faculty identify the deviation and facilitate use of the standards.

Nurses and faculty role-modeling the use of standards in clinical situations will help the student adopt standards as part of being a professional. Standards then serve as a safeguard that an acceptable level of nursing practice is being delivered.

BOARD OF NURSING

The nurse practice acts in each state that regulate the practice of nurses are legislative mandates that assure the safety of the public, protect the practice of nursing, and make nurses accountable for their actions. These acts establish state boards of nursing and define specific powers of the boards. Practice acts differ from state to state but have some common powers such as the power to grant licenses, accredit nursing programs, establish standards for nursing schools, and regulate nurses' scope of practice (Catalano, 1996).

Licensure is a function of the boards of nursing. Graduates of accredited programs of nursing must pass a uniform licensure exam given through the National Council of State Boards of Nursing (Catalano, 1996). The National Council Licensure Examination (NCLEX) is a test of minimum competency designed to evaluate graduates' abilities to provide safe and effective nursing care. The exam is based on the knowledge and behaviors necessary for entry-level nursing practice.

The content of the exam and practice regulations are other ways to establish accountable nursing practice. Nursing faculty must present material so that graduates can meet minimum requirements and pass the NCLEX exam. This content can be presented in a variety of methods so that students learn. Learning is an active experiential process; it is holistic and emphasizes meaning, principles, and relationships among phenomenon (Reilly & Oermann, 1992). Learning is an integrative process where new learnings are incorporated into a perceptual field causing a reorganization of the field. This transfer of knowledge or skill occurs when there is relevance in meaning between previous and new experiences (Reilly & Oermann, 1992).

Teaching, the facilitation of learning, involves a sharing of the perceptual field of both learner and teacher. Faculty seek to assist students to develop a sense of excitement, curiosity, and discovery about what is learned (Reilly & Oermann, 1997). Students need to be involved in the process by problem solving and thinking reflectively and intuitively. It is this total learning experience that will assist students in the pursuit of new knowledge and the skills to use that knowledge in practice within a humanistic context (Reilly & Oermann, 1992).

Developing a teaching/learning environment that supports individualized learning is a real challenge to nursing faculty, but by doing so students learn and develop accountability. A positive learning attitude assists students, once they are graduates, to continue to learn.

CONTINUING EDUCATION

Some Boards of Nursing also have responsibility over nurses maintaining their competence by continuing education. Continuing education programs take a variety of forms, ranging from intensive journal reading and completion of a post-test to formal programs lasting several weeks. The important aspect is to continue to learn and for nurses as professionals to be held accountable for the decisions they make and the actions they take to provide client care (Catalano, 1996).

As a new health care system is developed, there will be even higher demand for professional accountability (Catalano, 1996). Nurses will need to enhance their knowledge and skills through lifelong learning.

Nursing faculty develop the concept of lifelong learning by exposing students to the variety of educational opportunities available to them. By having multiple textbooks and articles both required and recommended for student learning, the faculty shows students what is current in the area of interest. Faculty plant ideas of continuing formal education programs by discussing possibilities with students. Faculty who share with students their excitement in learning new knowledge and skills enkindle in students the desire to learn more. Faculty who continue on in school and earn advanced degrees provide a tangible example of leadership development to students.

SUMMARY

Accountable nursing practice is essential for nursing to be a player in the health care industry of tomorrow. Students have many opportunities to learn how to be professional nurses and leaders throughout their educational experience. These opportunities include gaining essential knowledge and skills based on standards of practice and involvement in the application of standards of care to provide ethical care to all patients.

Creating a climate for accountability to flourish provides a challenge for nursing faculty. A paradigm shift that liberates and empowers both students and faculty will provide the context. This new climate must provide choices and flexibility. Students as partners in the learning process work with faculty in innovative teaching/learning experiences. As faculty and students become more invested in practicing together, they will empower each other, develop accountable nursing practice, and together will help lead nursing into the twenty-first century.

CRITICAL THINKING QUESTIONS

1. Obtain an institution's standard of practice and evaluate. How does it impact the actual care you have seen delivered in the institution?
2. Obtain a copy of your state's Board of Nursing's rules and regulations. What do you identify as the parameters for delivery of nursing care?
3. What are at least three ways that nursing faculty have stimulated you to be accountable? How did that make you feel?
4. Describe an unethical clinical situation you have witnessed. Why was it unethical? How could it have been handled in an ethical manner?
5. What are the characteristics of a competent accountable staff nurse? How can you become that nurse?

ACTIVITIES

1. Make a comparison study of the following documents:
    ANA's Code of Ethics for Nursing
    ANA's Care Standards
    ANA's Standards of Professional Performance.

    Discuss how these documents differ. Evaluate which area of your nursing practice/profession each document seeks to guide and direct. Determine how they are used by nurses, with nurses, and how they are enforced?

2. Obtain and read a specialty nursing organization's standards of professional practice. Discuss with your class how it differs from ANA's and how it is similar.

3. Read and discuss ethical situations with your peers, faculty, staff nurses, and others. Keep a Journal of these discussions exploring your own beliefs about the issues in relation to your colleagues' beliefs.

4. Talk to an interdisciplinary ethics team at your local or regional hospital. Explore how they function, who the team members are, and their credentials. If there isn't such a team, explore how ethical issues faced by patients/ families are handled.

5. Discuss with your class how and why nursing students are held accountable for their practice.

REFERENCES

Batey, M., & Lewis, F. (1982). Clarifying autonomy and accountability in nursing service: Part I. *Journal of Nursing Administration, 12* (9), 13–18.

Bosek, M.S., & Savage, T.A. (1997). Teachable moments: Integrating ethics into clinical education. *Deans Notes 18* (5), 1–4.

Catalano, J.T. (1996). *Contemporary Professional Nursing.* Philadelphia: F.A. Davis Company.

Gillies, D.A. (1994). *Nursing Management: A Systems Approach* (3rd ed.). Philadelphia: W.B. Saunders Company.

Hancock, C. (1983). The need for support. *Nursing Times, 79* (38), 43–45.

Hyde, P. (1985). Accountability. *Nursing Mirror, 160* (16), 24–25.

May, K.M., & Loyd, B.H. (1993). Academic dishonesty: The honor system and students' attitudes. *Journal of College Student Development, 34,* 125–129.

Montgomery, K.L. (1997). NIH clinical center nursing department: Nursing standards (on-line). www.cc.nih.gov/nursing/nsgstand.htm/.

Pellegrino, E.D. (1991). In search of integrity. *JAMA, 266,* 2454–2455.

Reilly, D.E. & Oermann, M.H. (1992). *Clinical Teaching in Nursing Education* (2nd ed.). New York: National League for Nursing.

Roberts, F. (1997). Nursing student dishonesty. *Ethics Forum, 7* (2), 1–4.

Snowdon, A.W., & Rajacich, D. (1993). The challenge of accountability in nursing, *Nursing Forum, 28* (1), 5–11.

Sullivan, E.J., & Decker, P.J. (1997). *Effective Leadership and Management in Nursing* (4th ed.). New York: Addison-Wesley.

ADDITIONAL SUGGESTED READINGS

Beauchamp, T., & Childress, J. (1994). *Principles of Biomedical Ethics* (4th ed.). NY: Oxford University Press.

Silva, M. (1995). *Annotated bibliography for ethical guidelines in the conduct, dissemination, and implementation of nursing research*. Washington DC: American Nurses Publishing.

Veatch, R., & Fry, S. (1995). *Case Studies in Nursing Ethics*. Sudbury, MA: Jones and Bartlett.

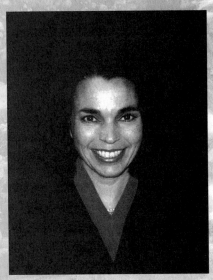

Photo courtesy of Robin M. Weingarten

Carol Toussie Weingarten,

PhD, RN

Carol Toussie Weingarten, PhD, RN, is associate professor at the College of Nursing at Villanova University near Philadelphia. Upon graduation from Barnard College of Columbia University with a BA in French Area Studies, she entered the generic masters program at the Graduate School of Nursing at New York Medical College. She later earned MA and PhD degrees in nursing from the Division of Nursing at New York University. During her 25 years as a nurse, her clinical practice has included work in parent-newborn settings, community and health promotion areas, and adult acute- and critical-care units. Dr. Weingarten's

publications include numerous articles, chapters, and co-authorship of the textbook, *Analysis and Application of Nursing Research: Parent-Newborn Studies and Nursing Care of the Childbearing Family*, now in preparation for its third edition. Her research focuses on birth defects and high risk parenting. Her own professional memberships include the: American Nurses' Association; Association for Women's Health, Obstetric and Neonatal Nurses (AWHONN); American Association of Critical-Care Nurses; Delaware Nurses' Association; National Association of Neonatal Nurses; Sigma Theta Tau, the International Nursing Honor Society, and the leadership and professional honor societies Phi Kappa Phi, Omicron Delta Kappa, and Phi Lamba Theta.

Dr. Weingarten's first contact with any student nurses' association was in September, 1983, when as a part-time instructor, she was asked by one of her students for some extra help for Villanova's chapter of the Student Nurses Association of Pennsylvania. The student, Sandra Myers Gomberg, was the chapter and state president whose recruitment efforts resulted in Dr. Weingarten's becoming advisor to SNAP-Villanova in September of 1986. Her efforts have been recognized by seven awards from Villanova's Student Development Program for outstanding guidance to a student organization, an award of lifetime Honorary Membership in the state SNAP, a state advisor of the year award, and by the first Leader of Leaders Award, given by the National Student Nurses' Association.

CHAPTER 5

The Role of Faculty in Developing Leadership in Students

INTRODUCTION

How many times have you heard someone say, "She is a born leader?" While this old cliché may apply to a few people, most successful leaders *learn* how to be leaders, develop as leaders over time, and find that the learning process never really ends. Leadership in nursing does not begin with graduation, but with nursing students' earliest days in their nursing programs. Leadership is a thread that should be drawn throughout nursing curricula, even when programs have special leadership courses designed for graduating seniors. Along with leadership comes the importance of political socialization—the process of gaining the norms, values, attitudes, and beliefs of political systems (Brown, 1996). These political systems include not only one's personal beliefs, but also the politics related to one's profession, employing organization, community, country, etc. Whether working on a small unit or with large groups, political awareness is needed to be an effective leader in all these areas. Brown notes that from the beginning of nursing education students must:

1. be empowered with the belief that they are the future of nursing
2. learn nursing's unique role within the health care team

3. visualize political influences upon that role
4. believe they have the ability to affect policy decisions and health care
    (Brown, 1996, pp. 120–123)

While leadership development is a complex process that begins early in life, nursing faculty members play a major role in the evolution of the leadership skills that will be needed by future nurses. Explore this chapter with your class, your faculty, and your SNA advisor. It will require each of you to stand outside the box of your curriculum and SNA and look in as a critical thinker.

WAYS FACULTY CAN HELP STUDENTS DEVELOP AS LEADERS

A classic Webster's dictionary definition of a leader—someone who shows the way by going first or directing by influence—applies well to nursing faculty. Whether or not faculty are consciously aware of their actions, they are role models who have enormous impact on fostering or squelching the development of leadership in future nurses.

Before and along with leadership development in students, faculty need to focus on their own continued leadership development. This goes beyond an assignment to teach a clinical or lecture course. Faculty are the professionals who have the first and the most contact with nursing students. Students come to their nursing programs with expectations of learning practice content from their faculty. Students also expect to develop skills that will allow them to negotiate the nursing profession and the world of health care successfully. For this reason, faculty at all levels bear a responsibility for leadership development in students. Faculty need to be aware of the trends and issues related to their own area of clinical expertise, as well as to the profession. They need to have a sense of nursing's progression and change over the years, and also a sense of vision that empowers others with the ability to look toward the future. Most students will not have this perspective and direction as they begin their nursing programs. Indeed, their views of nursing may be highly colored by characters in television shows, other media portrayals of nurses, their own diverse backgrounds, and varied opinions of relatives and friends.

In developing leadership in nursing students, faculty need to keep up with the newest literature and current nursing and health related events, and then discuss these with students in and outside the classroom.

Many changes in health care have altered traditional nursing roles and locations for employment. These changes have also given nurses unprecedented opportunities for practice and leadership in both alternative and traditional settings. One common complaint is that often non-nurses have made decisions that affect nursing. (Canavan, 1997). One solution is for nurses to prepare for, seek, and assume leadership roles. That begins with faculty fostering leadership skills in students who may one day become key decision makers in health care.

PROFESSIONAL INVOLVEMENT FOR FACULTY

Holding membership in professional nursing organizations is a necessity, not a frill for faculty. Today, there are so many nursing organizations that it is hard not to find a group in one's area of interest. Many national groups have regional and local organizations that search for members to become involved; some nursing organizations have begun working together toward meeting common political and educational goals. Faculty will often hold membership in more than one group, for example organizations such as the Association for Women's Health, Obstetric and Neonatal Nurses (AWHONN) and the American Nurses Association, which bring nurses from all areas together. Currently, many faculty serve as officers or committee members within their organizations.

Certainly, there are annoying as well as strong aspects to membership in any group. However, faculty learn about leadership development through the many opportunities available to them as members of professional organizations. Remember, just as it is hard for a three pack-per-day cigarette smoker to teach a credible class about the benefits of not smoking, so is it difficult for faculty who are not members of their own professional organizations to talk about leadership development to nursing students.

A ROLE MODEL FOR LEADERSHIP— ONE NURSE'S EXAMPLE

Nancy Sharts-Hopko, PhD, RN, FAAN, was president of the Alpha Nu chapter of Sigma Theta Tau, the International Honor Society of Nursing, as well as a member of the American Nurses Association and other nursing organizations. She makes time to serve as a distinguished lecturer for Sigma and attends several conferences. Back home at Villanova University, she shares her experiences and enthusiasm for her professional activities with students in her classes and also at a special, well attended meeting of the Student Nurses Association of Pennsylvania. Dr. Sharts-Hopko encourages students and outlines how they can actually become involved professionally. Beginning students are at first surprised to see their instructor doing and enjoying these activities. They see the connection between school and lifelong involvement, come to value this type of leadership development, and become or remain active in their SNA.

FACULTY ADVISORS

In many nursing programs, each student is assigned a faculty advisor. This advisor remains the student's faculty contact, advocate, and friend until his or her graduation. The advisor helps the student navigate the program. Some advisors also serve student nurses' organizations on local, state, and national levels. Students have personal responsibility for taking best advantage of their advisors. They need to make knowing their advisors a priority.

Whenever faculty can get to know students as individuals, opportunities to foster leadership as well as academic growth will develop. A recent survey at one nursing program revealed that students viewed faculty support and encouragement as major factors in their decisions to become members of student nurses' associations and to participate in leadership activities (Villanova, 1996). In another qualitative survey, McCabe identified high school students' perceptions of the most effective teachers (McCabe, 1995). These results were similar to what was valued by the nursing students. The students felt that personal qualities, along with subject competency, made for the most effective teachers and advisors (Krumberger, 1997). Table 5-1 lists qualities that students highly value in an educator or advisor.

Table 5-1: Qualities Students Value In Their Best Teachers/Advisors

Understanding of their subject matter/program/organization

Personal and professional qualities that identify the advisor as a role model for leadership/nursing

High but realistic expectations for students

Ability to negotiate the system well and orient students to the workings of the system

Ability to help students learn about professional behavior

Openness; willingness to listen and encourage diverse opinions

Respect for students' opinions; sensitivity to students' feelings

Caring about students; genuine interest in getting to know students

Sense of humor

Accessibility

Willingness to spend time with the students or organization—attending events or meetings

Enthusiasm and joy in their own work and in the role of advisor—a positive, "can-do" attitude

Ability to give appropriate praise during good times and support when students have difficulty

Willingness and ability to intercede on students' behalf when appropriate

Ability to demonstrate that learning and leadership go together

Ability to inspire others to attain personal best

Ability to make opportunities known to students and encourage students to feel confident enough to try for them (e.g. running for office in the SNA, authoring a resolution, applying for a scholarship)

STRATEGIES TO DEVELOP LEADERSHIP IN CLASSROOM SETTINGS

Faculty can help you make connections between leadership and subject content during regular class sessions. Emphasizing why leadership content is relevant to students' personal lives is an important factor in increasing students' motivation for leadership development (McCabe, 1995). As one student noted, "During our class on postpartum care, my professor spoke about shortened postpartum stays and their impact on women and newborns who did not have adequate follow-up. I found myself getting involved in this issue and writing to my legislator."

Small group projects and presentations require that students work together and assume leadership in planning and implementation. In most cases, students' grades depend upon it. In some cases, students within the group also grade each other in terms of leadership and participation. This is a very stressful, although frequently effective way to promote participation on the part of all group members. Such a learning activity requires students to look beyond themselves, make adjustments in personal schedules, make individual contributions, and yet work toward the good of everyone. To work smoothly, group members need to listen to each other, be conscientious about producing their contributions, and be flexible in terms of schedules and opinions. No wonder students often groan at the idea of group work. It is rarely easy or convenient. Due to conversation and group process, such projects tend to take longer than individual assignments. Conflict between such work-styles of people who start assignments immediately versus those who procrastinate until the last minute results in loud complaints that sometimes require faculty intervention. To the surprise of students, occasionally friends find they cannot work together, whereas people who could barely tolerate each other recognize that they can really get a job done well.

Many people have limited experience speaking in front of a group and feel anxious about doing so for a grade. However, by constructing assignments that require students to hold the attention of the class, faculty foster the development of leadership. One student leader fondly recalled the teacher who made her discover her own leadership skills. "I was always a very quiet student who sat near the back of the room. Not only did Ms. P rearrange the seating and divide us into work groups, she required everyone to take a turn leading the small group and giving presentations to the class. At first I was terrified; by the end of the course, I learned I could be good at this and enjoy it too."

Group projects should not be a substitute for classroom teaching. Indeed, students pay a lot of tuition and deserve to hear their expert faculty in classroom presentations. However, student presentations are a valuable adjunct to classes and enrich student leadership and content learning. Presentations don't need to be strings of oral sessions filling each class across the semester. Instead, such presentations can add interest and variety to one portion of a regularly scheduled lecture. In discussion of student presentations, faculty need to emphasize the leadership learning involved with this type of project. Students also have the responsibility of valuing their peers enough to remain through their presentations, even when the content will not appear on exams for the course.

Faculty can use alternate types of student presentations to foster leadership development. For example, in one community health course, students divide into small groups. Each group selects a nearby community and proceeds to do a thorough assessment, according to specific written assignment guidelines and in consultation with an advisor (who is one of the course faculty members). The presentations are delivered as a professional poster session held in the student center on campus. The poster presentations give students not only the community assessment experience, but also the chance to explain their work and the health needs of surrounding communities to faculty and fellow students throughout the day. With an attendance of nearly one thousand people who pass through the student center and stop to discuss the superb displays, the presenters are showcased for their leadership and expertise.

DEVELOPMENT OF LEADERSHIP IN CLINICAL COURSES

Despite leadership activities outside a clinical practice setting, students may still be anxious and unsure of themselves as they begin clinical nursing courses. With appropriate faculty support, this changes rapidly, and the clinical setting provides numerous opportunities for development of leadership. Again, students look to faculty, as well as other nurses on their units, for primary role models. Faculty with strong working relationships with the other health care providers in the clinical setting provide examples of ways in which networking, collaboration and negotiation, rather than confrontation, achieve patient-care goals.

LEADERSHIP DEVELOPMENT THROUGH INTERDISCIPLINARY COLLABORATION

In our first example, a nursing student was assigned to newborn Baby J. In performing an assessment, the student immediately noticed that the baby's arms and legs were a deep blue, although the baby appeared otherwise well. Was this an example of the normal newborn condition of acrocyanosis or was the baby developing a serious problem? The student at once called her instructor and the pediatric resident, who wanted to transfer the baby to the intensive care nursery. However, the student's instructor thought the condition was indeed acrocyanosis, although a very pronounced case. Transferring the baby would have been emotionally devastating to the parents, would have involved the discomfort and risks of intensive care evaluation, and would have been costly. The instructor, who got along well with the resident and had a long standing professional friendship with the Chief of Neonatology, instead asked to have her colleague come to the well baby nursery, which he was happy to do when the situation was explained. The neonatologist, who happened to have a photo of a similar newborn in one of his medical textbooks, indeed diagnosed acrocyanosis, which was explained to the relieved parents. The baby continued to do well, went home without incident, and the nursing student was able to learn how advocacy and leadership need not involve confrontation.

In our second example, the instructor from an affiliating nursing program noticed that the medical student appeared to be awkward in handling babies. The medical student was standing at the periphery of the nursing student group as the instructor began a demonstration of newborn assessment. The instructor, correctly identifying that the medical student knew little about real babies, invited her to join the student group, introduced her and the nursing students to each other, and oriented her to a newborn assessment as well as to basic newborn care. This initiated a friendly working relationship between the medical student, her medical colleagues, and the nursing students, who helped each other throughout their rotation. The physician faculty also welcomed the nursing students on teaching rounds with their medical students. The positive relationship among the nursing and medical faculty leaders and their interest in students, regardless of discipline, set an example that resulted in nursing and medical students working well together.

UTILIZING CLINICAL EXPERIENCES AS LEADERSHIP DEVELOPMENT OPPORTUNITIES

In clinical practice, mastery and leadership are closely allied. Faculty need to understand the level of their students to make patient assignments based on each student's unique level and learning needs. There is a large difference between providing challenging learning and overwhelming a student with patient assignments that would be difficult for a nurse specialist with years of experience on the same unit. Negative clinical experiences and experiences without faculty support derail interest in the clinical subject and also toward nursing.

Clinical Conferences

Pre- or post-clinical conferences provide an ideal setting for fostering leadership. Groups tend to be small (10 students or less), and it is feasible for everyone to have an opportunity to participate in discussion. Although some students will readily contribute their opinions, others will choose to remain silent and listen to their instructor's "words of wisdom." Some students do not have the courage to speak in front of someone they view as an expert, or worry about what other students will think of their opinions. Understanding that leadership can be developed through opportunities to speak in groups, faculty need to design strategies that will require students to present their beginning expertise. For example, while working with an especially quiet group, one instructor required everyone to contribute at least one comment during every post conference or risk being called upon. Within a few weeks, a strategy that was first met with snickers became an excuse for lively discussions in which even the "quietest" students actively participated. Other strategies require each student to lead a group conference. For example, the students' assignment can entail selecting an article related to the clinical area from a current nursing journal, presenting the article and topic to the group, and leading a discussion. This type of assignment allows students to explore a topic of their interest, actually retrieve an appropriate article from the current nursing literature, and have a real experience in planning and leading a small group conference.

Leadership occurs in clinical experiences on many levels. On the units, activities that promote leadership include one to one patient teaching or small group classes led by students. The old adage, "No one sits until everyone sits," is helpful in encouraging students with lighter assignments to help students and staff who need assistance. Teaching students to learn how to ask for help and to look beyond completion of their own assignments to the welfare of their fellow students and the staff helps them to gain a broader perspective of nursing care and life on the units.

Developing leadership does not mean abandoning students to figure out on their own what to do. Faculty need to remain an active and supportive presence on clinical units. For example, demonstrating a patient assessment or accompanying a student unsure of her own patient assessment should be viewed as a form of mentoring, rather than the more negatively viewed "spoon feeding." Even the best nursing arts laboratories do not prepare students for their first time working with real people. Faculty need to help students gain confidence, which in turn leads to a student's further development of leadership and independence.

Home and community settings for health restoration and promotion require leadership skills that may differ from acute care settings. Indeed, these settings provide unique opportunities for students to be independent. For example, in one school, health promotion and community health is a senior level nursing course that places students for seven week blocks in home health and then in wellness settings. One group affiliated with an inner-city elementary school, short on resources and greatly in need of health education for the children. The school's principal, herself an extraordinary leader, reached out to the nursing faculty and other members of the community to bring services and enrichment to the school that could otherwise not offer these services to the children. Over the rotation, in consultation with the clinical instructor and with the individual classroom teachers, the group of 10 students, working in pairs, taught over 90 classes on various health topics. The nature of their clinical placement required them to be leaders and role models for the children, and developing skills that many of the nursing students did not realize they possessed. An unintended and unexpected by-product of this experience is that many of the children voiced their determination to remain in school so that one day they could also become nurses. The rotation is so popular that nursing students vie for the chance to have one of the ten spaces, despite the heavy workload involved.

Respect for Diverse Opinions and Backgrounds

Students who do not feel their diverse opinions and backgrounds are valued or respected will often remain quiet, become angry, or simply turn off to a rotation. One aspect of leadership development is for faculty to address the potential for this situation to occur and strive for an atmosphere that accepts diversity, even when agreement is not possible. One assignment, for example, asks students to identify their own opinions about an issue and then present an argument from the opposing viewpoint. Nontraditional students can be encouraged to make connections between previous experiences, (for example in the business world), and current health care situations. Initiating discussions of why patients might not like particular situations or care arrangements and then identifying realistic ways in which the situation could be handled effectively promotes problem solving and leadership.

PROMOTING LEADERSHIP IN A STUDENT NURSES' ASSOCIATION

Student nurses associations are student run groups. However, the role of the faculty advisor is crucial to the success of the group. The strongest and most active groups in the United States tend to have advisors who care about them, are able to invest a considerable amount of time, and are also very involved. (See Table 5-1.)

SNA chapters attract the best students and bring out the best in students. As one former chapter officer observed, "It's hard to become involved and not learn about leadership." Many NSNA alumni credit their days as students for giving them a start in their development as leaders. One student warmly recalled being at her first convention as a freshman when her advisor, Judith Errickson, encouraged her to run for office. "Who, me?" she remembers asking while being surprised that she was even being considered. "Yes, you. You have the potential, and you could do a great job," replied her advisor, who identified the student as a possible leader and then informed her of the process of being a candidate. The student, Cynthia Rich Schmus, ran, won the election, became increasingly involved as a leader at the local, state, and national levels, and eventually was elected president of NSNA. Continuing her leadership in several professional nursing organizations and in her clinical practice in pediatric oncology, Ms. Schmus credits her advisor and involvement with the student nurses associations for her start as a successful nursing leader.

Nursing programs differ in selection of advisors. Deans or program directors appoint advisors in some places; in others, advisors are elected by the students. Some advisors may serve a certain term; others remain as advisors until they themselves, the students, or the dean or program director requests a change. Whatever the source of appointment, advisors need to be well informed about the SNA on the local, state, and national level. In most cases, the advisor's efforts are directed toward the care and development of the local chapter. The NSNA has several publications that advisors find helpful in learning about the organization. For example, *Getting the Pieces to Fit* is an excellent handbook, targeted toward state associations and school chapters. NSNA also maintains a New York City office, where staff is available to answer questions or help advisors get in touch with appropriate resource pesonnel. (NSNA at (212) 581-2211)

Chapter leadership development does not simply happen. Chapter leadership requires a vigorous approach to planning, implementation and evaluation of goals and events, a working partnership between advisors and student leaders, and an eye toward recruitment and retention of members. Students look to advisors for their unique perspectives on chapter development; seasoned advisors provide guidance, strengthened with experience of knowing and working with the student groups. New advisors face all the challenges of having to learn about a complex organization, while the group is carrying on a current agenda and evolving toward future goals. Occasionally, former or outgoing advisors will serve as mentors to new advisors in the same program.

However, in many cases the new advisor is the only advisor. A major benefit of NSNA and of the state SNAs is a network of advisors. Faculty consultation about leadership and chapter development has taken place over the telephone, at individual meetings in the advisors' geographic areas, and in advisors' meetings at state and national conventions. A list of advisors is compiled each year by NSNA, although this list does not identify length or nature of advisement experience. A call to the state consultant or NSNA can help a new advisor identify a colleague for consultation.

Being an effective advisor is a large and challenging job that definitely becomes easier and increasingly satisfying with experience. Time and access to students is necessary. The advisor should anticipate this, and the students can expect this to be provided by their advisor. Regardless of experience, advisors do need to be in regular contact with the student officers. Although students handle their own organization, during the academic year, advisors of active chapters may speak with the group's president daily or several times per week. In addition, advisors need to attend SNA chapter meetings and events. "Being there" for students fosters a strong student-faculty relationship, allows for trouble shooting, and makes for some very special memories.

Without financial support from their programs or due to other commitments, faculty may not be able to attend state or national conventions. However, other advisors are always present and are sources of support and advice to individual students or student groups attending. In a recent situation, one student from a particular school wanted to attend NSNA's national convention. The student did not know anyone else and would have had to travel alone. Her advisor was not able to attend, but contacted another local advisor who was accompanying a large delegation from her school to the convention. The student was then able to travel in the company of a group of nursing students, who welcomed her as a new and valued friend. She was included at dinners and events attended by the larger delegation, assisted by the chapter's advisor, and was able to learn a great deal about chapter building and leadership through her networking. Without such an opportunity, the student said she might not have gone to the convention and would have missed out on a learning opportunity.

Some advisors worry that giving any opinion when asked by students or offering any advice will interfere with the students' leadership. A complete hands-off attitude can give students the impression that the advisor does not care to be involved or that asking for advice is useless. Students ultimately make decisions for their chapters. In a strong advisor-student chapter relationship, the students turn to their advisor for advice in leading the chapter, but never feel "forced" into following the advisor's ways of thinking. For example, a charitable organization contacts the SNA advisor to ask whether the group will help with a "walk" event to raise awareness of heart health and raise money for research and patient care. The advisor knows the students would probably be excited to help this group whose event is perfectly timed, accessible to them, and an opportunity for community service. Nevertheless, such a commitment will require the students to spend their own time and work with a group they have not affiliated with in the past. The advisor, therefore, tells the director of the charity that she first needs to speak to the chapter's president, who will then contact the charity. The students decide to participate, the student leader follows up the contact, and both the SNA and the charity benefit from a well-staffed event.

In another situation, the chapter is planning to pay for a group of members to attend the NSNA convention, a plane ride away from the school. The advisor learns of a special fare on a legitimate airline; this fare is $100 per seat less than the best fare the group has been able to find. However, due to the ever changing fare rules in the airline industry, the special fare needs to be confirmed that day. Knowing that the group will be saving a great deal of money for transportation on a major airline to a convention they already intended to attend, the advisor, whose signature is needed for any payments, authorizes the Student Development Office to purchase the tickets. The group then uses the savings toward other chapter priorities. Ultimately, the advisor needs to keep a delicate balance between encouraging students' creativity and leadership, providing needed advice, and avoiding the need to "run the show."

Advisors, as well as chapter officers, need to ensure continuity of goals and activities from one academic period to the next. This can be problematic for a group when student leaders graduate or when elections for student officers are held just as the school year is closing and students take new leadership positions. One school addressed this difficulty by holding elections for student officers at the end of the first semester, in December. The outgoing president, usually a senior, remains on the board in the position of immediate past president; this individual also leads the school's delegation to the NSNA in April. In addition, members of the "old" student board remain accessible. August brings the return of a seasoned board of student leaders, half way through their terms. This arrangement works well in three or four year programs. Shorter programs and those which span the calendar year may need alternate strategies. For example, an "Old Board-New Board" meeting, held after elections, allows the new student leaders to be oriented by outgoing chapter officers.

Orientation handbooks, created by student leaders, are very helpful to future leaders, particularly when they do not have easy access to former leaders. Information in these booklets should include brief job descriptions for student officers and the faculty advisor, budget deadlines, room assignment issues, sample schedules and agendas for meetings, the names, addresses, and phone numbers of important contacts, and any other relevant tips for the successful running of the organization. Once prepared, such booklets need only periodic updates.

THE SNA CHAPTER

In working with student leaders of the SNA chapter, advisors need to make certain that the following topics are addressed: Short and long range chapter planning, leadership of the chapter, leadership development for students who are not chapter officers, schedule planning, budgeting, relationship with state and national SNAs, professional behavior, addressing financial concerns related to membership, and visibility.

Short and Long Range Chapter Planning

By helping students to create and implement a strategic plan for the chapter, faculty help students realize that leaders need "to avoid getting lost in the detail and the chaos of the present, but to instead look for the 'big picture'" (Frymier, 1995). Well developed chapters implement activities that include education, professional development, community service, and socializing. By having a good knowledge of the chapter's history and past issues, the advisor can help students learn from the experiences of students who have already graduated. Chapter archives, kept in a secure place and including a copy of all "paper" related to the organization, provide access to information not available from students no longer at the school. Accompanying computer disc archives can also be important, particularly for copying and updating annual reports, related to the SNA. However, rapid changes in technology may make current discs obsolete in the future; an actual printout better ensures that records will be accessible. Advisors also foster leadership by encouraging documentation through minutes of meetings, an end-of-year student and advisor's report, and copies of budgets and correspondence.

Leadership of the Chapter

In some chapters, student officers form a core Board of Directors that meets regularly as a steering committee and then presents the outcomes of their work to the general membership. Students appreciate the advisor's presence and guidance at these meetings, particularly in identifying solutions to potential problems and workable strategies for realizing goals. Such meetings give the advisor an opportunity to serve as a leadership mentor and to help students as they plan to run meetings and events. In many cases, the advisor is the only individual who stays with the organization over the years and beyond the graduation of present student leaders.

Leadership Development for Students Who Are Not Chapter Officers

Learning how to delegate responsibilities and inspire others to want to make their own best contributions is an important characteristic of leaders. However, in being responsible themselves, student officers may try to do every task without knowing how to involve their peers. Faculty advisors can work with student leaders to develop student committees that will include any members interested in a particular project. The advisor can then help student committee leaders identify the importance of communicating an agenda for the committee's tasks and making sure that students who indicated interest are actually contacted and given credit for their contributions. As one student remarked, "I signed up to help with a community service project, but nobody ever called me. I assumed I wasn't needed and lost interest." Another student recalled being recruited for the chapter's Resolutions Committee at the first meeting she attended. "I signed up for this committee, although I didn't know anything about resolutions, and the committee chair called me and included me. I had some responsibility but was not overwhelmed. With the help of the student chairperson and our advisor, I learned a lot and just wanted to continue being involved." This student eventually became legislative coordinator and then president of her chapter. With her growing experience and confidence, she authored a resolution and presented it on behalf of the chapter to the Houses of Delegates at the state and national conventions.

Student nurses' conventions are superb opportunities for leadership development in all students. Indeed, students who attend simply as members later find themselves running for office. One chapter holds a lottery for convention. Although student officers earn a place as part of the school's convention delegation, any member who wants to go submits his or her name. A lottery determines the rest of the delegation. This method ensures that potential leaders are not turned away because they are new or not close friends with the advisor or chapter officers.

Schedule Planning

Crucial to the success of any chapter, schedule planning is a fundamental leadership activity. Ideally, schedule planning for the next year takes place before the end of the academic year and is done by the student Board of Directors in consultation with the advisor. The year's agenda can then be presented to the general membership for approval or modification. Scheduling involves planning for regular meetings as well as for special events. For example, when meetings are not scheduled for the night before midterms or during hours when major courses are held, more students attend. In programs where someone always seems to have a class conflict, varying meeting times encourages members' participation. As one school found out, planning a health fair one day before Thanksgiving resulted in only a handful of people attending. Scheduling a similar event during an otherwise quiet March of the following year drew a large crowd. The student leaders also learned that explaining the volunteer and community service aspects of the event to the facilities management supervisor and to the head of the student center resulted in a donation of the services of the maintenance crew, tables, and trays of food for the health fair. Such items alone would have strained the budget for the project.

Planning questions to be addressed include: When and where meetings will be held? How is the best meeting space negotiated? Who at the school needs to be contacted for meeting space and how far in advance must this be done? What restrictions (for example, no food in certain meeting rooms) or requests (for example, audiovisual materials) need to be considered? Are there fees associated with meetings and events, and what are the best ways to address these financial concerns? What will take place during each meeting or event? How can meetings be made interesting? How can goals for each meeting be met within a well defined time period?

No one wants to attend a long, disorganized meeting. Time management for all the SNA events is crucial. In some programs, meetings, which do not exceed one hour, include both chapter business and a guest speaker. While some chapters have funds to pay guest speakers, many others do not. Successful alumni and other health care professionals are usually pleased to give a short talk about their specialty to students. Such programs, selected according to students' interest, introduce students to local leaders and experts and also reinforce the educational goals of the group. Student leaders tend to become leaders within their community and the nursing profession. Indeed, students have identified mentors, as well as their lifetime specialties from such meetings. Students often look to their faculty advisor to suggest speakers for meetings; advisors who are involved in their own professional activities and have a wide network of contacts usually have no difficulty in suggesting speakers.

Budgeting

Many students have not had experience in planning budgets for organizations; however, proper budgeting and making sure that budget deadlines for programs and schools are met will be necessary. Although SNAs may get some financial support from their institutions, most groups need to raise funds through sales or income-generating events. Advisors can guide students in selecting appropriate fund raisers and in making certain students understand what fund-raising involves and how income needs to be planned and handled.

Relationship with State and National SNAs

Membership in the state and national organizations is a major benefit of membership in an SNA. Faculty advisors can help students identify and strengthen connections between their local chapters and the state and national groups. A growing trend is for faculty to support students in efforts to make membership in the SNA a regular part of tuition and fees. Simply through the many publications, students learn about important issues facing students and beginning nurses and receive a dimension of leadership and professional development they would not have without membership. Based on their experience and knowledge of the profession, faculty make decisions about what is needed for clinical content. Many students will not automatically know about the benefits of membership. Indeed, students who have become active late in their nursing student days often regret not becoming involved sooner. By supporting membership in the SNA, faculty build into the program a commitment to lifelong professional involvement and leadership.

Professional Behavior

SNAs provide excellent settings for learning about professional behavior, for example in going to interviews, running for office, or attending convention. Despite diversity, students do not automatically understand how to connect leadership with professional behavior. As one student noted, "Someone from my school ran for office at the convention. Following our advisor's suggestion, the group decided that the whole campaign would focus on our candidate's strengths and ability to do the job well. We also decided to avoid bad-mouthing any of the other candidates, no matter what happened. This was a pretty new idea for some of us, particularly when the candidates for U.S. political office say and televise such bad things about each other. . . . Long after the election, we ended up working well on projects with the opposing candidate."

Addressing Financial Concerns Related to Membership

Belonging to a chapter, state, and national organization requires a fee. While many consider these charges modest, any fees are burdensome for others. Students should never be denied membership in an SNA simply because they cannot afford to join. Faculty can make membership possible for students in such ways as: hiring students to provide a few hours of research or other professional assistance; seeking grants that would cover the cost of membership for students with financial need or, ideally, all students.

Visibility

In addition to student efforts in promoting meetings and events, sponsored by the SNA chapter, faculty can make certain that the group remains visible. In some nursing programs, each committee chair provides a written e-mail report prior to each faculty meeting, and SNA chapter advisors should always contribute an SNA chapter update. In addition, requesting the chance to make announcements on behalf of the chapter at faculty meetings, recruiting other faculty to speak at chapter meetings and assist with special events, and making certain that faculty all receive copies of any chapter newsletters help promote the chapter as a leadership learning priority for the program. Advertising such important dates as state and NSNA conventions and requesting faculty cooperation in not scheduling major tests and assignments during those periods allows students to become involved.

Other faculty may need help in accepting the great value of student nurses' conventions as educational opportunities for leadership and career development. Many chapter advisors and students have had to deal with narrow focused views of other faculty who contend that a clinical day is sacred and cannot be missed, even for an equally important but different experience. During a time of great changes in health care and the nursing profession, students cannot afford to be denied the chance for professional development by the very faculty whose reason for hire is to educate students in the scope as well as practice of nursing. Indeed, classes or clinical time can be made up in a variety of ways, limited only by faculty and student creativity. Dealing with stubborn faculty is a major challenge, but one that can be overcome with time, persistence, and a good power base.

CHANGING FACULTY PERCEPTIONS

What problems I encountered from other faculty in 1986, the first year I became advisor to our program's SNA! It seemed like the students and I were constantly battling one or another of my otherwise highly regarded colleagues. Other faculty could not seem to understand that participation in leadership development at the state and NSNA conventions could really, *really* be accepted as valid learning experiences and not just chances to avoid getting up early for clinical. With the backing of the dean, the faculty grudgingly allowed an ever increasing group to go. Things changed. The students who attended conventions tended to stay active in the group and became the school's most outstanding leaders. They in turn recruited more students, ran for state and national offices, became highly involved in other school activities and ultimately brought a great deal of positive recognition to the nursing program. Faculty also gradually began to become more involved themselves; many volunteered to help with the SNAs special events and took a few moments to announce SNA meetings at the start of their classes. Attendance at conventions for students in good academic standing is no longer an issue, and the SNA chapter is a source of conversation and pride to the faculty as well as the students. I felt we had really arrived when a faculty member actually telephoned me to apologize for accidentally scheduling an exam during a convention and to promise that alternate arrangements would be made for the students who were attending.

LEADERSHIP DEVELOPMENT AND SNA SUPPORT BY THE DEAN OR PROGRAM DIRECTOR

Successful SNAs usually have the support of their deans or program directors. As heads of the nursing programs, these individuals set a tone that can foster leadership development in students. Strategies to promote leadership development include:

1. encouraging student participation on various faculty committees; scheduling program meetings to allow students to attend

2. announcing SNA meetings and special events at each faculty meeting and encouraging faculty to support the students and advisor in these activities

3. voicing support for the development of leadership qualities in students and voicing support for the student nurses association

4. accepting students' invitations to attend SNA meetings or special events when possible

5. providing or supporting students' efforts to identify office space for their SNA "headquarters," if possible

6. if feasible, providing tangible support, which might include sponsorship of students to state or national conventions, approval for some secretarial assistance, and office supplies

7. in programs where advisors are appointed, selecting faculty who can work well with students and have power positions within the program. Part time or junior level faculty certainly do an excellent job as advisors to thriving chapters. However, when the advisor is a full-time faculty member with a strong power base, a commitment to students and a knowledge of effective working within the system, leadership development for students in the SNA is facilitated. Unfortunately, being a chapter advisor is a heavy time commitment that not all faculty in the prime of their careers can make. Such strategies as counting SNA advisement as a committee assignment and including SNA advisement in faculty load (where this is feasible) can make the role of advisor possible for faculty who otherwise would need to decline.

Providing Support for the Advisor

Attending state and national student nurses' conventions has many benefits for advisors and the programs they represent. For example, advisors learn how to foster leadership development in students, learn more about state and national student issues, and, of course, can provide guidance to their students. Deans and program directors can help faculty attend by excusing them from meetings at the home program, permitting them to reschedule or arrange coverage for classes they will miss, and providing financial help to make attendance possible. In attending conventions, advisors represent their programs and travel on school business. Their attendance should not have to come from their personal budgets.

SUPPORTING A NEW ADVISOR IN LEADERSHIP DEVELOPMENT

The late Judith Errickson, former advisor to Villanova's chapter of the Student Nurses Association, was an "advisor's advisor" and herself a superb leader. When she gave a year's notice before leaving to become a captain in the United States Army Nurse Corps, Dean M. Louise Fitzpatrick appointed me, at the students' request, as a second advisor to Villanova's chapter of the Student Nurses Association of Pennsylvania (SNAP). My own nursing program did not have an SNA. Although eager to work with the students in this role, I was truly "clueless." However, Judy Errickson provided a splendid orientation. Her great support through the year's activities at Villanova and through the state and national student nurses' conventions allowed me to become independent and to then help the students develop the chapter and meet their own leadership goals. Finances are a concern at every nursing program. However, Dean Fitzpatrick's investment in SNAP has paid off many times over.

SUMMARY

Nursing leadership development begins with students' first days in their nursing programs. Faculty have the earliest and the most contact with students. As advisors and as classroom and clinical teachers, faculty have major impact on promoting or suppressing leadership in students. Faculty are role models, whether or not they choose to be. As such, they need to be aware of their own professional activities and their responsibility in helping students learn to navigate effectively in nursing and health care.

Regardless of content area, faculty need to devise classroom and clinical strategies that help students develop as leaders. As academic and student nurses' association advisors, faculty have the opportunity to help students identify leadership opportunities that meet their unique needs. Students likewise have responsibility to accept the opportunity to know their advisors and share their own perceptions of leadership development needs.

Membership in the student nurses' associations provides superb opportunities for leadership development. While faculty advisors have key roles in leadership development for students within the associations, all faculty can support students' becoming active and successful members. Deans and program directors are the primary leaders within their nursing programs, and their commitment to the student nurses' associations and support for students and faculty advisors will help ensure that leadership development is a priority that pervades an educational program from the most basic to the highest administrative levels.

In a time of great change in health care, nursing faces unprecedented challenges and opportunities. Future nurses must learn to be leaders and decision makers in every aspect of health care. Faculty can help and empower students as they travel along the critical path to leadership development.

CRITICAL THINKING QUESTIONS

1. How does your faculty foster leadership development in students? How have they fostered leadership in you? What are your own responsibilities for your leadership development as a future nurse?

2. In your opinion, in what ways do faculty and other students impede leadership development in students? How could that be changed?

3. What strategies could be used by faculty in your own setting to develop leadership in students who are not officers of your SNA, or other groups? How does leadership development begin?

4. How could faculty foster the development of a SNA chapter in your program? What obstacles would need to be overcome?

5. How do you think leadership development strategies can be designed to acknowledge and build upon the diverse backgrounds of nursing students and nurses?

ACTIVITIES

1. Select and read at least one copy of *Imprint,* the journal of the National Student Nurses' Association (NSNA) and one copy of your state's student nurses' association's newsletter. Outline ways in which these publications promote learning and leadership development for nursing students.

2. Interview nursing students who are leaders in your school chapter, state SNA, or NSNA. How do they feel the organizations are helping their leadership skills develop?

3. Interview a faculty member who is a leader. Discuss what participation has meant to him or her. What advice does this person have for developing leadership in the next generation of nurses?

REFERENCES

Brown, S.G. (1996). Incorporating political socialization theory into baccalaureate nursing education. *Nursing Outlook, 44* (3) 120–3.

Canavan, K. (1997). When nursing jobs are on the line. *American Nurse, 29* (3), 1,13.

Frymier, A.B., & Shulman, G. M. (1995). What's in it for me? Increasing content relevance to enhance students' motivation. *Communication Education, 44* (1), 40–50.

Krumberger, J. (1997, June). Krumberger says courage will keep the dream alive. (National Teaching Institute's NTI News, Post Meeting Issue). *American Association of Critical Care Nurses,* 1–2.

McCabe, N. (1995). Twelve high school 11th grade students examine their best teachers. *Peabody Journal of Education, 70* (2), 117–126.

Villanova Chapter, Student Nurses' Association of Pennsylvania. (Spring, 1996). Unpublished survey of nursing students.

ADDITIONAL SUGGESTED READINGS

Davidhizar, R. (1991, September/October). Ten strategies for increasing your self-confidence. *Imprint,* 105–109.

Joel, L. A. (1997, July). Editorial: The leader-follower connection. *American Journal of Nursing,* 7.

The Bill of Rights and Responsibilities for Students of Nursing. (Rev. 1991, pp. 1–8). New York: National Student Nurses' Association, Inc.

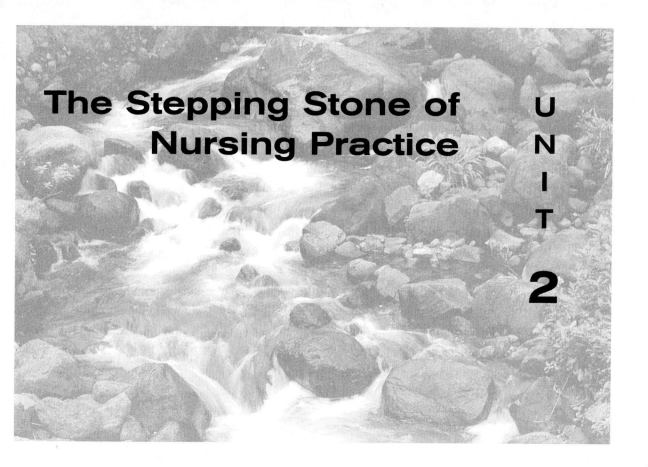

The Stepping Stone of Nursing Practice

UNIT 2

As you begin your nursing education, you will soon have the wonderful opportunity of experiencing the heart of nursing—patient care. In recent years, staff nurses have seen first-hand many significant changes that have impacted patient care. Those nurses have developed as leaders through continuing to advocate for quality care, often under challenging conditions. As a future nurse leader, it will be important for you to seek leadership development opportunities wherever you enter practice, and to understand nursing roles and the outcomes that nursing care provides.

Chapter 6 shares one *staff nurse's leadership development* during these changing times. Chapter 7 looks at *nursing's role and outcomes in practice and advanced practice*. Recognizing that better patient outcomes occur when all members of the health care team work together effectively, Chapter 8 discusses the important process of *interdisciplinary socialization*. Finally, to help you understand various patient advocacy efforts in nursing, Chapter 9 outlines *the rights and opportunities of workplace advocacy, shared governance, and collective bargaining*.

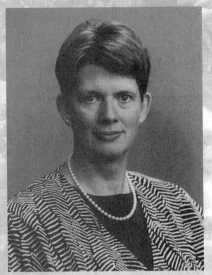

Mary E. Foley,

RN, MS

Mary E. Foley, RN has been a registered nurse for over 20 years. She received her basic nursing education in Boston, attended a public health administration program in New York, and obtained a Master's degree in Nursing from the University of California, San Francisco. Since late 1997, Mary serves as Director of Nursing at Saint Francis Memorial Hospital in San Francisco, where she has been employed as a medical surgical direct care staff nurse for over 15 years.

Mary was elected First Vice-President of the American Nurses Association in June 1996, after completing a term as Second Vice-President. The American Nurses Association (ANA) is the only full-service professional organization representing the nation's 2.2 million registered nurses. Previous to this office, Mary served two terms as president of the California Nurses Association. She is an active and supportive member of the new ANA affiliate in California, the ANA/C. She continues to be involved at her hospital as a member of the Professional Practice Committee and Safety Committee.

Mary is a professional consultant on a NIOSH Grant entitled: Training for the Development of Innovative Control Technology, which is dedicated to connecting the frontline health care worker with the designers and manufacturers of health care equipment.

In addition to her occupational health, direct-care nursing, and professional association activities, Mary is a part-time clinical faculty member at San Francisco State University School of Nursing and is the faculty advisor for the nursing student association at the school.

Mary has been active in the health care policy arena for many years. Her belief in nondiscrimination in the provision of health care and interest in and knowledge of occupational health issues led to participation in the San Francisco HIV Task Force in the late 1980s, and as a nurse representative on the California Department of Health Services Task Force for the Elimination of TB. She has presented testimony for ANA in opposition to proposed Medicare cuts, and on behalf of ANA/C she has lobbied in support of legislation to assure safer needle design in California.

CHAPTER 6

Developing Leadership as a Staff Nurse

INTRODUCTION

I am pleased to have the opportunity to tell my story. I enjoy telling any ready listener, or reader, what it is like to be a clinically active nurse employed in a hospital, part-time clinical faculty, and at the same time, an elected officer of the American Nurses Association. The roles have a lot in common, such as using the nursing process to assess a problem and make decisions that may have a lifelong impact on a person, family, or association. I want to tell you a little about how I was so fortunate to attain these roles, what they mean to me as a professional nurse, and hopefully, provide each of you with some inspiration as you enter your new career.

ORIGINS OF INVOLVEMENT

I attribute my professional involvement to my early positive role modeling, which started in my initial diploma nursing program and with the Massachusetts Student Nurses' Association. I became interested in the student association because of some very supportive nursing faculty who were active in nursing associations and encouraged student participation. I was interested in the politics of health care funding and worked to support funding for nursing scholarships and a national health plan for the United States (we are still working on that goal, regretfully). In 1973, the year I was to graduate from the Diploma program in Boston, the governor of the state decided to reduce the cost of regulations in Massachusetts by doing away with the licensing body for many professions, including nursing. The implications of that decision quickly became obvious to nurses—no one would have an individual license to practice and health care institutions could hire anyone that they wanted, to do anything they wanted! The profession had been on the alert for a model of health care regulation like this—known as institutional licensure—and was prepared to oppose it in the interest of public protection. I was scheduled to graduate in June and was informed that if the governor's proposal passed none of the graduating nursing students in the state would be able to take the licensing exam. We would be unable to practice in Massachusetts, or any other state. This was the first example of the personal becoming political, or as Catherine Dodd RN, Executive Director of ANA/California states in her *10 Commandments of Politics,* "each of us is just one personal or professional injustice away from becoming involved in politics!" My participation in the response to the governor's proposal changed my life forever, as well as my belief about what nursing can accomplish when it works together! Organized by their respective associations, students, registered nurses, licensed vocational/practical nurses, and the professional groups rallied together, literally, to proclaim their objection to such a proposal. Huge events were held in Boston and other cities throughout the state to call the public's attention to the danger of this idea. Hearings were held, and I had my first opportunity to present testimony on behalf of the student association. This would be my first, but not my last public and political event. It sure was a grand initiation. The proposal was defeated, we all had the privilege of taking the licensing exam, and the practice of nursing in Massachusetts survived another close call by well intentioned but poorly informed politicians. I became a convert and vowed to be professionally and politically active for the rest of my professional life.

As a result of the Massachusetts experience and my excitement, I ran for an office at the National Student Nurses' Association convention and was elected to the Board of Directors as Director of Legislation. The following year, I had the privilege of being elected President of the National Student Nurses' Association (NSNA). I had never been on a plane before, or out of New England until my NSNA experiences. I was nervous, excited, and as I look at pictures from that time, no fashion statement. But I learned a lot, and experienced many leadership development opportunities. Those early board meetings and conventions helped form my beliefs about involvement, leadership, and responsibility. One person who especially deserves mention here as a mentor is Mary Ann Tuft. Mary Ann was Executive Director of NSNA during my tenure in the 1970s and has remained active in health care and nursing associations. She took each of us in NSNA under her wing, gave us the benefit of her expertise, and pushed us to flourish and thrive in our new roles as association leaders. I am pleased to say I made some important friendships, many that endure to this day.

Many of those friends are nurse leaders who continue to contribute as professional leaders across the country.

The NSNA President always attends the conventions of the American Nurses Association (ANA), and my term coincided with the 1974 ANA convention in San Francisco, California. That meeting became a sentinel event in forming my career path, although I didn't know it at the time. The San Francisco/Bay Area was in the middle of a nurses strike, led by the California Nurses Association, then a member of ANA. Over 30 hospitals were on strike, and they were striking for professional principles: issues of critical care qualifications and the role of the nurse practice committees in each hospital. I was indelibly impressed by the professional stance the nurses were taking, and eventually, I followed a path back to California to become one of those active staff nurses.

I completed my Bachelors of Science in Nursing and had more exciting and career shaping opportunities while doing so. I had the honor of attending a summer internship in Washington D.C., working on health issues such as second opinions for surgery in the Medicare program and preventive care for children in the Medicaid program. As a result of those interests, I moved to New York City and worked for a federal health review agency and studied public health administration. I worked as a per diem staff nurse to pay for the New York lifestyle, while I was in the public health program. I was active within the New York State Nurses Association, helping to found a state political action committee and in local politics through the district nurses association. I attended ANA conventions as a delegate from New York and maintained my interest in national nursing issues and politics. In 1980, I moved to San Francisco with friends who were relocating at the same time. As I started my job search, two important factors influenced my choice. First, President Reagan had cut the funding for public health planning and programming to a virtual zero, and my public health aspirations were not likely to find an employment opportunity in the Bay Area. Second, my skills as a staff nurse were still sound, and I was interested in working in a hospital represented for collective bargaining by the California Nurses Association (CNA) and ANA. My only knowledge of collective bargaining for nurses was theoretical. I wanted a firsthand experience to make me more informed and to help expand my ideas of collective action by nurses beyond the political arena. I believed in the multipurpose function of a professional nurses association, and that a professional nurse could be represented by a nurses association for collective bargaining to advance professional standards of patient care. I also wanted a health care facility in which I would be empowered, like those nurses I had seen in 1974, to make nursing decisions and work with other nurses to advance patient care and the economic and general welfare of nurses through a contract.

I had no trouble finding a staff nurse position, and I became a part-time night nurse at Saint Francis Memorial Hospital in San Francisco. I am now completing my 16th year at the hospital as a staff nurse. I can say without hesitation that the opportunity to work in a professionally organized work setting has affected me deeply. My theories were put to the test, and I still believe that nursing and patient care can be assisted by the presence of a collective bargaining agreement—sometimes! Not all institutions need a collective bargaining unit to recognize nursing's roles and contributions. I refer you to the ANA work on Magnet Hospital recognition, both the work from the 1980s (*Magnet Hospitals: Attraction and Retention of Professional Nurses,* 1983) and the present program in the American Nurses Credentialing Center that establishes the criteria for ideal nursing environments and awards institutions for meeting that criteria.

In my first summer, I became a member of the nurse negotiating committee and tried to fill the large shoes left by a nurse who has been an inspiration to many at Saint Francis and in San Francisco, Fely Horanzy. Fely had been the nurse representative and negotiator for Saint Francis during the 1970s, and I was honored to work with her. Although I assumed the role as nurse negotiator and contract representative, I never took her place. During those long summer sessions in 1981, we were able to negotiate one of the first clinical ladders to be offered in a nursing contract. The clinical ladder was designed in response to the challenge of nurse retention—how to provide a promotional opportunity for the staff nurse who wants to remain clinically grounded. It has always been true that the expert staff nurse had no growth opportunities unless he or she accepted a position in administration or inservice education. It is essential that the nursing workforce retain the talents of the expert nurse as resource, clinician, and role model. The opportunity to participate as nurse negotiator in 1983, 1985, and 1988 allowed me the firsthand view of a nurse watching the volatile health care sector adapt and change. In the mid 1980s, nursing experienced a temporary surplus of nurses when the Diagnostic Related Groupings (DRGs) were introduced to control Medicare costs, and health care institutions struggled to meet a tighter budget. Hospitals closed floors and consolidated units as the financial incentive shifted from long lengths of stay to more efficient care in the hospital and a growth to alternative settings such as home and ambulatory care. It wasn't long before hospitals realized that even with fewer patients in the hospital, and the length of stay reduced, the patients were sicker and the demand for the registered nurse outgrew the supply. By 1988, the United States was in the midst of the latest, and not the last, nursing shortage. Contract negotiations shifted back to finding incentives to keep nurses in the hospital, and to reward the expert nurse. Longevity pay was introduced to help the experienced nurse keep up with the salaries that newly hired nurses were attracting, and nurses with 10, 15, and 20 years of service began to be rewarded. At the same time, serious concerns were expressed about safe staffing, and constructive remedies were introduced to address patient safety during this time. The potential to make a direct difference for patients and nurses was a very positive feeling, and I felt the empowerment I had hoped for when I first moved to San Francisco.

Another critical event for nursing and health care occurred in the mid-1980s when the AIDS crisis arrived in hospitals and throughout society. As a direct-care nurse in a San Francisco hospital that had some of the early AIDS patients, I developed an interest in AIDS education, health care worker safety, and working to prevent discrimination in health care or social policy because of a particular diagnosis. I turned this interest into a nursing degree in occupational health and nursing administration and presently work in a project to develop safer health care equipment, especially needles and syringes.

While working at Saint Francis, I became actively involved in the Golden Gate Nurses Association, Region 12 of the California Nurses Association. I served as committee member, board member, and treasurer of the Region. In those roles, I was exposed to organizational finances and issues of budgeting, personnel management, and investment. Local politics led to statewide nursing involvement. I was elected to the statewide policy body for collective bargaining issues, and from there was elected to the state nurses association board as Treasurer, and eventually, President for two terms. The dual role of staff nurse and association officer allowed me to participate on city and statewide policy bodies that enhanced the role, and voice of nursing. I had the chance to serve on the Mayor's HIV Task Force in San Francisco, the California Board for Nursing's Advisory Task Force on the Nursing Shortage, and the California Health Department Task Force on the Elimination of TB. I was proud to be asked to share my knowledge of the real-life issues of nurses in practice and the patient populations we are trying to serve. I know that nurses in other roles could have well served on these committees, but the direct care perspective was unique, and offered a special opportunity to showcase the contributions of nursing care.

My state involvement led to national committees on the workplace and collective bargaining, as an elected officer representing the body of state presidents and executives on the ANA Board (Chair of Constituent Assembly), and eventually to election as First and Second Vice-President of the ANA Board of Directors. Many of the current state and national leaders in nursing are on similar tracks, and started their professional involvement as staff nurses. Whether nurses continue in staff nurse/direct care roles or have changed positions, their knowledge of and love for direct care nursing influences their decision making and makes nursing a richer profession for their perspectives.

STAFF NURSE CAUCUS

During the 1980s and 1990s, staff nurses in California and throughout the country were using their collective skills and voices to be sure the state and national associations reflected their issues and concerns. At the national level, committed staff nurses started the Staff Nurse Caucus within ANA. The staff nurse caucus is a network to inform nurses of the national issues of nursing and to prepare staff nurses for state and national office. The caucus recently celebrated a ten year anniversary. One of their tangible accomplishments was to assure that ANA designate four seats on the board of directors for nurses in direct practice. An outstanding staff nurse who deserves mention here is Mary Ellen Patton, a nurse from Ohio, who epitomizes a lifetime of commitment and leadership. She has recently been honored by the naming of a national staff nurse award, a much deserved honor.

Let me outline for you the leadership that staff nurses can bring to nursing, and how the nursing profession will be stronger with the staff nurse presence. Let me also illustrate how all practicing nurses, in all settings, can be strengthened in their work by professional involvement.

DIRECT CARE NURSES AND THE ASSOCIATIONS

Every opportunity I have had in regional/district, state, and national nursing associations have been possible because of two important factors: having the time/making the time for involvement, and learning to talk about nursing as well (or better) than I do it. Let me address the time issue first, since I know it is often the obstacle that nurses tell me precludes them from involvement.

Making Time

I fully understand that each of us at some point in our lives will be too busy, or committed to other priorities, to throw ourselves into professional involvement. I respect that reality, and because of that, ask that every one of us do a little of the work on a regular basis. But what will help is to pace the involvement. When the smoke clears, and time permits, each of us should assume a part of a project, a committee assignment, or an appointment or election to a board. When each of us contribute, it can all get done. It is always reaffirming to experience how much joy and satisfaction nurses get when they talk together and work on projects to advance nursing and health care. I have been told over and over how much energy nurses get when their work is acknowledged by peers and in the community. And in-between activities, or at unexpected moments that life can bring, each of us may need a break or time-out to recoup our strength. It is as important to learn how to say no to unrealistic assignments as it is to volunteer. Just like at work on the nursing units, we get our work done by dividing the assignment, taking turns at the difficult patient or family, relieving each other to take a coffee or lunch break, and taking vacations and holidays to renew and refresh ourselves.

Talking About Nursing

Nurses involved in direct care spend a lot of their time talking—to each other, to doctors and other health team members, and to the patient and family. The most successful nurse is able to translate complex terminology into a language understandable by the frightened, confused, angry, and the hurting. In fact, other than telling my students in clinical to touch patients, I spend most of my time helping students to interpret the medical lexicon into lay terms.

It became obvious to the nursing profession during the health reform discussions of the early 1990s that the general public and policy makers actually wanted, and needed to know, what nurses think. It was an opportunity to tell our story. The policy makers during the AIDS crisis had no idea what caring for a patient sick with a high fever and a mysterious disease needed. As a nurse, I had the chance to tell a congressional committee that AIDS patients did not need nurses and other staff isolated from them in high-tech space suits, or quarantined from the general population. I was able to explain, in scientific and human terms, the tangible ways to fight the infection, not the people with the infection. I was able to describe appropriate necessary equipment, such as gloves and needle disposal systems, and reinforce the need for more education about AIDS.

As a staff nurse and officer of the state nurses association, I had the chance to work with community and business leaders in opposition to a state ballot initiative that was proposed by the statewide medical association to satisfy very narrow insurance goals—payment for medical services! I had credibility as a nurse that proved effective in public education. I was active in the statewide debate and appeared on panels, radio, and television. I even had the chance to have a speaking role in my own TV commercial. One of my fondest memories is of a Sunday evening shift before the election. I was in a room with a patient who just woke from a nap—she kept looking at the TV, and then at me. The commercial was on at that very time, and I had to assure her that she wasn't dreaming, that her nurse was indeed on the screen.

Other nurses utilize their special knowledge to reach out to communities and policy makers. Nurses in cancer care work to increase screening awareness; public health nurses work to educate about family planning and immunizations; cardiac nurses teach CPR and nutrition classes; burn unit nurses teach fire safety, and thousands of other examples exist. But, more communities beg our involvement, and policy makers need our practical advice as they struggle to design health care coverage for the uninsured, and start to reform the current out-of-control insurance driven system.

Current examples of staff nurse voices making a difference further confirm the importance of staff nurse involvement. Nursing budgets have undergone another round of administrative cuts as institutions responded, and over-reacted to the financial pressures of a managed care environment. Direct care nurses have been telling Congress, the President's Commission on Health Care Quality, state legislators, and the public about the danger to patient safety that results when inadequate numbers of registered nurses are in place to provide the essential level of care. Staff nurses wouldn't be able to tell these stories without the access provided by the professional associations, and the associations wouldn't have the same relevance or accuracy they do without the nurses who give the care speaking out for patients and nursing.

WHAT THE NURSING ASSOCIATIONS PROVIDE THE STAFF NURSE

As a professional nurse, I believe it is important that I understand my role in the bigger picture of health care. Thanks to my work with the state and national nursing associations, I have been fortunate to have access to a lot of information about health care trends. I know that what I may experience at my unit level, at my hospital, my city, and in my state has a relationship to the trends in technology, society, economics, and politics. I am aware of the cause and effect of reduced Medicare reimbursement or other insurance issues, such as what laser surgery could mean to my patient's length of stay. I believe I must be informed about the world around me, or I won't be as effective in my patient care, whether it is providing pre- and postoperative teaching, advising a family about home care or hospice options, or helping decide the wisdom of a new staffing model.

I believe a professional nurse is an informed nurse, who can integrate the influences of the outside world on her or his daily life. In this way, we can better assist the patient as we explain not just the science of our care but the structure and process of the environment that influences care. Many nurses were taken by surprise by the recent changes in health care, and found themselves unprepared, professionally, personally, and emotionally for change. As institutions started to close beds, and care shifted to other settings, some nurses could not believe their job security could be in jeopardy. The American Nurses Association has been advising nurses for a number of years to plan for career security instead.

I believe that nurses should belong to at least two organizations—the specialty association that most closely matches their area of practice, and the professional nurses association—the American Nurses Association. I have surmised that nurses who excel only in their clinical expertise have compromised their care by ignoring the other factors that affect their care, and the settings in which it is given. The specialty organization provides extensive clinical practice information and support and can advocate well for that specialty area. Information about the policies and politics of the broader health care arena can best be obtained from associations like the SNA and ANA. I urge nurses to be become trend watchers, to predict the changes in health care, and acquire the skills that will be required to succeed in the new settings. Nurses who are trend watchers are readying themselves for the shifts from inpatient to outpatient surgery, and are revising their skills to the long-term care, rehab, or home setting. Much of the care that nurses traditionally gave in hospitals are given in other settings now—and those patients need the skills of expert nurses!

The important message here is that it is the job of associations to keep their members abreast of current events and to assist in the transitions that nurses must make. Because nursing organizations are in the business of trend analysis, trend reporting, and policy advising they can help the nurses feel less alone as change occurs, and less victimized. It was a critical moment in the history of ANA when the campaign "Every Patient Deserves a Nurse" was announced. (See Appendix B). Nurses throughout the country were being laid off and unlicensed personnel were brought in to substitute for the registered nurse. Patient care was jeopardized, and nurses were frightened and angry. The campaign has taken a multi-prong approach—public relations and media, career development for nurses, regulatory and legislative work to address issues of public and worker protection, and a research initiative to document the positive outcomes that adequate numbers of nurses are directly responsible for. The excitement that is generated by finally getting the data that proves what nurses have said all along—we are essential providers of care in all settings—will grow as the project expands in acute care settings and on into community-based settings. The ANA *Nursing Report Card for Acute Care* (March, 1995) led to the *Nursing Quality Indicators* (1996) and is a prime example of the extraordinary work that a nursing organization can perform to help each nurse succeed in their individual clinical setting.

SUMMARY

It is my hope that I have stimulated professional involvement by explaining how symbiotic the relationship is between the staff nurse and professional associations. I want to challenge the common misconception that nursing organizations are led by nurses with lots of titles who don't know about nursing. When nurses continue their education, or obtain a credential through certification, they deserve to be recognized. The true test of a nurse's leadership (nurse educator, staff nurse, advanced practice nurse, nurse administrator, nurse entrepreneur, nurse attorney, nurse legislator) should be what they believe about nursing, and how hard they work to make it possible for every nurse to practice the best nursing they can! Only when staff nurses give their support and active involvement to professional associations will that myth become a reality.

I believe that the professional nursing association is the unifying common ground for nurse involvement. Try to think of a personal topic you care strongly about. What health-related issue do you wish you could change? It may be your area of practice, teen smoking, seatbelt safety, or a related area of interest that you deeply care about. In professional involvement you will find others who share your fervor, or maybe you'll attract people to your cause. You will definitely attain new skills for making changes happen, and you may just find expertise and resources that can be directed to your issue. I urge you to fulfill your professional goals with a lifelong commitment to learning, being proud that you chose nursing, and finding time to financially support and whenever possible become involved in the professional association. Like a hard day at work, the satisfaction gained by trying to make the profession stronger, and our care better, will make you a better, and happier nurse! I look forward to working with you in future projects.

CRITICAL THINKING QUESTIONS

1. What role do mentors and role models play in professional development? How can you recognize opportunities to be assisted?

2. What opportunities do you have as a student to become involved in your school and/or the local or state student nursing association?

3. When you select your first nursing position, what organization will you select to support your clinical area?

4. What health issue are you really interested in and would like to make better?

5. How will you revise your personal schedule to allow for professional development and participation?

ACTIVITIES

1. Through a literature search, explore the role of a staff nurse in the 1950s, 1970s, and 1990s. Compare and contrast the strengths and weaknesses described in various published accounts of those staff nurse's roles.

2. Talk to your local or regional hospital's nurse recruiter. Explore what career ladders, options, and upward mobility plans are in place for the hospital's nurses.

3. Determine whether the hospital has a Clinical Nursing Practice Committee. If so, ask to sit in on one of the meetings to explore their purpose and functions.

4. Review the ANA brochure *Nursing Facts: RN Demographics* reprinted in Appendix E of this book. Ask the nurse recruiter or representative from your state's hospital association to come and talk with your leadership class about staff nurse opportunities in your state.

REFERENCES

American Academy of Nursing. (1983). *Magnet Hospitals: Attraction and Retention of Professional Nurses.* Washington, DC: American Nurses Association.

American Nurses Association. (1995). *Nursing Care Report Card for Acute Care.* Washington, DC: ANA.

American Nurses Association. (1996). *Nursing Quality Indicators: Definitions and Implications.* Washington, DC: ANA.

American Nurses Association. (1996). *Nursing Quality Indicators: Guide for Implementation.* Washington, DC: ANA.

ADDITIONAL SUGGESTED READINGS

Anati-Otoing, D. (1977). Team building in a health care setting. *American Journal of Nursing, 97, (7), 48–51.*

American Nurses Association. (1996). *The Acute Care Nurse in Transition.* Washington, DC: American Nurses Publishing Company.

Joel, L. (1997, October). Moral compromise revisited [editorial]. AJN, (10), 7.

Kany, K. (1997, September/October). ANA quality indicators applied to unit search. *The American Nurse,* 18, 23.

Nursing Facts from the American Nurses Association. *Managed Care—challenges & opportunities for nursing,* PR–27 33M 12/95. Washington, DC: American Nurses Publishing.

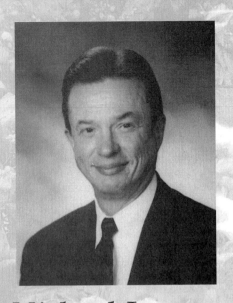

Michael L. Evans,

PHD, RN, CNAA, FACHE

Dr. Michael Evans has been a registered nurse for over twenty years. His career has included the roles of staff nurse, nurse manager, and nurse educator. After earning a degree in English, he received his basic nursing education at Northwest Texas Hospital School of Nursing in Amarillo, Texas. He then completed a Bachelor of Science degree in Nursing at West Texas State University and a Master of Science degree in Nursing Administration at the University of Texas Health Science Center at Houston. Dr. Evans completed his Doctor of Philosophy degree in Nursing Systems and Administration at the University of Texas at Austin.

Dr. Evans has held several important elected positions in professional nursing. As a nursing student, he was elected President of the Texas Nursing Students Association. He was later elected to the board of the National Student Nurses' Association as *Imprint* editor. Using that student experience as a foundation, he has served as President of the Texas Nurses Association and has been serving as an officer on the Board of Directors of the American Nurses Association since 1992.

Since 1995, Dr. Evans has been serving as Vice-President for Nursing Services at Presbyterian Hospital of Dallas. Prior to that time, he was Vice-President for Operations at St. David's Medical Center in Austin, Texas for 7 years.

Dr. Evans' nursing research interests involve outcome studies on the use of registered nurses and advanced practice nurses in the delivery of quality patient care.

CHAPTER 7

Nursing's Role and Outcomes in Practice and Advanced Practice

INTRODUCTION

The changes in health care over the past 10 years have dramatically underscored the role of nursing and nursing care in meeting desired clinical and financial outcomes. The health care industry is relearning that nursing care is central to America's health care delivery system. Nursing practice, both basic and advanced, is an important precursor of cost efficiency, desired clinical outcomes, and patient satisfaction. The American Nurses Association has established a program aimed at validating the strong conceptual link between nurse staffing and specific patient outcomes (ANA, 1997).

HISTORICAL PERSPECTIVE

The shift to managed care has had dramatic implications for virtually all aspects of health care (ANA, 1996). Nursing services within hospitals and health care systems have been changed to ensure highest overall quality at an appropriate cost. Health care institutional providers have had as a primary priority the imperative to reduce costs to be able to compete for managed care contracts. There have been successful and unsuccessful approaches to reducing costs for institutional nursing services.

Nursing is at the heart of the services that are provided by a health care organization. Nurses comprise the largest number of individual employees in health care systems because of the patient's needs for nursing care. Nursing costs are generally at least half of the overall personnel budget within a hospital or health care system. Periodic and cyclical nursing shortages during the 1970s and 1980s caused by increased needs for nursing care contributed to the increase of nursing salary and benefit structures as health care organizations sought to attract and retain registered nurses during those periods.

HEALTH CARE INITIATIVES TO REDUCE COST

There have been differing approaches to reducing costs in health care systems. Many hospitals across the country embarked on a complete redesign of the work nurses do in an effort to redefine roles, consolidate care activities closer to the patients, and reduce costs. Many health care organizations called this approach "patient focused care," which actually came to mean many different models. The one attribute that the patient focused care models shared was the presence of a cross-trained, multiskilled, unlicensed assistive role within nursing services. The actual role of these workers has differed widely from one model to another. In some models, they are conceptualized as the caregiver with a nurse overseeing a number of unlicensed assistive personnel. In other models, the nurse was conceptualized as the caregiver, and the assistive person was there to assist the nurse as the nurse cared for a group of patients. These two differing conceptualizations are very important. The latter has been found in most health care organizations to be a more successful approach based on long-term financial outcomes, as well as clinical outcomes.

Many health care organizations have learned that while an unlicensed person can be taught to perform many of the manual tasks nurses have done in the past, the cognitive connect between what the nurse does and what the nurse knows is vital. That connection between theory, science, and practice is central to the quality versus cost issue in health care. That connection becomes clear with the measurement and analysis of patient outcomes.

DISCUSSION

Replacing the role of the registered nurse with an unlicensed person has not been found to be an effective answer, although the presence and the appropriately defined role of the unlicensed worker is vital. Some health care organizations have sought to reduce nursing costs without a full appreciation of the contribution of the registered nurse to patient care. Replacing nurses with unlicensed workers may seem to be a sound strategy if one believes that the unlicensed worker can be trained to do all of the "work" nurses do. But we have relearned that the work nurses do goes far beyond the tasks nurses do. The art and the science of nursing practice were lost as unlicensed workers were introduced into some systems to replace nurses. The replaced nurses often became supervisors of these unlicensed personnel.

There is renewed value in the role of the registered nurse in health care as the link between quality and cost has become more clear. Quality and cost are the flip sides of the same coin, instead of two separate but related topics. Health care leaders have learned that there is no cost-efficiency to low quality care. That which seems less expensive over the short-term usually proves to be far more costly when satisfaction, complications, and return rates are factored into the delivery system.

Managed care has created many changes. One of them is a continually decreasing length of stay for patients in the inpatient setting. Lengths of stay for some diagnoses have been reduced by half compared to what they have been in the past. Placing a major emphasis on teaching patients self-care has become imperative for maintaining patient wellness and satisfaction. However, it is rare that nurses have the time to be able to just teach and nothing else. Teaching by registered nurses often occurs during the provision of care itself. If an organization has reassigned the nursing care tasks to unlicensed personnel, the teaching is less likely to occur because the overall contact with a nurse may be nearly nonexistent. The result is lower care quality, lower patient satisfaction, lower physician satisfaction, higher readmission rates, and higher costs.

Reassessment of outcomes during the managed care revolution has taught many health care organizations that registered nurses are the best bargain in health care. Appropriate registered nurse to patient ratios are linked to lower medication error rates, lower patient injury rates, lower nosocomial infection rates, lower skin breakdown rates, lower mortality rates, lower readmission rates, and decreased patient length of stay (Lewin-VHI, 1995). All of these outcomes are huge cost savers. Care delivery models have been developed which appropriately use the cross-trained, multiskilled unlicensed worker in an assistive role to the care provider—the registered nurse. Staffing models are carefully monitored to be certain that the appropriate ratios of registered nurses to unlicensed personnel are maintained.

A central construct of many of the most successful nursing service delivery systems has been nurse satisfaction. Nurse satisfaction is linked with and is a precursor of patient satisfaction. Nurse satisfaction is measured and compared longitudinally. Higher nurse satisfaction leads to increased retention and lower turnover, which is valuable in that nurse turnover greatly increases the cost of nursing services in a health care organization. Satisfied nurses with longer tenure who view their engagement with the health care organization as a career and not just a job are more likely to be able to move from the novice to the expert level of nursing practice. Expert nurses are better able to provide the level of care that is likely to reduce length of patient stay while maintaining patient satisfaction during the care experience.

ADVANCED PRACTICE NURSES

Another important event in the health care transition to managed care has been the changing role of the advanced practice nurse. Advanced practice nurse or APN is usually an umbrella term that encompasses the role of nurse practitioner, certified nurse midwife, clinical nurse specialist, and certified registered nurse anesthetist. These nurses in advanced practice usually hold a graduate degree in their specific clinical specialty, and often certification is another requirement for their role.

The clinical nurse specialist (CNS) has become a valued role model in health care organizations. The models in which the CNS practices vary, but the CNS usually functions in a clinical educator/preceptor/consultant role for nurses practicing in various clinical specialties. They also encourage and facilitate nursing research utilization projects and research based practice. Moving nurses from the novice to the expert level occurs with the assistance and guidance of the CNS.

The nurse practitioner (NP) is proving to be a vital role in American health care. The role of NP is becoming more prevalent in both inpatient and outpatient/clinic settings. In the inpatient setting, the NP provides care for patients in a clinical specialty area, working in collaboration with nurses, physicians, and others. The NP in the outpatient or clinic setting is usually in a primary care role. Studies have shown that the NP role is very successful in these types of settings. The nurses provide more health promotion activities than their physician counter-parts and nurses scored higher than physicians on quality of care measures. In addition, NPs spent more time with their patients than physicians. Patient satisfaction with the NP was overall higher than satisfaction with physicians (Brown & Grimes, 1993).

Certified registered nurse anesthetists (CRNA) function in the oldest advanced practice nurse role. These advanced practitioners administer the majority of anesthesia given in rural settings, and have extensive roles in urban settings as well. Their expertise and quality outcomes have been well documented (ANA, 1995).

Certified nurse midwives (CNM) have varying levels of independent practice determined by state laws and the nurse practice act where they provide care. CNMs provide well gynecological and low-risk obstetrical care including prenatal, labor and delivery, and post-partum care (ANA, 1995). Debate over requirements for certification eligibility, especially in this role, are ongoing.

All advance practice nursing roles and the educational programs preparing nurses for these roles are undergoing extensive growth and transition in these late 1990s. As the United States works to provide quality health care that is affordable, with equal access for all citizens, advance practice nurses are serving valuable roles in many settings.

SUMMARY

Health care organizations have a delicate and important relationship with patients, physicians, and their payers. The best way to reduce nursing care costs is through building, nurturing, and fortifying a nursing service organization. Even though that may not yield the dollar savings from next month's financial statement, the yield is there over time and the relationship with the patient, payer, and physician are enhanced as patient care satisfaction from all groups grows stronger.

It is vital that all nurses—those who have been in the profession as well as those who are new to nursing—understand the powerful role they play in creating positive outcomes through their practice. The careful identification of desired outcomes, collection of data, analysis of data and sharing of results with nursing staff and others is very important. Many health care organizations perform these functions in a program labeled continuous quality improvement, quality management, or with a similar title. Whatever it is called, the programs depend on nurse volunteers to assist with collection, analysis, and dissemination of information. Nurses should volunteer to participate in this very important affirmation of the value of nurses and nursing practice.

Advanced practice nurses are making an important difference in American health care. These nurse pioneers are gaining the respect of nurses, the public, physicians, and other health care colleagues as their unique contributions are being acknowledged and valued.

The role of the registered nurse, both basic and advanced, is proving to be vital to American health care. A new emphasis on the value of nurses and nursing care is evolving as the link between patient outcomes and overall cost in the health care delivery system is being better understood. Past, present, and future research activities aimed at better delineating and defining that link will further increase the understanding of the vital role of nurses and nursing practice in contemporary American health care.

CRITICAL THINKING QUESTIONS

1. What are some examples of unsuccessful approaches to reducing costs in health care?

2. What are some examples of a successful approach to reducing costs in health care?

3. Why has managed care created the imperative to reduce costs and increase quality?

4. Research suggests that registered nurses in appropriate numbers and with appropriate roles have what effect on clinical outcomes?

5. What outcomes are suggested in research stemming from the nurse practitioner in a primary care delivery role?

ACTIVITIES

1. Invite the nurse manager or nurse administrator from the hospital, long-term care facility, and home care agency (where you will be doing clinicals) to come and participate in a panel discussion for your class. Ask them to explain how they each determine and allocate staffing patterns. Also have them explain FTEs (full-time equivalents) and how they use them in staffing. Ask them to address how they factor in acuity levels; any facility, state, or federal staffing level requirements that impact their staffing; or any other factors that affect staffing at their facility.

2. Invite a Continuous Quality Improvement (CQI) or Quality Management Nurse to come and talk to your class about CQI and some of the studies their facility has looked at in the past. Negotiate with your preceptors in clinicals and your instructors to provide you with some clinical time, in at least one of your classes, to assist the facility where you do clinicals to accomplish a part of one of their CQI studies.

3. After graduation, when you begin work as an RN, volunteer to be your unit's or group's CQI Coordinator. If you accomplished Activity #2, you already have some expertise and experience to bring to the role.

4. Explore legislative development in your state, and nationally, related to advanced practice nursing over the past seven years.

5. Perhaps most important, learn to articulate what nursing is and does. Study and accomplish some outcomes research. Communicate the difference that nursing care makes on outcomes, in whatever setting you practice. Seek to publish what you have learned.

REFERENCES

American Nurses Association. (1995). *Advanced Practice Nursing: A New Age in Health Care.* Washington DC: American Nurses Publishing Company.

American Nurses Association. (1996). *The Acute Care Nurse in Transition.* Washington, DC: American Nurses Publishing Company.

American Nurses Association. (1997). *Implementing Nursing's Report Card: A Study of RN Staffing, Length of Stay and Patient Outcomes.* Washington, DC: American Nurses Publishing Company.

Brown, S.A., & Grimes, D.E. (1993). *Nurse Practitioners and Certified Nurse-Midwives: A Meta-Analysis of Studies on Nurses in Primary Care Roles.* Washington, DC: American Nurses Publishing Company.

Lewin-VHI. (1995). *Nursing Report Card for Acute Care Settings.* Prepared for the American Nurses Association. Unpublished.

ADDITIONAL SUGGESTED READINGS

Levitt M., Stern N., Becker K., Zaiken H., Hangasky S., Wilcox P. (1985). A performance appraisal tool for nurse practitioners. *Nurse Practitioner,* August, Volume 8, pp. 28–33.

Malone, B.L. (1986). Evaluation of the clinical nurse specialist. *AJN,* 86 (12), pp. 1375–1377.

Titler, M.G. and Stenger, K.M. (1994). Role evaluation of the critical care clinical nurse specialist. In Gawlinski and Keyn (Ed.). *The Clinical Nurse Specialist Role in Critical Care.* Philadelphia: W.B. Saunders, pp. 275–292.

Walker, M.L. (1986). How nursing service administrators view clinical nurse specialists. *Nursing Management, 17* (3), pp. 52–54.

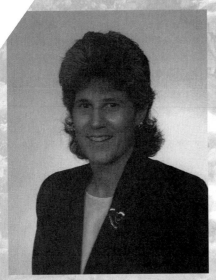

Photo courtesy of MUSC Graphic Art and
Medical Photography

Pamela F. Cipriano,

PhD, FAAN

Pam Cipriano began her involvement in NSNA as a local Breakthrough To Nursing chair for the Philadelphia area. She was elected First Vice-President in 1974 from the floor at her first NSNA national convention. She then was elected president in 1975. In her role as NSNA President, she served on the American Nurses Association's (ANA) Commission on Nursing Education and later chaired the Titling Work Group during the efforts to achieve the baccalaureate as the requirement for entry into practice.

Pam's first elected position within ANA was to the Congress on Nursing Practice in 1980. In 1986, she was elected to the ANA Board of Directors and then was elected as Treasurer in 1988. Since her graduation from nursing school, Pam has continuously held a national level elected or appointed position within ANA. She is currently completing a four-year term on the ANA Congress on Nursing Economics and is the Chairperson. She has also served on three state nurses association Board of Directors and in various other local and state SNA positions.

In addition to roles as staff nurse, head nurse, clinical nurse specialist and nursing director, Pam now serves as the Chief Operating Officer and Chief Nursing Officer at the Medical Center of the Medical University of South Carolina in Charleston; she is also an associate professor in the College of Nursing where she has taught health policy and nursing administration.

Her research interests include study of nursing workforce issues such as compensation, supply and demand, and transition of workers out of the hospital setting. She has been an American Nurses Foundation Scholar and was funded by the National Cancer Institute to plan and execute a conference on prevention—early detection and screening of women at risk for breast cancer in South Carolina. Pam is also a Fellow of the American Academy of Nursing and a Distinguished Lecturer for Sigma Theta Tau International.

CHAPTER 8

Interdisciplinary Socialization

INTRODUCTION

In recent years, an interdisciplinary team approach to care has become synonymous with providing comprehensive care designed to anticipate and meet patient and family needs across the continuum. While it may sound simple, possessing the skill and ability to work well with individuals from other professions does not come naturally to many. To practice in an interdisciplinary manner means, "combining or involving two or more professions" (Flexner, 1983, p. 993). Interdisciplinary socialization is the process of establishing relationships with members of other disciplines or groups. Nurses have enjoyed a long tradition of practicing in an interdisciplinary environment. However, more attention has been paid to the power and image of the nurse than to the relative value of the nurse's contributions. Even less attention has focused on helping the nurse acquire the knowledge, confidence, and skills needed to be a successful interdisciplinary team player.

STUDENT SOCIALIZATION

NSNA has enjoyed a rich tradition of reaching out to other disciplines through its relationships at the national level with other student professional associations. For many years, there was an exchange of information and participation among the elected leaders of the American Student Medical Association, the Student Dental Association, as well as student Optometric, Podiatric, and Pharmacy associations. Positions on issues such as unionization for nurses and physicians, the rights of students and ethnic diversity of both the student body and future workforce were common topics to name a few. We exchanged convention speakers, attended each other's board meetings, and shared significant association actions for support from the other groups.

The process of socialization, however, is one that has not been addressed in any direct manner. A few health professions universities have offered courses attended by students from multiple disciplines, focusing on understanding each others' roles and contributions to the health care team. Schools may offer electives open to students from multiple disciplines but the content does not address the process of working together with others who offer a different focus and expertise with patients. So how does one learn or become exposed to interdisciplinary socialization, let alone learn skills to become successful?

TEAMWORK

Performing in interdisciplinary teams is an every day occurrence in many health care delivery systems. Hospitals, in particular, have many teams focused on meeting the needs of patients and families, addressing performance improvement projects, meeting to solve problems and completing time limited ad hoc projects. Socialization to working with colleagues from other disciplines is the first step to making these teams successful.

Nurses, for many years, were subordinated to physicians. A nurse would customarily serve in the role of team member—in deference to the physician "captain of the team" role with its resulting designated power, control, and status. The imperatives for constant and rapid change and reducing the costs of care appear to have been catalysts in the transition to the use of teams to make and drive decisions. Teams are larger, membership is interdisciplinary, and they are used for multiple purposes. Frequently teams drive quality improvement activities and participate in organizational governance. Registered nurses often serve as leaders of interdisciplinary teams because of their breadth of knowledge and skill in facilitating groups.

No one discipline can have all the information needed to make good nonroutine decisions. Often there are many stakeholders in a decision, and each must demonstrate the ability to compromise and support any change; no single individual can take on that role. Teams with the right members and trust of one another can be highly effective in these situations (Kotter, 1996).

Trust is an integral part of defining our interdependence with others, the dependence varying with the task, situation, and person involved. Trusting behaviors increase mutual trust and lead to improved communications.

A COMMON PURPOSE AND GOALS

There is little disagreement with the axiom "the whole is greater than the sum of its parts." This applies well to the coming together of interdisciplinary team members in health care. Individuals bring their personal values to work. Today we see values changing in the work environment due to the increasing levels of educational achievement, increased interdependence, and rapid rates of change. Many people believe work is no longer the focal point of their lives. New social values are emerging including the desire for a higher quality work life, for more balance between work and leisure activity, for meaningful and motivating work, and for empowerment to utilize one's special skills, talent, and creativity. In response to changing values, organizations have migrated from traditional punishment and reward management to believing people are basically good. Differences are accepted as opportunities for growth and creativity, and risk taking and collaboration are expected and supported (Barker, 1992). Diversity also brings richness to the world. In the workplace, diversity is the background pattern in the fabric that defines the nature of a group. Like diversity, high-performance participation must value the uniqueness each person brings to the organization (Senge, 1994). Groups must understand diversity and help each member work together more effectively. A new model of relationships that supports this approach is one where individuals:

1. openly share (not hoard) information
2. share the credit for work well done and accomplishments
3. role model, recognize, and praise honesty and openness
4. encourage and acknowledge active partnering
5. critique, refresh, and renew relationships within a group on a routine basis

Clarification of expectations of one another's role is the first step to understanding and valuing professionals from another discipline. Organizations are social systems in which everyone assumes a particular role. Each person has expectations that become the basis of trust of other individuals in the system. Clinicians expect other clinicians to be competent in their role performance; they must bring a level of expertise, knowledge, and skills. We have studied the relationship between physicians and nurses for many years and continue to discuss the interface in the care of patients. Physicians and nurses have a common ground and share a commitment to patient welfare. With the pressures to reduce costs, decrease the length of hospital stays, and reduce resource consumption in general, a more collegial, unified relationship between nurses and physicians can only lead to improved care and protection of the best interest of the patient (Gianakos, 1997). Seeking a common goal allows nurses and physicians the opportunity to share authority and power. Together they move from a position of self-interest to pursuing a common end. The enabling forces in this interdisciplinary work are communication, respect, and trust for one another. In the process, professionals educate one another to their respective clinical, physiologic, social, and emotional knowledge. Shared knowledge can only lead to an increased probability that a patient's and family's needs will be met. This collegiality and teamwork is particularly evidenced in the hospital setting where "doing more with less" or caring for increased numbers of patients while trying to decrease costs "appeals to the spirit of teamwork" (Moderow, 1996, p. 138).

Another imperative driving the need for interdisciplinary socialization is the Joint Commission on Accreditation of Healthcare Organizations' (JCAHO) standards for accreditation of hospitals. Since many nurses still find employment in hospitals, it is important to be familiar with the expectations in this area. The JCAHO standards address many different aspects, but in particular standard TX. 1.2, Care of Patients states, "Care is planned and provided in an interdisciplinary, collaborative manner by qualified individuals" (JCAHO, 1996). Other standards address requirements for an interdisciplinary nutrition therapy plan, a collaborative and interdisciplinary patient and family education process, and the hospital's assurance of coordination among health professionals and services or settings involved in a patient's care. As a recognized authority for quality, these standards are an important tool to establish interdisciplinary efforts to achieve desired outcomes.

SOCIALIZATION PROCESS

One of the ways to appreciate the need for interdisciplinary socialization is to use the analogy of a jazz band. A jazz band leader selects the music, finds the right musicians, and schedules public performances. The result—the effect of the performance—however, depends on the environment, the players in the band, and the need for everyone to perform as individuals as well as members of the group. The leader is also dependent on the group members and their ability to play well (DePree, 1993). Similarly, this is how our health care organizations operate. We are interdependent, rugged individualists within our own profession. Yet, we perform best when we work together and complement one another.

You are probably not going to find instructions in a book that will tell you how to work most effectively with individuals from other disciplines. It involves common sense and draws on what you know about developing interpersonal relationships. The underlying principles are shared values, communication, trust and an appreciation or valuing of the other person. These principles are basic to human interaction and developing relationships.

Articulating and establishing shared values are the first steps for a group to work toward defining its purpose and vision. Group members should discuss their values openly and see what is most important to everyone. Adopting a set of core values common to the group establishes an important foundation.

Communication among health professionals is an essential part of all relationships and takes on many forms. What is most important in interdisciplinary relationships is a commitment to communicate that includes both listening and giving effective messages. Almost every step of the process of caring for patients involves either written or oral communication, and therefore is a mainstay of productive relationships with other professionals. Besides listening, expression of messages determines how co-workers of all disciplines will respond. You must ensure you express the intended thought, use words and phrases that are free of judgment as well as control nonverbal behavior.

Trust is something that is usually earned over time. Because health professionals believe everyone is committed to the common goals of serving the patient, there is an automatic sense of trust in the work setting. This trust cannot be violated but instead should be validated by one's behavior over time. You establish trust through demonstration of truthfulness, sharing knowledge, following through on your word, and establishing credibility. By trusting one another, we increase our vulnerability. Great consequence arises if vulnerability is abused.

Valuing another individual comes from appreciating one's unique contribution. Just as nurses want to be recognized for their individuality and special contribution to a patient's experience, so do professionals of all other disciplines. Expression of valuing other individuals is accomplished through actions such as active listening, soliciting information, making a conscious effort to include the other professionals in sessions when decision making will occur, and acknowledging their contributions appropriately.

Depending on the practice setting, interdisciplinary relationships are established between nurses and any number of other groups. These interdisciplinary groups or teams most often include nurses, physicians, pharmacists, therapists (physical, respiratory, occupational), mental health specialists, dieticians, social workers, administrators, as well as a host of technicians. Others may include clergy, law enforcement officials, attorneys, educators, researchers and advocates for the patient and/or family, and in strong advocacy settings, whenever possible, the patient themself.

Members of teams should offer complementary skills. These include technical or functional skills, problem-solving and decision-making skills, and an array of interpersonal skills. The interpersonal skills include effective communication, constructive conflict and conflict resolution, risk taking, helpful criticism, objectivity, active listening, giving the benefit of the doubt, support for one another, and recognizing the interest and achievements of the other (Katzenbach & Smith, 1994).

Collaboration among individuals, either separate from or part of group behavior, is actually a conflict minimization or resolution activity. The impetus for collaboration and use of teams is in part due to the focus on total quality management where the involvement in decision making and actions occur with frontline workers. In team managed environments, staff nurses must possess the skills to succeed in building and leading effective teams (Barker, 1995). Decision-making around quality service issues in team environments is superior to decision making reserved for individuals at the top of a hierarchy. In order to foster the advance of nursing's role in quality decisions, nurses need to have excellent collaboration skills and be comfortable operating in teams.

MEASURING SUCCESS

There are several ways to know you have arrived with interdisciplinary socialization. These can be thought of as group norms achieved by all members and include:

1. Comfortable relationships exist with active ongoing communication.
2. All stake holders are invited to the table when anticipating a decision or solving a problem.
3. No one points a finger to blame another when success is not achieved.
4. Vested interests are left at the door and the common good prevails in decision making.
5. Recognition is given freely to one another among disciplines.

Nurses are stars when it comes to interdisciplinary socialization and collaboration. Perhaps this is because we demonstrate greater humility than many other professional groups, or because we have always been inclusive, not exclusive, in our holistic approach to care. Regardless, nurses are able and willing to acknowledge the contributions of others and work toward the common end, for the good of the patient and family in all situations.

INTRADISCIPLINARY NURSING RELATIONSHIPS

The paradigm for teams in nursing was a variety of nursing personnel, primarily registered nurses, licensed practical nurses, and assistants to nurses. The teams were asked to care for a group of patients for a given period of time or shift. The new paradigm is interdisciplinary teams. Registered nurses have long focused on appreciating the specialty knowledge of other nurses. The new focus is expanded to appreciate and value contributions to providing or managing care across the continuum.

Within nursing we still have many intraprofessional relationships. These relationships may be with a specific specialty area such as psychiatry, with a specialty team, with academic colleagues, across systems, or with provider groups. Within an integrated delivery system nurses relate to other nurses at affiliated hospitals, satellite institutions, in-service settings across the continuum of care such as home health and extended care, or with case managers. Nurses have always coordinated the care of patients across services, among different professionals, and across the continuum of care. The formal evolution of the case manager role in the last decade has its roots in the early public health system of nursing. Today it takes on greater elements of resource utilization and monitoring. Case manager roles exist in many acute care and community based settings. Since other professionals also function as case managers, the skill sets are not unique to nursing. The case manager must have both intra- and interdisciplinary skills.

HINTS FOR LEADERSHIP DEVELOPMENT

Creating opportunities for interdisciplinary socialization is an important basis for establishing your desire to be successful in today's organizations. Honing your personal skills to be an effective team member will assist your maturation from participant to leader. Just as team members have expectations of one another, there are added performance expectations of those who assume the role of leader.

Nurses bring a patient-advocate perspective to any interdisciplinary effort. Nurses also have the capacity to be effective coordinators of information, an important aspect of participation in interdisciplinary teams. Other professionals with a more narrow scope of practice recognize the broader, holistic, and inclusive range of responsibilities that rest with the registered nurse. The nurse must demonstrate the accountability that accompanies the responsibility.

To grow as a leader in an interdisciplinary environment, broaden your knowledge base of the roles and expertise of other professionals who contribute to the team. Be an eager learner and listener. Encourage synergy among team members by fostering creative cooperation (Covey, 1989). Keep an open mind and refrain from judging others. Actively demonstrate your support for other team members. Express yourself through your professional competence. Extend the olive branch when needed, and above all keep the patient first. By focusing on achieving optimal patient outcomes, leaders can guide groups to make the right decisions.

SUMMARY

Nurses must seek interdisciplinary socialization in order to work effectively with professionals of other disciplines. Nurses are positioned well to not only be effective team members but also leaders. The development of key interpersonal skills such as active listening, sharing constructive feedback, developing trust, valuing others, and giving support and recognition is important for personal success in an interdisciplinary environment.

CRITICAL THINKING QUESTIONS

1. What barriers have you identified that might hinder interdisciplinary socialization? How would you remove them?
2. What are the most effective methods for teaching or developing interpersonal relationship skills? Why?
3. When you observe professionals interacting in a clinical setting, what skills are easily demonstrated? What skills require greater development?

4. Compare and contrast the skills necessary for interaction with patients, with those necessary for successful interactions with other professionals. What is similar? What is different?

5. How can nurses best maintain a balance between individuality and being a successful team player?

ACTIVITIES

1. Create a personal skills inventory as a self-assessment of your ability to succeed in interdisciplinary socialization. Rate your interpersonal skill readiness. Ask a peer and mentor (supervisor if employed) to rate items such as:

   • communication skills (listening and sending messages)
   • developing trust
   • resolving conflict
   • demonstrating value for others

2. Identify a good role model for interdisciplinary socialization. Interview her or him to determine her or his pointers for success.

REFERENCES

Barker, A.M. (1992). *Transformational Nursing Leadership: A Vision for the Future.* New York: National League for Nursing Press.

Barker, K. (1995). Improving staff nurse conflict resolution skills. *Nursing Economics, 13*(5), 295–298.

Covey, S.R. (1989). *Seven Habits of Highly Effective People.* New York: Simon and Schuster.

DePree, M. (1993). *Leadership Jazz.* New York: Dell Publishing.

Flexner, S.B. (Managing Ed.). (1983). *The Random House Dictionary of the English Language (2nd ed., unabridged).* New York: Random House.

Gianakos, D.. (1997). Physicians, nurses and collegiality. *Nursing Outlook* (45), 57–58.

Joint Commission on Accreditation of Health Care Organizations. (1996). *1997 Comprehensive Accreditation Manual for Hospitals.* Oakbrook Terrace, IL: Joint Commission.

Katzenbach, J.R., & Smith, D.K. (1994). *The Wisdom of Teams.* New York: Harper Business, Harper Collins Publishers.

Kotter, J.P. (1996). *Leading Change.* Boston, MA: Harvard Business School Press.

Moderow, R. (1996). Teamwork is the key to cutting costs. *Modern Healthcare.*

Senge, P.M., Kleiner, A., Roberts, C., Russ, R., & Smith, B. (1994). *The Fifth Discipline Fieldbook.* New York: Doubleday.

ADDITIONAL SUGGESTED READINGS

Covey, S.R. (1989). *Seven Habits of Highly Effective People.* New York: Simon and Schuster.

Katzenbach J.R. & Smith, D.K. (1994). *The Wisdom of Teams.* New York: Harper Business, Harper Collins Publishers.

May, C.A., Schraeder, C., & Britt, T. (1996). *Managed Care and Case Management Roles for Professional Nursing.* Washington, DC: American Nurses Publishing.

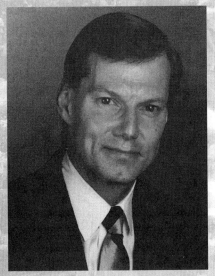

Photo courtesy of Tim Porter-O'Grady Associates, Inc.

Tim Porter-O'Grady,

EdD, PhD, FAAN

Dr. Tim Porter-O'Grady has been involved in health care for 27 years. He has served in many positions from staff nurse to both hospital and health service executive. He is currently senior partner of an international health care consulting firm specializing in organizational innovation and health service transformation issues. He also serves on the graduate faculty of Emory University in Atlanta.

Dr. Porter-O'Grady has a graduate degree in nursing and business administration and holds a doctorate in learning behavior. Tim had completed postdoctoral studies in aging and is a certified clinical specialist in gerontology. He has recently completed a second doctorate in health systems.

Tim has written over 130 articles and book chapters, and has published nine books, and is completing a tenth. He has consulted with over 500 institutions and has spoken in 1300 settings in the United States, Canada, Europe, and Asia. He logs about 350,000 miles a year. Dr. Porter-O'Grady is listed in seven different categories in Who's Who in America, serves on seven editorial boards, is a member of the New York Academy of Sciences, and a Fellow in the American Academy of Nursing.

Tim has served on a number of community and national boards and has been an elected officer in a variety of health related agencies and organizations. He has been a health systems expert for the National Health Policy Council and is on the governing board of the National Franciscan Health System.

Tim has focused his practice on systems innovation and creativity as applied to the delivery of health services. He works to lead health care systems to more effectively create their own futures. Tim challenges all leaders to develop new ways of thinking, knowing, and doing. In this, he hopes, we will renew our commitment to creating truly healthy communities.

CHAPTER 9

Workplace Advocacy, Shared Governance, and Collective Bargaining: Rights and Opportunity

INTRODUCTION

When compared to the long history of nursing, workplace advocacy and collective bargaining are relatively recent experiences. In much of the industrial age the worker has been looked at as a subset of the work (Rosenfeld, 1994). Historically, the work essentially takes more priority in an industry's life than does the worker. It is only during the last half of the industrial age that issues around worker rights and worker participation have predominated in discussions related to the workplace (Belasco, 1996). Workplace advocacy and collective bargaining processes have been a part of the development of human resource approaches in workplaces for the last 70 years in the business community and the last 30 in health care services (Bluestone, 1993).

It has only been in the last 30–40 years that nurses have focused on workplace advocacy processes and collective bargaining. Collective bargaining in health care, as a more recent undertaking, has been emerging quite slowly as a fundamental part of the health care service experience (Scott, 1994). Since the 1960s, the American Nurses Association has been instrumental in driving both workplace advocacy processes and collective bargaining as a fundamental right for the professional nurse. Indeed, much of the formative and subsequent activity in collective bargaining in nursing has been undertaken through the leadership of the American Nurses Association. Many position statements, advocacy processes, and active collective bargaining developmental and implementation processes have been led on behalf of nurses by the American Nurses Association and undertaken by state nurses associations across the country. Through their efforts, much of the general economic welfare of nurses has advanced reflecting the American Nurses Association's commitment to workplace advocacy and collective bargaining processes. Because of the lucrative and sizable pool of nurses in the United States, many other labor unions have been active in organizing nurses for purposes of collective bargaining over the past 20 years.

WORKPLACE ADVOCACY

All American citizens have basic rights. The fact that an American citizen is at work should not in any way abrogate the rights that person has under the constitution. However in the industrial age, it has been the historic experience of workers that the minute they enter the work site, individual rights and privileges they imply somehow appear to be diminished. The company takes control, the decisions of the company predominate, and the worker simply becomes one of the functional elements of the decision-making engine of the organizational system (Ryan, 1991).

This scenario is no less true for health care. Indeed, there are many who might argue that the health care hierarchical and organizational bureaucracy have many more components that challenge the rights of individuals than any other workplace format (Belasco, 1996). Decisions affecting practice are affected by others; control over decisions affecting the direction of clinical activity are influenced by non-clinicians; work for which registered nurses are responsible is undertaken by other providers; and the relationship between disciplines is subjugated to the administrative control of the operating environment. These and a host of other circumstances work in concert to reduce the ability of the individual to control his or her own decisions, to influence his or her life, and to control the elements of professional practice (Pinchot, 1994).

In some instances, the disparity that exists in organizations is of such intensity that it actually impedes the individual nurse in practice to undertake his or her work. The control of decision making, authoritarianism, bureaucracy and hierarchical nature of the organization, and the overwhelming and overreaching control of administration and management into the practice issues of a profession, all create the conditions and circumstances limiting the ability of the individual professional to practice his or her profession (Porter-O'Grady & Finnigan, 1984). Nurses can certainly elucidate a host of anecdotes in a number of different settings representing these circumstances and conditions that limit the ability of the nurse to function as a coequal part of the health care team.

While many health care systems are changing, the nature, content, and character of the changes are not always driven in the best interest of those at the point-of-service (Goldsmith, 1996). Indeed, in many organizations, decisions about changes are not often arrived at in consultation or in relationship with those upon whom the changes would have an impact.

Many practice changes, point-of-service adjustments, and patient-care decisions that occur in the workplace are often determined and arrived at by those who do not provide patient-care services and are not located at the point-of-service. Some of those decisions indicate the lack of necessary wisdom when they are not made by those at the point-of-service or involved in patient-care delivery. Many such decisions and the negative impact they have on patient care could have been avoided if those who are involved in patient care were consulted or incorporated into the decision-making processes. An organization whose management is the sole arbitrator of decisions affecting patient care is not only grossly negligent with regard to its commitment to service, but severely handicapped in its management skill set and its operation of a clinical organization (Wilson, 1991).

Workplace advocacy processes relate specifically to the development of mechanisms and structures in an organization that make it possible for the relationship between the organization and the workers to be facilitated, advanced, and enhanced. Workplace advocacy processes relate to worker-workplace committees, councils, task forces, forums, and work groups. Workplace advocacy relates to building and strengthening the relationship between those who do the work of the organization and those who manage it. Advocacy means espousal for the services, purposes, direction, and work of the organization and the relationships necessary to sustain it.

Much of the work of the emerging age is to build relationships between a number of different players. Workplace advocacy demands that the structures and interactions that facilitate relationships impacting the quality of patient care be the focus of the organization's work and be developed in a consistent and meaningful way for the sole purpose of benefiting those who the organization serves.

Here again, the American Nurses Association, the American Organization of Nurse Executives, and others have provided much leadership in the development of workplace advocacy processes. Employer-employee committees, practice groups, councils, problem-solving groups, continuous quality improvement committees and work groups, unit-based decision making models, service pathways and integrated delivery teams, team-based decisional structures and service frameworks all represent elements of the work advocacy process now essential to the integrity and effectiveness of most workplaces. It is recommended that every nurse, upon employment, seek opportunities to be members of the various decisional groups that affect and improve the quality of work life, patient care, and relationship in the organization. The purpose of workplace advocacy activities is to enhance the relationships necessary to sustain the commitment on the part of organization and profession in undertaking the critical work they do in relationship to patient care.

There are several characteristics that workplace advocacy groups should evidence in the formation and structuring of their functions and activities:

- Equal representation between management and staff around issues of mutual concern
- Advocacy groups that focus on the point-of-service at the unit level. Advocacy for patients can occur best in the places where providers and patients relate
- Problems (regarding the ability to do the work, decisions related to the work, and the structure of the organization which facilitates the work) are discussed in workplace advocacy groups
- Staff sharing equal roles in deliberations and decisions related to patient care, relationships, and professional interactions at the point-of-service; staff lays out on the table issues related to management's support, behavior, and interaction with the staff in a way that facilitates the development of improved and effective relationships between staff and management
- Staff involvement in workplace advocacy processes regarding decisions about the kind of work to be done, how it is to be done, work expectations, roles, and functions of the staff in contributing to the design and development of good patient care processes; decisions are not made solely by management
- Equity is required in order to assure that the contribution of each member of the workplace advocacy process has value to the process; each member makes a contribution, and that contribution is valued by the system; problems between management and staff, workplace and worker, process and practice are appropriate issues of concern in the workplace advocacy committees or work groups; problems are solved by the people who own them and in the places in which they are located
- Workplace advocacy and patient advocacy are essentially the same thing; workplace advocacy groups have patient-care issues and all of the elements necessary to facilitate and promulgate good patient care at the center of their consideration process

Workplace advocacy efforts and activities should be formalized and organized as an ongoing part of the decision-making structure of an organization. Practicing nurses and managers should see that those kinds of activities and forums are an effective and essential part of the decision-making structure of any health care organization. All professionals need a framework for problem solving and decision making. Professional activities of nursing are affected if nurses cannot play a role in making decisions that affect the quality of care, relationship between the profession and the organization, and the relationship between disciplines and individuals. Workplace advocacy activities should ensure that these issues are addressed, and that a framework and format exist in the organization for that to occur.

Any organization that does not, at a minimum, have a basic foundation for workplace advocacy processes is positioning itself for increased difficulty in the relationships between staff and management and in the problem-solving processes associated with the delivery of good patient care. New staff nurses in employment interviews should ask questions related to the presence of workplace advocacy processes and the elements of decision-making and problem-solving that exist in an organization, including the role of the staff in leadership and in making decisions.

SHARED GOVERNANCE

Perhaps no organizational process has been as dramatic or had as far-reaching implications for the organization as have shared governance activities. While collective bargaining activities have unfolded in under 10 percent of the hospitals in the United States, shared governance activities have unfolded in well over 60 percent of the health care organizations in the United States. Shared governance is an organizational model of empowered decision making that involves the practicing nurse in decisions affecting practice, quality, competence, and the nurse's role within the organizational system. Shared governance is the framework for organizing nursing decision making. The concept dates from the early 70s. As a format for defining the nursing organization as an operating system, shared governance began to unfold seriously in organizations in 1980. Since 1980, a vast majority of organizations have implemented some component of shared governance as a part of their operating system.

Shared governance as a structure ensures that the practicing nurse participates at both the point-of-service and in the organizational structure in decisions that affect the delivery of care, financing of that care, relationships necessary to promulgate that care, and decisions that ensure the facilitation of patient care across the continuum of services. Shared governance structures address the whole organizational system for nursing, as well as every individual component. It provides an opportunity for individual nurses to fully participate in decisions affecting their practice and moves the locus of control and authority for those decisions from the management structure and from the higher echelons of the organization to the point-of-service and into the hands of the professional practicing nurse.

Of the vast number of health care organizations that have implemented shared governance, only a handful have successfully and fully implemented all of the components of shared governance. There is a high degree of risk to the organization to make the commitments necessary to truly empower the staff to make decisions that they should already own. The risk to the organization is imbedded in the requirement that management move its locus of control to the staff, give up much of the authority and need for control, and learn new skills of facilitating, coordinating, and integrating decision-making rather than directing and controlling decisions for the staff. This skill set change, the organizational structures that must shift, and the implications that it has on the relationship between staff and management is tremendous. Often these implications are more challenging than many leaders can see themselves implementing and sustaining in the organizational system.

Much work, implementation, documentation, writing of shared governance models, and related research that underpins the mechanisms for evaluating shared governance have unfolded in the past 15 years. Many organizations that have implemented shared governance have used it as the framework for building further integration in the health care system. Often shared governance is used as a template for building relationships within the discipline of nursing as well as between nursing and other disciplines in the organization. Whole system shared governance has now become a framework for integrating multidisciplinary organizational systems. Driven by nursing's leadership, the success of the model as applied to organizational decision-making forms the basis for broader development. Entire health systems are beginning to look at it as the model and framework for linking and integrating a transdisciplinary organizational system.

New nurses, upon employment, should be asking the organization whether shared governance decision-making structures are in place. This question helps determine if the staff has been empowered, if authority for decision-making has been generated to the staff, if professional nursing has control over clinical practice, and if nurses can fully participate in decisions affecting their practice within the shared governance framework. At this stage staff should have a right to expect that, at a minimum, those processes are in place in any health care workplace in the United States.

The shared governance structures of an organization (to varying degrees) have the following elements in place:

- An overall organizational structure where nurses may participate fully in making decisions about their practice
- A counsel, forum, congress, etc., where nurses participate fully in decisions affecting the strategy, direction, financing, and application of the priorities of the organization and nursing's role in relationship to it
- A decision-making structure at the point-of-service (unit, or service place in the organization where the majority of nurses practice) is evidence that the decision-making process is ongoing, operating, and effective; nurses should be a part of the evaluation process of the system
- An expectation that all nurses participate in decisions affecting their practice; a rotating of the authority for making decisions on councils, forums, and congresses between and among all the nursing staff; full participation is evident
- A format linking decisions made at the system level, organizational level, service level, and the unit level of the organization; The mission, purposes, and objectives of the organization, and the principles and priorities of the profession are linked and integrated along the decision-making pathway; This seamless integration of decision making is one of the fundamental characteristics of effective shared governance systems.

Shared governance and empowerment strategies are no longer the exception in many health care organizations, they are the rule. While there are a number of organizations that are still autocratic, narrow, rigid, and unilaterally management-driven, their ability to sustain is decreasing as changing models of health care emerge. Increasingly, collaborative, horizontal, interdisciplinary, professional processes of deliberation, collaboration, and decision making are becoming the necessities for thriving in any health care organization. Shared governance creates both a format for making such processes possible and a structure which sustains them. Most nurses should at least be aware of the elements of shared governance, have many of the components already in place in their workplace, and be working diligently to strengthen, advance, and improve the models of empowerment, shared decision making, staff leadership, and collaboration within a transforming health care system.

PATIENT ADVOCACY

Nurses cannot be empowered to advocate for the patient if they are not empowered to advocate for each other and for the profession. There is a direct relationship between patient advocacy and advocacy of the profession. Advocating for the patient is advocating for the profession. Being positioned to make a difference is critical for the success of advocacy. There is no more impotent role than to be an advocate for a group and be without political, organizational, or professional power. Unfortunately, this circumstance often exists for the nursing professional.

It is the obligation of every nurse to advocate for his or her patient. The safety of the patient, the ability to assure that the patient's needs are met, the ability to obtain outcomes, and to promulgate in advance the conditions and circumstances supporting the patient are the fundamental foundations of the work of nurses. Patient advocacy is an outflow of professional obligation. The processes of shared governance and workplace advocacy should ultimately be directed to advancing the relationship of the nurse with the patient. Patient advocacy also means strengthening the relationship between the disciplines. It means advancing the decisions made in each of the disciplines in the way that will support decisions made in all disciplines. It means building an interdisciplinary relationship for the team, configuring its work around the patient, to fulfill its mutual obligations required to provide good patient care and meet the demands of good service.

Every nurse is called to be an advocate. In order to successfully advocate for the patient, each nurse must be willing to undertake the following obligations:

1. Assertively represent their own role and position as a professional nurse as well as decisions affecting the patients they care for

2. Participate fully on shared governance councils and in other activities resulting in decisions affecting how care is delivered; move forward the relationship between providers; further the practice and processes associated with patient care

3. Join in the processes associated with clarifying the activities and contributions each professional makes to the continuum of patient care. Tying nursing practice to specific outcomes and identifying the contribution that each makes to the process is critical to creating sustainability in service and promulgating continuous and improved outcomes

4. When the safety of the patient is compromised, when the defined clearly enumerated standards of patient care or outcomes for patient care are compromised, the nurse should advocate clearly, articulately, and competently for the patient in a way that closes the gap between the behavior expected and the standards of performance identified

5. Identify deficits in the system and in practice, at the individual level and the systems level; advocate for the patient by following up on the questions, problems, concerns, issues, and deficits in the delivery of patient care.

When nurses fail to be assertive in identifying and following up on problems in the provision of patient care, they advance the perception that nurses do not respect the professional obligation or commitment to the delivery of good patient care services. Every nurse has an obligation to take on those issues that demand corrective action no matter where the organization is regarding the level of its awareness and commitment to the consumer. Advocacy requires courage.

Patient advocacy is tied into the professional activities of every nurse at every level of decision making. Good workplace advocacy processes and shared governance structures create dynamics and mechanisms in the system providing a format for advocacy. Within those processes the issues of concern regarding patient care, safety, and relationship are important elements of consideration and deliberation. Indeed, they are the work of advocacy and shared governance. Each nurse, however, has a responsibility as a patient advocate to fully participate in advocacy to assure that nurses are used in the best interest of advancing patient care and improving both the quality of work life and the quality of health.

NURSES AND COLLECTIVE BARGAINING

Collective bargaining is a fundamental and basic workplace right in the United States. Every individual has a right to pursue activities of collective bargaining for any reason he or she determines. Collective bargaining provides an opportunity for every individual to be represented in an organized approach to the issues affecting work and its activity. Collective bargaining assures that the rights of the individual worker are maintained and that due process is placed in motion through collective action. This provides mechanisms of response to inadequacies or inappropriateness in the workplace within the context of a negotiated collective bargaining agreement.

Collective bargaining originated in the earlier part of the twentieth century in the United States as a response to horribly inhuman and inadequate conditions of work. The fundamental rights underpinning collective bargaining exist regardless of the conditions in the workplace. Collective bargaining as a right can be promulgated by any individual in the workplace regardless of the urge or need to pursue it. Collective bargaining does not need to be stimulated by poor management or inadequate working conditions. It can be pursued and undertaken by the workers simply because of their desire to be represented collectively. Furthermore, staff does not need to experience the conditions that initially drove the movement towards collective bargaining in order to initiate it. Around World War II, there were basement sweatshops, management beating staff, unsafe conditions in the workplace, 16-hour workdays, limited child labor laws, and a host of unhappy and inappropriate workplace conditions. While most of those have not existed in America for well over 40 years, the right and need to organize collectively has not dissipated. The partnership created through positive, well-designed, and well-utilized collective bargaining processes can assure a mutual understanding between workplace and worker that can be clearly articulated in the context of a contract.

Every worker, regardless of whether a collective bargaining agreement is in place, has a right to expect the following behaviors and processes from management and leadership in the hospital or health care organization:

1. A support of clear and well-developed policies that are consistent throughout the organization

2. Good morale and a strong commitment from the organization for its members and staff

3. Good benefits representing the specific needs of the employees and advancing their present considerations and future opportunities

4. A commitment to improvement of efficiency, effectiveness, and quality of patient-care services

5. A clear commitment to promoting economy, preventing waste, and supporting good utilization of scarce resources

6. Promulgation and promotion of the highest possible standards for patient care and patient safety

7. Enforcement of the highest practice of all safety obligations, rules, and regulations for the health care entity

8. Protection and preservation of the environment, resources, and property within which workers operate in the course of doing their work

9. Creation of a cooperative and collaborative environment supporting the relationships and decisions necessary to improve patient care

10. Clear, detailed, well-informed, knowledge-based, and appropriate instructions, processes, orders and directions

11. Follow-up of all reports of occurrences and inappropriate behavior, inadequate conditions and situations, and the appropriate corrective actions necessary to resolve them

12. Acting on the suggestions for improvement, advancement, and the correction of errors

13. Facilitation, coordination, and integration of the activities and work of the professional and clinical staff in a way that helps them meet the needs of those they serve

ELEMENTS OF LABOR LAW

Collective bargaining is protected at the federal level by a body of law assuring and promulgating the right of individuals to organize for purposes of collective bargaining. It is important that the individual nurse understands the basic elements of labor law that promulgate the right to collective bargaining. This provides an opportunity through the collective bargaining process for people to respond to the conditions and elements of work and to have specific activities that are protected by law.

The Wagner Act, the first federal labor law, was passed in 1935. This law has been amended through periodic amendments such as Taft-Hartley, Landrum-Griffen, and recent incremental shifts and adjustments in the law. The recent amendments were intended to make the laws more relevant, current, and balanced in the context of changing work conditions.

In the Federal Labor Relations Act, there are protected activities that unfold and assure the benefits of any group of employees who gather together for any purpose concerning their working conditions. The law guarantees the following rights:

- Right to self-organize
- Right to form, join, or assist labor organizations
- Right to bargain collectively through chosen representatives
- Right to engage in concerted activities for the purpose of bargaining as a group and for mutual protection
- Right to refuse to join, form, or assist labor organizations at any time

Under the federal labor relations laws there are also prohibited activities. The prohibited activities specifically address the employers and supervisors in the process of collective bargaining activities. These prohibitions are:

1. Any interference with the rights of employees to collectively bargain
2. Assisting or interfering with the formation of a labor organization or contributing money to it as an employer
3. Discriminating against any person or group in hiring, firing, or business practices in order to discourage their union membership
4. Punishing an employee for giving testimony regarding any factor related to collective bargaining
5. Refusing to bargain with the selected legal, chosen representative of the employees.

Any violation of the protective or prohibitive activity is called an "unfair labor practice." Unions may also contribute unfair labor practices just as well as employers can.

There are a number of unfair union labor practices that are prohibited as a part of the union's activities. Such unfair union labor practices are:

1. Restraining or coercing employees in exercising their protected rights
2. Attempting to cause an employer to discriminate against employees
3. Refusing to bargain with the employer
4. Engaging in secondary boycotts—trying to get an employer or his employees to stop dealing with another employer
5. Extorting or charging exorbitant fees and other matters related to inappropriate charging of fees or exorbitant rates to employees and members of the union

The staff nurse must remember that an employer has the right to hire or fire for any reason as long as it is not on account of union activities or on the basis of an individual's race, sex, religion, or disability. Sometimes union organizers will tell employees that they can't be fired if they belong to a union, or during an organizational campaign. Sometimes organizers will also tell an employee to notify his or her supervisor if he or she is engaging in union activity for two reasons: (1) to put the hospital or health care system on notice of such activities so that any firing can be tied to union activity, (2) in order to "bait" the supervisor into firing that employee. These activities are not protected, and are against the law. Staff should be careful that they are not involved in these activities when they are involved in organizing for the purposes of collective bargaining.

Any firing or layoff during any organizational activity is subject to question and should be cleared very carefully with administration. Except in specific circumstances, such as insubordination, drunkenness, serious violation of safety rules, inadequate patient care, or failure to report to work there are three reasons for making sure that you do not fire during labor union organizing activity:

1. Unions will sometimes work to "drum up" discharge cases to aid the organizing efforts.
2. Unions can sometimes take credit if it is finally determined the firing was discriminatory and inappropriate.
3. Unions can be recognized as representatives of employees without an election if it is determined that the firing was discriminatory and the act created an atmosphere of fear among the employees so that a fair election cannot be conducted. Caution, therefore, should be exercised around the issue of hiring and firing during a union organizing campaign.

As the staff is participating in the processes of beginning an organizing effort, they have the right to convince their fellow employees to join them, and the employer has no right to prevent them from having representation for purposes of collective bargaining and grievances. Unions can attempt to organize employees in a number of ways that are appropriate and valid. They can:

1. picket the health facility to advertise.
2. pass out leaflets outside the health facility to advertise.

3. contact employees in their homes or by telephone.

4. provide leaflets and other materials to sympathetic employees who campaign inside the health facility.

If the union or employees secure sufficient number of signed cards authorizing them as representatives of the majority of the employees in a group with common interest, it can demand to be recognized by the employer as the bargaining agent for all the employees in that group. The employer can voluntarily recognize the union and bargain with it. Or if the employer has "good faith doubt" that the union actually has the full support of all the employees, the employer can refuse to recognize the union. If the employer refuses to voluntarily recognize the union, the union will submit a request with the regional office of the National Labor Relations Board asking the board to certify the union as a representative of the employees. In this case, the union will be required to show that it in fact represents a majority of the employees in the unit, and that the employer has no good faith doubt as to its majority status.

Generally, however, the union files a petition for election. Upon the employer's consent for an election, an election is scheduled to take place usually within 30 days. At the election, the union must get a majority of the eligible employees to vote in its favor. If the numbers are not sufficient or the vote is a tie, no majority has been established and the union does not win the election. If a majority has been established then the union wins the election and the right to represent the employer for purposes of collective bargaining.

During the election period both the employer and the union campaigns to the employees, trying to convince them to vote either for or against the union. There are many limitations on the part of both union and employer with regard to what behavior they can exemplify during the collective bargaining process. The employer and the staff, in an organizing effort, must be careful not to violate the standards of behavior essential to good, responsible action in the collective bargaining organizing effort.

UNION REPRESENTATION

Often nurses are not fully aware of what union representation means legally. Collective bargaining is a right that must be accessed carefully and understood fully so that it can be utilized appropriately in the best interest of those to which it is directed. The following are legal implications of union representation:

1. All employees in the elected bargaining unit, except for those designated as supervisors, have transferred to the collective bargaining unit all of their rights to negotiate with the health facility officials and the supervisors about wages, holidays, hours, schedules of work, vacation, insurance, overtime, and conditions of work, and every other thing related to wages, hours, and conditions of work consistent with their agreement.

2. Representation will continue for at least a year, and likely longer (as long as the contract is in force).

3. The union will represent all employees in the bargaining unit, whether they voted for the union or not.

4. Designated or elected employees will be determined by the union to a assume a leadership position of officer, steward, or leader in all matters. Therefore, all issues must go through this individual(s) whether they be complaints, requests, or other activities.

5. Employees will have to conform to the national or central union policies.

6. Those who are members will have to pay dues out of their salaries and wages every month.

7. Special monetary assessments, requests, and per capita taxes can be made for designated funds, strike funds for other organizing efforts in other health facilities, for politics, and in the other reasons the union may seek to solicit additional funds.

THE COLLECTIVE BARGAINING AGREEMENT CONTRACT

The collective bargaining agreement is the product of deliberations and negotiations between an employer and a union elected to represent the employees. This contract governs the terms of employment for organizing employees in such areas as wages, hours, working conditions, and benefits. These contracts are highly variable depending on the culture, concerns, issues, focus of individual institutions, and the environment and circumstances surrounding deliberations and negotiations. Each contract has unique characteristics. However, there are essential conditions and circumstances that are common to all union contracts. There are several basic articles in each union contract, some of them are as follows:

- Article One—Recognition of the Collective Bargaining Unit
- Article Two—Union Security
- Article Three—Check Off
- Article Four—Union Activities
- Article Five—Management Rights
- Article Six—Nursing Practice Committees
- Article Seven—Grievance Procedures
- Article Eight—Arbitration
- Article Nine—Strikes and Lockouts
- Article Ten—Discipline and Discharge
- Article Eleven—No Discrimination
- Article Twelve—Seniority

- Article Thriteen—Transfers and Change in Status
- Article Fourteen—Employee Personnel Files
- Article Fifteen—Health and Safety
- Article Sixteen—Hours of Work
- Article Seventeen—Unpaid Leaves of Absence
- Article Eighteen—Vacations
- Article Nineteen—Holidays
- Article Twenty—Sick Days
- Article Twenty-one—Bereavement Leave and Jury Duty
- Article Twenty-two—Wages
- Article Twenty-three—Overtime
- Article Twenty-four—Shift Differential
- Article Twenty-five—Variable Pay Processes
- Article Twenty-six—Insurance Benefits
- Article Twenty-seven—Separability
- Article Twenty-eight—Conclusions
- Article Twenty-nine—Duration

Each Article of the Collective Bargaining Agreement carefully and considerately enumerates the elements and issues of concern to the collective bargaining process. Each one of the contracts creates a binding agreement between employer and union related to those particular articles. Every member of the union must abide by the articles of the contract, just as the employer must. No independent, unilateral, or non-aligned action can be undertaken by any member of the collective bargaining unit out of context of the collective bargaining agreement signed by the union and the employer. The contract becomes both the parameters and constraints, as well as the protections and enumeration of the rights of employment, for every covered employee of the hospital or health system. Therefore, while it is certainly clear that the collective bargaining agreement does protect within the context of the elements agreed to in the contract, it also prohibits the independence, individualism, unilateral, and unique, sometimes creative adjustments and changes that can occur through action, assertiveness, forthrightness, or independence.

While collective bargaining protects, it also constrains. Both of these elements should be understood by individuals prior to making choices for collective bargaining. The collective bargaining process is a fundamental right that should not be precluded, prohibited, or suspended in any way. In exercising this right, certain other actions are precluded very much like any other aspects of human dynamics and interaction. The gift of collective bargaining is that it legally mandates the relationship between employer and employee and protects that relationship by weight of law. No other workplace advocacy, shared governance, or empowerment process in the organization extends the same degree of legal right as articulated specifically and functionally in a collective bargaining agreement.

Collective bargaining is the strongest, most significant, and specifically defined delineation of rights, obligations, and expectations of any of the workplace advocacy processes available to nurses. While shared governance and other specific workplace advocacy processes have specific legal implications that can protect their presence once they are in place and operating, those rights are not as clearly and specifically spelled out as is required in collective bargaining agreements. On the other hand, not having specifically detailed parameters can provide a broader range of creativity, innovation, and change driven by the staff as the opportunity and need for change occurs. In a collective bargaining agreement, the ability to adjust and change the collective bargaining agreement can be limited by timing, availability, and the legal constraints defining the appropriateness of the collective bargaining process. Each of those limit the opportunity to make changes that may meaningfully position nurses to move creatively and immediately adapt and adjust to the changes that are occurring in the marketplace or the health care system. On the other hand, the collective bargaining agreement prohibits the employer from being capricious and arbitrary regarding inappropriate change. The downside of collective bargaining is the sense of entrenchment, slowness of mobility, and the requisite for agreement among everyone before changes are incorporated into the process of adjusting the collective bargaining agreement.

These processes are sometimes time-bound, politically influenced, power-based, and subject to the requirement of broad-based consensus before shifts and changes in the collective bargaining agreement reflect the environmental, contextual, and system shifts required by an organization to remain viable and sustainable. The ability of an organization to be fast, fluid, flexible, and mobile can be constrained by the individual's lack of ability to adjust, alter, change, and adapt quickly. In the future, more flexible approaches to contracting will be in order to continue the value, viability, and essential contribution that the union movement has made to the improvement of the workplace in America.

TURNING THE PAGE—A TIME OF CHANGE FOR UNIONS

Nurses need to be aware of the fact that the workplace is changing dramatically. While there has been much change driven by constraint of resources, much more significant transformation is occurring in the health care system. We are inexorably and slowly moving towards early engagement health care. This changes the focus on treating late-stage illness and begins to address the needs of health and illness in earlier stages of determination. This reduces the total amount of cost for delivery of service and begins to have a broader and more significant impact on the health and status of the community as a whole. The focus on reducing costs, raising the quality of the community's health care, and responding to the technological impetus to less intensive or decentralized services form the foundation for a fundamental change in the delivery of health care. This change is having an impact on how work is done, what work is valued, where it is done, the whole process of patient care, the decentralization and de-institutionalization of care services, the portability of technology, and the mobility of the provider. All of these circumstances joined together create the conditions for a transformed and shifting health care system. Much of this impact has a dramatic and direct affect on the practice of nursing.

For the past 100 years, nursing in America has been essentially institutionally located and bed-driven. Much of the care and services that have been provided for 75 percent of those we serve has been bed-related services. Technology, economics, and social and political considerations have now moved the focus of delivering service away from bed-based strategies and institutional models.

The practice of nursing has been radically altered through integrated organizational systems, horizontally aligned networks, decentralized service structures, multidisciplinary team approaches, high-tech low-invasive innovations, the movement to primary care services, and the creation of systemic approaches to the delivery of health services. The journey toward these new arenas, unbundling nursing activities, and functions away from predominately bed-focused processes creates a great deal of "noise" and trauma in the practice of nursing and the application of the future of the profession of nursing. The conflicts that come from being on the cusp between an age when bed-based services predominated, and an age where decentralized, mobile, fluid services predominate, create much tension, anxiety, and issues around viability, future practice, and patient advocacy in the current workplace environment.

These changes create an impact on work advocacy and collective bargaining processes. Some of the old mechanisms of collective bargaining can no longer be sustained if the future is going to be promulgated in a meaningful way. As we create highly functional points-of-service that are team-driven and interdisciplinary in terms of their interaction and work processes, unilateral, individualistic, institutional, and fixed-site approaches to work and to the collective bargaining rights and protection are no longer sustainable. In order to better position nurses for the future and to make the collective bargaining process more viable, sustainable, and to assure its continuing key role in protecting the rights and conditions of those it represents, nursing leaders of the future will need to look at some of the changes that must occur in the advocacy process. The following circumstances are creating the conditions which will require unions and workplace advocacy processes to be radically altered:

- The change in the American economic circumstances have created a specific change in the way in which health care is financed and paid for. Fiscal shifts in operation have affected the whole service framework for providing health. The way health care services are paid and the emergence of the capitated and managed-care marketplace change the conditions and structures for paying for health care and health care professionals' services.

- The attitude and approach of unions in the '70s, '80s, and early '90s are not always in the best interest of the sustainability of the business of health care and have even threatened the viability of institutions to respond and to change quickly to this changing social environment for the delivery of health care services. In the '80s, the change in the workplace environment driven by President Reagan's behavior with the air traffic controllers set in motion a series of activities and impressions of collective bargaining that threatened the union movement in many unfortunate and inappropriate ways.

- The technology associated with how work is done, where it is done, and why it is done has shifted the way in which work is unfolded in the health care system. As a result, changes in work force numbers, allocation, service content, job descriptions, locations, and others have created much challenge in the operating system and threatened the viability of many collective bargaining agreements. It creates the conditions of untenable sustainability for some union contracts and makes it challenging for unions to adequately respond to the changes in reality.

- Unions have sometimes been caught up in their own intransigence and lack of responsiveness. The changes that are occurring in the social, political, and economic milieu affect unions as much as they affect any other component of the system. The methods of collective bargaining, the content of collective bargaining, even the processes associated with collective bargaining may have less and less viability as more of the social structure changes.

Listed below are a number of specific and identifiable changes that will be required on the part of unions and collective bargaining processes in order to maintain their sustainability and their viability as important contributing members of the health care system and promulgators of essential change for their members.

1. Unions must understand that they must incorporate into their strategic activity the fact that the workplace is changing and changing dramatically. The radical changes in the workplace are inexorable and inevitable. The contract cannot prevail against those changes. The union must be actualized and incorporated in the process of facilitating their own change with dialogue centered on how the union can be benefited by making those changes and how the union can benefit the system's need to change. Staff and union members must be a part of building creativity and innovation into the change process as members of the union.

2. The individual and personal perceptions of the collective bargaining member regarding what she or he needs is changing. This requires a deeper understanding of the emerging needs of the worker and a higher level of dialogue within the context of the work system. The demands on the worker are becoming increasingly high tech, the performance expectations for the worker are becoming increasingly mobile, fluid, and flexible moving away from fixed and finite work circumstances and structures. The collective bargaining process must now be supportive and facilitative of the changes necessary to assure the viability of the worker and of the union. The longer the collective bargaining process insulates the worker from the essential change in role

expectation the less viable that individual becomes in the changing and evolving workplace structure. The union, providing leadership in making decisions about worker's response to the changing environment, needs to incorporate more flexibility and fluidity in job definitions, expectations, and performance conditions of members of the collective bargaining unit.

3. Increasingly, clarity between role functions is becoming less defined in new system models of work. In the old industrial age, all work could clearly be defined as fixed, finite, and functional. The delineation of descriptors of work, including those outlined in collective bargaining agreements, reflected this characterization of work. In the new work environment, work is becoming fluid and flexible. Skill sets must become much more mobile. No longer can the rigid parameters of workplace, department, and institutional structures be the only delineations of work. Contracts that contain such language, and only identify work within that context, are no longer viable and do not address the real issues of concern for the future of nursing practice. More fluid approaches to the definition of work, a recognition and support of mobility in the skill set, and continued protection will be critical on the part of union leadership. Contracts in the future may not identify particular sites of work, but will instead identify specific considerations and conditions of work regardless of where that work is carried out. This flexibility will be critical to the future viability of collective bargaining agreements.

4. As integration occurs in the health care delivery system and interdisciplinary models of care unfold, there may actually be conflicts between collective bargaining agreements outlined for different professions within the same work setting. These conflicts will create conditions of nonviability. Therefore, it will be increasingly required for collective bargaining units to dialogue and interface with other collective bargaining units representing different unions, different disciplines, and professionals within the same institutional framework. Identifying common frames of reference, even common contract elements and processes may become an increasingly frequent requirement for the collective bargaining process in a number of organizational systems. Integrated transdisciplinary activities and team-based approaches will increasingly be a part of the content of the health care delivery system affecting the viability of collective bargaining agreements.

Partnership is now the characteristic principle that is undergirding much of the change at every level and in every place in the health care system. Forming partnerships between disciplines, organizations, systems, and components of the systems along with the continuum of care will create new kinds of relationships, and new kinds of practice interfaces. While some are covered by collective bargaining agreements, some dealing with the same professionals are not covered by collective bargaining agreements or are covered by other agreements. This conflict addressing the same level of professional person in a different context can create some difficulties in assuring work decisions are appropriate, work constraints and possibilities exist in the organizational system, whether elements are covered by the collective bargaining agreement, and for whom are they covered. Increasingly, the partnership delineation for relationship will create conflicts with regards to who is covered, what is covered, and what coverage means within a collective bargaining agreement. The agreements themselves must become more fluid, less narrow in content, more context driven, much more reflective of the environment into which we are moving. They must be much more individual in terms of their application to specific cultures and sites, unique vagaries, and variables found at the point-of-service. Making them fluid and flexible will be critical to their viability over the long-term.

There is nothing that is of greater importance to the worker in the long-term than the protection of rights, processes, and practices that are fundamental to their ability to contribute in the workplace. Collective bargaining has a long and noble history of addressing these specific issues. If it is able to continue to do so, and to remain viable, it will also have to adapt and adjust its way of addressing these issues so that they, too, are more flexible, appropriate, and amenable to the issues of concern that they address in a changing workplace.

The union movement is essential to the democratic process in America. The future of democracy requires that unions be strong and effective. In order to maintain strength, unions, like all the other components of the social enterprise, must make the necessary changes and adjustments essential to their own health and viability.

Just as collective bargaining must shift, so must other workplace advocacy processes and shared governance designs shift and adjust to adapt to a broader-based, continuum-driven, multifocal health care delivery system. The cost constrained components of the health care system now move nurses from making best judgments to making wise decisions. Wisdom incorporates the issue of resources, quality, and the variability of work. For the first time in our history, within this generation of nursing professionals, the issue of value drives the choices that we make in rendering patient care. When there were unlimited resources and there was no concern for such constraints, value was not a significant issue. Best choices were made under all circumstances. With the introduction of value in decision making the professional nurse now must consider several variables in undertaking patient care, cost, the outcome of the choices that he or she makes, and the mix of activities that must be adjusted and changed in order to bring a tightness-of-fit between what he or she does and achieves.

SUMMARY

At the foundation of all of the efforts related to workplace advocacy, shared governance or collective bargaining is the commitment on the part of each individual nurse to fully participate in the activities of his or her profession. The attitude that is often promulgated of "just doing my job" is no longer sufficient to create sustainability and viability within the profession and in the health care delivery system.

The changes, the drama of transformation, the impact on the profession, and the future of nursing demands the commitment, involvement, and ownership of every practicing nurse, whether that be in the arena of workplace advocacy, in the full participation of shared governance decision-making, or in undertaking the responsibilities and obligations of the collective bargaining process at every level of the organization. The nurse has an obligation to give evidence of full commitment and participation. No nurse is exempt from that obligation.

Increasingly, the value of the discipline will be measured by the degree of leadership it provides in making decisions around the positive impact of change on nursing and patient care. Advocacy for the patient cannot unfold unless there is also advocacy on behalf of nursing and on the part of the nurse.

Advocacy requires ownership and investment. Every nurse that passes from education into practice inherits the obligation to fully participate in decisions that affect the future of the profession of nursing, of health service, and of patient care. Patients expect nurses to advocate in their interest and on their behalf utilizing the best of what is available to advance their care and safety. In order to do that, every nurse must be involved in those decisions that assure that the practice of nursing is protected, advanced, and positioned to continue to make a significant difference in the lives of those we serve. Every nurse is an advocate, every workplace is an opportunity for advocacy, and every patient has a right to expect that the nurse will fully engage in those activities that advance the patient's best interest.

CRITICAL THINKING QUESTIONS

1. What is the nurse's primary responsibility in relation to workplace advocacy?
2. What is the one common element that threads through workplace advocacy, shared governance, and collective bargaining processes?
3. Identify at least three specific contributions the practicing nurse can make in workplace advocacy processes?
4. What is the single most unique circumstance of the collective bargaining process as a most significant workplace advocacy vehicle?
5. What talent, gift, or contribution will you make to workplace advocacy processes? What will be your personal commitment to exercising it where you work?

ACTIVITIES

1. Explore with your State Nurses Association (SNA) how they function to assist nurses in the state with workplace advocacy, collective bargaining, and shared

governance issues. Invite the executive director of the SNA to come and talk with your leadership class about these issues.

2. Read and discuss the article titled "Long-awaited providence ruling upholds the right of charge nurses to bargain." (Bich-Quyen Nguyen, J.D. (1997, September–October). Long-awaited providence ruling upholds the right of charge nurses to bargain. *American Nurse,* 1, 14.

3. If in your future nursing practice you are faced with employment practices that place your patient's health and safety at risk, how will you strive to correct the problem? Discuss your answer with a classmate.

4. In 1990, the National Student Nurses' Association passed a resolution titled Nurses' Trade Unions vs. Representation by the American Nurses Association. It was submitted by the Iowa Association of Nursing Students, Inc. The resolution actively supported the American Nurses Association acting as the collective bargaining agent for nurses who elected to be represented. Discuss with your class why nurses should represent nursing, and what workplace advocacy process you feel will be most widely used in the twenty-first century.

REFERENCES

Belasco, J., & Gorham, G. (1996). Why empowerment does not empower: The bankruptcy of current paradigms. *Seminars for Nurse Managers, 4* (1), 20–27.

Bluestone, B., & Bluestone, I. (1993). *Negotiating the Future: A Labor Perspective On American Business.* New York: Basic Books.

Goldsmith, J. (1996). Burning the seed corn. *Healthcare Forum Journal, 39,* (2), 18–25.

Pinchot, G. E. (1994). *The End of Bureaucracy & The Rise of the Intelligent Corporation.* San Francisco, CA: Berrett-Koehler Publishers, Inc.

Porter-O'Grady, T., & Finnigan, S. (1984). *Shared Governance for Nursing.* Rockville, MD.: Aspen Publishers.

Rosenfield, R. (1994). Replacing the workshop model. *Topics in Healthcare Management, 20* (4) 1–15.

Ryan, K., & Oestreich, D. (1991) *Driving Fear Out of the Workplace.* San Francisco, CA: Jossey-Bass.

Scott, C., & Lowery, C. (1994). Union election activity in the health care industry. *Health Care Management Review, 19* (1), 18–27.

Wilson, C. (1991). *Building New Nursing Organizations: Visions and Realities.* Gaithersburg, MD: Aspen Publishers.

ADDITIONAL SUGGESTED READINGS

Block, P. (1992). *Stewardship,* Barrett-Kohler Publishers.

Huber, D. (1995). *Leadership and Nursing Care Management:* W. B. Saunders Company.

Porter-O'Grady, T. (1992, May–June). Of rabbits and turtles: A time of change for unions, *Nursing Economics, 10* (3), 177–182.

Porter-O'Grady, T., Hawkins, M., & Parker, M. (1997). *Whole Systems Shared Governance: Architecture for Integration:* Aspen Publishers.

Porter-O'Grady, T., & Wilson, C. (1996). *The Leadership Revolution in Health Care:* Aspen Publishers.

Wheatley, M.J., & Kellner-Rogers, M. (1996). *A Simpler Way:* Barrett-Kohler Publishers.

The Stepping Stone of Professional Nursing Involvement

In Unit Three, I invite you as a future nurse leader in Chapter 10 to review the history of *the development of nursing's collective identity,* and our efforts to develop a unified voice. For many nursing student leaders in the country, *the march into professional involvement begins with NSNA* (The National Student Nurses' Association). Chapter 11 will discuss that march. Then in Chapter 12 you'll look at some of the leadership opportunities that are available to you within organized nursing as you review the importance of *political action for nurses: the vision, the path, and the roles.*

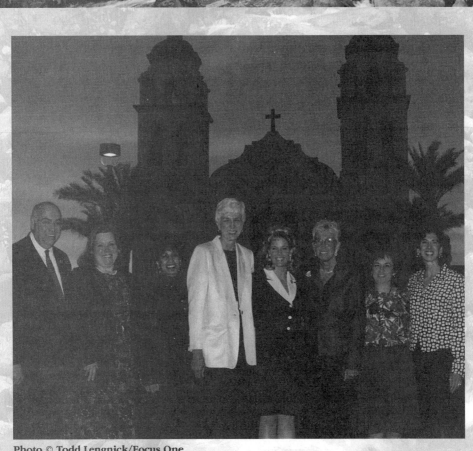

Photo © Todd Lengnick/Focus One

A Biography of Carol A. Andersen, BSN, RN is featured on page 2.

Pictured at the 45th Annual NSNA Convention in Pheonix, Arizona, from left are: Dr. Robert V. Piemonte, RN, CAE, FAAN, Immediate Past Executive Director of NSNA, Carol A. Fetters Andersen, BSN, RN, a Past President of NSNA; Dr. Beverly Malone, RN, FAAN, President American Nurses Association (ANA); Eunice Cole, BS, RN, NSNA Consultant and a Past President of ANA; Sharon Brigner, 1996/97 President NSNA; Dr. Margretta Madden Styles, RN, FAAN, Immediate Past President of the International Council of Nurses (ICN); Florence Huey, MA, RN, a Past President of NSNA; and Dr. Diane Mancino, RN, CAE, Executive Director of NSNA.

CHAPTER 10

Nursing–The Need for a Collective Identity

INTRODUCTION

Graduate nurses at the turn of the twentieth century found themselves in a society undergoing enormous changes. Those changes brought both opportunities and challenges. Women were entering the work force in record numbers. It is remarkable to review descriptions of that era for the parallels to today's nursing environment. They are evidenced by increased levels of change—changing women's roles, and the strong need for a unified voice in nursing.

Our rate of change in the United States today is greater than ever before. In the midst of these changes, two income families and single parent families are increasingly prevalent. As one of nursing's future leaders, I invite you to look back with me and explore the development of nursing's voice. As we learn how and why nursing's voice developed, understand our recent nursing demographics, and broaden our vision to include nurses around the globe, we can build the foundation for nursing's unified voice of tomorrow.

THE EARLY DAYS OF NURSING'S COLLECTIVE IDENTITY

Nurses at the turn of the twentieth century, being predominantly female, were interested in and influenced by developing changes for women and changes in society. This time brought the birth of the National American Women's Suffrage Association and the Temperance Crusade. Health care was also changing with the discovery of the germ theory and advances made in surgery. These led to an increase in patient populations and a boom in hospital construction. That boom also impacted nursing. The results included opportunities for advancement, new roles, and also exploitation of nurses. This new movement towards hospital-based care meant training nurses to meet that role. The problem was that the training was unstandardized, in both length and content, and the hospitals were often staffed by student nurses as a cheap form of labor. There was no assurance to the public of the knowledge level of the care provider treating them or the safety of that care. The need for a strong advocate voice began to emerge.

Nursing leaders of the day, Isabelle Adams Hampton, Adelaide Nutting, Lavinia Dock, and many others were actively working for woman's rights, standardization of nursing education, and the development of nursing's voice. In 1893, nurse educators joined together at the Chicago World's Fair to address these concerns. They were committed to nurses coming together to protect their communities from untrained nurses, and to protect their own jobs. At that meeting of the International Congress of Charities, Correction and Philanthropy, a visionary paper was presented by Edith A. Draper, then superintendent of the Illinois Training School for Nurses. She empowered her audience to recognize the necessity of an American Nurses Association by stating, "The difficulties to be encountered, one must truthfully admit, will mainly be of our own manufacture. What we need is energy of purpose, enthusiasm, a spirit of philanthropy, and ambition to lift our profession to a height to which the eyes of the nation shall look up. To advance we must unite!" (Draper, 1893) The priorities of the profession set by the International Congress were:

1. To develop a code for nurses (which became a long-term goal)
2. To get licensure laws passed for nurses
3. To form an organized association of American nurses

ASSOCIATIONS OF AMERICAN NURSES

The third priority of the International Congress was the first to be accomplished. Three years later, ten nursing school alumni associations came together to form the Nurses' Associated Alumnae of the United States and Canada on September 3, 1896. Fifteen years later the name would be changed to the American Nurses Association, as it is known today.

Isabelle Hampton Robb was the first president of an association that she had envisioned for years. As president, she oversaw the efforts by the states to have licensure laws established for nurses, and she also spoke publicly and published works regarding the need for nursing licensure. Nursing's success in this area was indeed remarkable when we consider that women did not even have the right to vote at this time.

GETTING LICENSURE LAWS PASSED

A great deal of credit for organizing the efforts on passage of licensure laws belongs to those who worked to develop effective communication channels in nursing. Considering that letter writing was the main avenue of day-to-day communication for most nurses in different cities and states, something more efficient and effective needed to be created. In 1900, many nurse leaders organized the formation of a private company that started the American Journal of Nursing (AJN). The magazine, funded by nurses and for nurses, had significant impact on disseminating information to nurses all over the country, thereby strengthening nursing's voice. Sophia Palmer, AJN's first editor-in-chief, personally accomplished much of the effort through her editorials and work at AJN over the next 20 years (Donahue, 1985). She wrote and spoke on the need for registration of nurses in the magazine, to women's groups, politicians, and anyone who would listen. She was known for her frankness and vision on this issue as well as many other pertinent nursing issues from those first days of the journal until her death in 1920.

These efforts have special meaning today as we've struggled to maintain the identity of registered nurses, maintain leadership by RNs in practice settings, and educate the public to the quality impact that RN care has on outcomes. As nursing's future leaders, we would be well served to review Sophia Palmer's editorials, those written by Editor Mary Mallison, BSN, RN from 1981–1993, other AJN editorials over the years, and recent editorials in AJN written by Lucille A. Joel, RN, EdD, FAAN, the magazine's current Editor-at-Large. How informed are you about national and international nursing issues? Keep reading.

PUBLIC HEALTH NURSING

Nursing, firmly grounded in the concept of service, disease prevention, and health promotion for individuals and communities, continued the work of Florence Nightingale as new nursing care innovators emerged. In 1893 Lillian Wald helped start public health nursing in New York City, out of the movement of social reform to meet communities sanitation and health needs. Nurses who worked under Wald's direction were educated in disease prevention, culture, diversity of people, political systems, as well as general nursing practice. In 1912 she was pivotal in the development of the National Organization of Public Health Nursing (NOPHN) promoted curriculums at universities to prepare nurses for these roles, and served as the association's first President. Her nurses functioned with a great deal of autonomy and clinical decision-making skills.

Unfortunately, with nursing's movement back to the hospital, we gave up much of that autonomy. Today, as care moves back again into the community, what can we learn from public health nursing's beginning?

MEETING DIVERSITY NEEDS

Black American nurses or "Colored nurses," as they were called then, faced even more challenges both from society and from within nursing. In educational and practice settings, these nurses were often segregated to separate facilities or living quarters, as was the practice of society at that time. Although, some did belong to the American Nurses Association (ANA) through their alumni associations, ANA did not address issues of discrimination at that time. Martha Franklin, a black nurse leader from Philadelphia who was dissatisfied with inaction on this issue, communicated on her own with other black nurses to research acts of discrimination. In 1908, in New York City, she called a meeting of black American nurses and 52 came. Together they held the founding meeting of the National Association of Colored Graduate Nurses (NACGN). The organization's mission was to fight discrimination in nursing. They developed objectives in the areas of education, employment, and within organized nursing. NACGN became even more important to black nurses in 1916, when the ANA adopted a federation model made up of district and state associations. This resulted in black nurses no longer being eligible to belong to ANA through their alumni associations. Then 16 southern states plus the District of Columbia moved to refuse membership to black nurses.

More challenges occurred during World War I when black nurses were not allowed to serve. In World War II, although some black nurses served, they were segregated to different living quarters and served mostly black soldiers. Then in 1948, with the establishment of the United States Cadet Nurse Corp, things began to change. The Corps created the provision of free education to 65,000 nurses the first year, which included over 3,000 black nurses. After WW II, the military was finally desegregated. But it was not until 1950 when the American Nurses Association opened membership to *any* registered nurse, without discrimination to race, color, or creed, that the NACGN voted to join their efforts with ANA. With their goals and vision now shared by ANA, they looked towards what could be accomplished with all American nurses together in caring.

Over the years, many national and world leaders in nursing have been people of Color. As we develop nursing's voice and nursing practice in the twenty-first century, it must reflect, recognize, and support diversity in all areas, just as it must recognize the health care needs of all our world's citizens through the continued development of transcultural nursing care. It is absolutely essential that we be united in respect of our differences, for only then can we truly embrace the development of nursing's collective identity.

MOVEMENT TOWARDS A CODE OF ETHICS

During World War I, nurses were given a heroic image for their involvement in the war effort. In total, eight million lives were lost during that war. Our country celebrated with a short time of prosperity in the early 1920s as our country tried to forget the horrors of the war to end all wars, as it was termed. Other changes were happening in society as women were *finally* given the right to vote. During the roaring twenties while much of the country celebrated good times, nursing leaders made good on their moral commitment to begin developing a code of ethics for nursing. The first priority of the 1893 International Congress was at last being addressed.

In the Foundation of the National Student Nurses' Association video *To Advance We Must Unite,* Marsha Fowler, PhD, RN talks about this first attempt of nursing to develop a code of ethics. She shares that this first code was "a beautiful document, written in a Victorian style." But, although eloquent, the code was "considered too flowery in expression to be enacted in that form." Even though the authors did not pen the format of the code that would be finally adopted in 1950, they certainly gave nursing strong cornerstones for its development. They charged us with "keeping alight the flame of nursing for humanity." This early group of nurses went on to describe the "central moral motif of nursing, in that, the nursing professions most precious gift was that of service, extending even to the sacrifice of life itself" (Foundation of the NSNA, 1996).

Nursing's Code of Ethics, adopted by the American Nurses Association in 1950, has served as a guidepost for the ethical practice of nursing and helps to broadly define our practice in all settings. The code has been revised through the years. At the American Nurses Association's House of Delegates meeting held in Washington, DC, in June, 1997, impassioned speeches were given as the code is again under revision. Through the years critics of nursing, and the code, have challenged what they call the "lack of enforcement" of the code (DeYoung, 1985, p. 89). However, the guidance that the Code of Ethics gives has been quoted in various State Board of Nursing reviews of nurses, in peer reviews and in grievance procedures both of nurses and nursing students, as well as courts of law. The Code of Ethics has also been quoted with pride by nursing professionals, as they recognize their colleagues for exceptional nursing service. I encourage you to stay informed about, and involved in the current changes to our Code of Ethics, an important document that helps define our profession.

MOVING TOWARDS A UNIFIED VOICE

In 1952, nursing found that there were a multitude of professional nursing organizations, much like we see occurring today. Because nursing recognized the need to act with a strong unified voice, rather than duplicating efforts, nurses came together in 1952 and voted to incorporate the nursing organizations of the day. Two major nursing organizations remained: the American Nurses Association, and the National League for Nursing. The National Student Nurses' Association was also formed that year. The profession recently experienced a similar movement for unification of nursing's voice. In 1991–1994, as nursing worked to define its role in the changing health care environment and entered into the discussions about unlicensed assistive personnel, organized nursing came together and voted to have the profession speak to congress and individual legislators with one voice—and that voice was the American Nurses Association. Nursing is the largest provider group in health care. Can we, in the next century of nursing, commit to developing one voice as nurses speak for and with our patients and their families?

UNDERSTANDING WHAT NURSING LOOKS LIKE

As with any patient scenario, the efforts to strengthen nursing's voice should begin with assessment. As a future nurse leader, you must keep abreast of what the current picture of nursing looks like. To help you begin, the American Nurses Association has granted us permission to reprint their summary publication about the 1992 study done by the U.S. Department of Health & Human Services, Public Health Service, Division of Nursing. It is included in Appendix E for your review.

The summary covers areas such as statistics on nursing (the largest segment of the health care workforce), ethnic and racial demographics of nurses, age statistics for nursing, family status, education level statistics, financing of nursing education, where nurses are working, in what roles they are working, and regional demographics including salary ranges. This is a valuable reference for you to use as you make your own career choices and negotiate for employment. It can also assist you in recruiting efforts with high school students and in communities during projects that you or your student nurses' association might undertake to promote nursing. As we consider the diverse populations we serve as nurses, it becomes more critical that we have diversity in the profession. These statistics show that we have work ahead of us to meet nursing's diversity needs.

BROADENING NURSING'S VOICE—THE INTERNATIONAL COUNCIL OF NURSES

The next step in our assessment, now that we have begun to understand what nursing looks like, is to understand some of the width and breadth of nursing's voice of yesterday and today. There is perhaps no one more qualified today to address this area than Margretta Madden Styles, RN, EdD, FAAN. Dr. Styles is the immediate Past-President of the International Council of Nurses (ICN), and President of the American Nurses Credentialing Center. She is a strong advocate for leadership development of nursing students and gave an empowering keynote address at the National Student Nurses' Association (NSNA) 45th Annual Convention in April, 1997, in Phoenix, Arizona. Dr. Styles wrote an article to future nurse leaders and published it in *Imprint,* NSNA's magazine in 1997, April/May titled "Marching for Global Change." In the article, she shares her experiences as president of ICN. She states, "ICN, a worldwide federation of 120 national nurses associations, is the vehicle whereby millions of nurses from a thousand different places come together as a unified force marching for global change" (p.28). She goes on to share that it is wise for us to be aware of the strategies and objectives of the march so that we can identify our place in the effort. ICN moves along three major courses:

1. Professional and clinical developments
2. Developments in nursing and health care regulation
3. Workplace advocacy

The ICN has a strong commitment to nursing education because they recognize two essentials to nursing's voice and strength in world health—unity and quality. Nursing students from all areas of the globe participate in the ICN's Quadrennial Congresses. The most recent took place in Vancouver, British Columbia in June, 1997. Perhaps one of you will be one of ICN's future presidents. The need is there for your involvement. Future efforts to move us towards health for all will certainly require each of us to maintain a global perspective and remain an active participant in nursing's march.

SUMMARY

Together, we have looked at the growing development of nursing's collective voice during the past 100 years. We've discussed an assessment of what the nursing profession looks like demographically (See Appendix E), and we've broadened our assessed view of nursing to include a global perspective. These are important steps. But, they will render us, as nursing's future leaders, impotent towards empowered change and the visionary development of nursing's twenty-first-century voice unless we internalize these steps, think critically, and move forward as changed leaders. There will always be new issues that challenge our collective action, as well as old issues that are yet unsettled. But the key will be that, as nurses, we move forward together. For it's by strengthening both our collective identity as nursing professionals and our collective voice that we *can* and *will* make a difference.

Edith A. Draper again calls to us from the 1893, International Congress. "The difficulties to be encountered, one must truthfully admit, will mainly be of our own manufacture. What we need is energy of purpose, enthusiasm, a spirit of philanthropy, and ambition to lift our profession to a height to which the eyes of the nation shall look up. To advance we must *unite*" (Draper, 1893).

CRITICAL THINKING QUESTIONS

1. What do you see as the greatest threat to nursing developing a unified collective identity in the twenty-first-century? What do you see as nursing's strengths as we continue to develop nursing's voice and nursing's vision?

2. If membership is less expensive in specialty nursing professional organizations, why should nurses belong to their State Nurses Association first? (Note: The American Nurses Association [ANA] uses a federation model of membership. This means that when you join your State Nurses Association, membership to ANA is through your state association.)

3. What do you consider essential nursing functions, skills, and expert roles? Do they apply to nursing in other countries also?

4. Is your definition of nursing applicable to nursing around the globe? In the future, if and when space travel becomes commonplace, how will nursing be defined?

5. You are a nurse in a third-world country where financial support and supplies are limited. How would you use unlicensed assistive personnel, meet cultural needs, and train the population to meet its own public health needs after you are gone?

ACTIVITIES

1. Nursing leaders such as Lillian Wald who helped to establish the practice of public health nursing, Jane Delano who was Chief Nurse of the American Red Cross in WW I, and Martha Franklin who helped form the National Association of Colored Nurses are wonderful examples, to us as future leaders, of nurses who spoke articulately and acted with vision and passion to address needs in nursing and society. The Foundation of the National Student Nurses' Association produced a tribute video for ANA's Centennial Convention in Washington, DC, in June of 1996, titled *To Advance We Must Unite!* I encourage you, your student group, or your school to obtain a copy. Contact NSNA at (212) 581–2211 for more details. These nursing leaders and many others who were pivotal in developing nursing's voice are included in the video.

2. As an individual or group project for your nursing leadership class, nursing issues class, or for your own leadership development, get current copies of the ANA Code of Ethics for nursing. Talk with the president of your State Nurses Association to stay informed about the current revisions to the code. Take this opportunity to get informed and involved with this important part of your profession.

REFERENCES

DeYoung, L. (1985). *Dynamics of Nursing* (5th ed., p. 89). St. Louis, MO: C.V. Mosby.

Donahue, M.P. (1985). *Nursing the Finest Art: An Illustrated History.* St. Louis, MO: C.V. Mosby.

Draper, E.A. (1893). *The Necessity of An American Nurses Association.* Paper presented at the International Congress of Charities Correction and Philanthropy, Chicago, IL.

Foundation of the National Student Nurses' Association. (1996). *To Advance We Must Unite [Video].*

Styles, M.M. (1997, April–May). Marching for global change. *Imprint,* p. 98.

ADDITIONAL SUGGESTED READINGS

Christy, T. E. (1971, September). The first 50 years. *American Journal of Nursing, 71* (9), pp. 1778–1784.

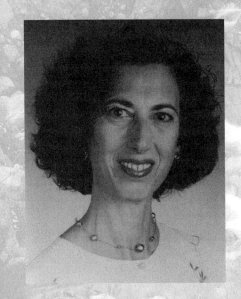

Diane J. Mancino,

EdD, RN, CAE

Diane J. Mancino has held the position of Executive Director of the National Student Nurses' Association, Inc. (NSNA) since April, 1996. First employed by NSNA in 1981, Dr. Mancino has served the association in several capacities including Director of Program, Director of Constituent Affairs, and Deputy Executive Director. Prior to joining the NSNA staff, she held the position of Director of Program and Education with the New York Counties Registered Nurses Association (District 13 of the New York State Nurses Association) in Manhattan. As a community and public health nurse, Dr. Mancino has practiced in both rural and urban New York locations.

Dr. Mancino entered the profession with a diploma from Middletown Psychiatric Center School of Nursing, Middletown, New York. Her Baccalaureate Degree in Nursing was earned at the State University of New York at Buffalo. Dr. Mancino graduated with a Master of Arts degree in nursing from New York University. In 1995, she completed a doctoral degree at Teachers College, Columbia University in New York City. The history of the National Student Nurses' Association is the topic of Dr. Mancino's doctoral dissertation.

Dr. Mancino serves in elected and appointed positions in nursing and association management voluntary organizations. She has published several articles and served as the executive producer of the video "To Advance We Must Unite!—100 Years of the American Nurses Association 1896–1996." Dr. Mancino views her NSNA's Executive Director role as one of mentor, educator, manager, and leader. She is currently implementing a five-year plan for the NSNA to celebrate its 50th anniversary in 2002.

CHAPTER 11

NSNA–The March Along the Critical Path Begins Here

INTRODUCTION

. . . we must prepare our nurses . . . to take their places in the onward march of our profession.

(F. E. Carling, 1915)

What would compel hundreds of the brightest nursing students to put aside their books, suspend their classes, reschedule their clinical time, and take exams early? And why would their faculty not only support these actions but also encourage them to spend their limited resources to travel far and wide to participate in debates, group problem-solving, decision making and self-governance? It is likely that these students and their teachers recognize that attending a National Student Nurses' Association annual convention cultivates future leadership—leadership for the onward march of the nursing profession.

NSNA: A PRACTICUM FOR LEADERSHIP BEGINS

Learning and practicing leadership skills beyond the boundaries of classrooms and campuses has the potential of accelerating the development of leadership in students. The National Student Nurses' Association (NSNA) serves as a practicum for learning leadership skills and developing future leaders. In NSNA, students can experience the "unified spirit" of the profession they will soon enter.

The NSNA officially joined the onward march of organized nursing in 1952. At that time, nursing leadership consolidated five nursing organizations into two: the American Nurses Association (ANA) and the National League for Nursing (NLN). Many of the leaders involved in these nursing organizations recognized that they shared the same core values and societal mission. They divided the responsibilities according to nursing education and practice. They also restructured their staff and shifted the positions of top executive leaders. They hired consultants to guide the reorganization, and new programs evolved to address the challenges of the day.

THE STUDENT ASSOCIATION HAS COURAGE TO STAND INDEPENDENTLY

Important to the discussion of the history of nursing organizations is the fact that one of the two organizations had the foresight to offer nursing students the privilege to be part of their organization. The students bravely exercised a different option by forming an independent organization. In this endeavor, they received the "blessing" and promise of support and cooperation from both the ANA and the NLN. These promises were honored. Today, NSNA remains an independent forum where nursing students prepare to join the onward march of the nursing profession.

Over the years, NSNA leaders developed a governance model with bylaws, policies, and procedures to ensure stability of the organization. The governance structure offers students an opportunity to examine and address health issues that are important to the profession. Through its programs and activities, the NSNA develops students as responsible and accountable leaders of the nursing profession. Involvement in NSNA helps students to see the parade, hear the band, and get ready to join the march.

THE CHALLENGES OF PREPARING FUTURE LEADERS

The challenge that NSNA faces in preparing students to be future leaders is arduous. The parade we march in today with leaders and followers is shifting form and direction. Futurists theorize that leadership for the next millennium will not be limited to individuals who head hierarchies. Instead, decision-making and accountability will be shared by those who recognize that they all play a role in moving an organization or a profession forward. Leaders will move in and out of the leadership role like migrating geese flying in formation. Every nurse will be a leader. Thus, every student nurse must learn leadership. It may be helpful to your leadership development to explore skills and attributes required of a leader in Table 11–1 that follows.

As we consider these attributes, we recognize that most individuals drawn to the nursing profession are determined to improve the health of society, comfort the sick and dying, and engage in satisfying work. Although most nursing services are delivered at or in proximity to the patient's bedside, nursing is one of the first professions to recognize that influences beyond the bedside impact health. Florence Nightingale's legacy remains as important today as it was in the last century. Nightingale initiated, influenced, and catapulted unprecedented institutional changes in the delivery of nursing care and public health during the nineteenth century. Having established the ideological core of the profession, she set in motion a new generation of leaders with common values and shared goals. This continuum of leadership is NSNA's mission— preparing nursing students to be future nurse leaders who accept the challenges of

Table 11–1: Leadership Attributes Needed by Future Leaders

- **Intellectual capacity**
- **Critical thinking**
- **Effective communicator**
- **Empathetic listener**
- **Adapts quickly to new situations**
- **Ability to identify global and local trends**
- **Acceptance of high moral and ethical standards**
- **Ability to facilitate group process**
- **Capacity to interchange leadership/followership roles**
- **Ability to mentor future leaders**
- **Respect and acceptance of all human beings**
- **Desire to strive for an inclusive society**
- **Ability to balance professional responsibilities and personal life**
- **Acceptance of responsibility and accountability for decisions**
- **Commitment to lifelong learning**
- **Advocates and practices cooperation**
- **Ability to balance high tech with high touch**
- **Creativity in problem-solving**
- **Capacity for deep introspection and reflection**
- **Capacity to connect with the spiritual nature of human beings**

tomorrow. Nightingale's words "No system can endure that does not march" continues to inspire nurses to move the profession forward.

The NSNA makes it possible for students to connect with nursing's core mission and to experience the unified spirit of the profession. Like most organizations, members join for different reasons. Many students join NSNA to contribute their time and energy to reach common goals and add their voice to the collective chorus of nursing. These students recognize the advantage of broadening their perspective beyond the classroom. They volunteer to serve on committees and task forces where they learn new skills, meet people, and build confidence.

Astute faculty who recognize the necessity of building future leadership often encourage and make it possible for talented students to hone their skills. Students with the intellectual capacity to maintain good grades and have both the time and energy to do volunteer work find their way to the march quickly. There are many leadership opportunities available in NSNA. (See Table 11–2.) Those who make it to the elected and appointed positions in the NSNA demonstrate high potential for making a significant contribution to the advancement of the profession. Through its ongoing interaction with other organizations and institutions, NSNA fosters the potential of future leaders working together to improve the health of society.

NSNA zealously embraces the challenge of preparing nurses to lead the profession beyond the transitional nature of institutions as we know them today. If we step away from the march for a moment and watch from the sidelines, we see an intense period of transition and transformation taking place locally and globally. Institutions and organizations are experiencing an unprecedented generation and dissemination of information via advanced communication vehicles. In addition to keeping pace with rapid change, nurses must anticipate and address health-related human responses to the technological revolution. Herein lies the paradox: using the information generated by the technological revolution to effectively address the health-related problems associated with living in a technologically advancing society.

Nursing students of today must demonstrate the intellectual capacity to keep pace with and manage an ever-expanding volume of information. The knowledge base of the nursing profession is expanding at an unparalleled rate. Research in nursing and other disciplines influences the way nurses practice and the outcomes of that practice. Leaders must know how to find and process research data to support their actions and plans. Every nurse must make a commitment to lifelong learning to keep up with the information age.

OPTIMIZING LEADERSHIP THROUGH EFFECTIVE GROUP PROCESS

To balance the expanding volume of information and advancement of technology, future leaders will facilitate group work to solve problems and explore new possibilities. They will create an environment that maximizes the dynamics of group process and builds interpersonal relationships. Collective critical thinking will be necessary to

Table 11-2: Leadership Development Opportunities in NSNA

- Run for elected office
- Serve in elected positions
- Serve on committees
- Serve in appointed positions
- Participate as a delegate in the House of Delegates
- Plan and implement Community Health Projects
- Participate in Breakthrough to Nursing Projects (recruitment of under-represented populations into the nursing profession)
- Plan and implement political education activities
- Write for publication in *Imprint* magazine, state, and school publications
- Participate in fundraising campaigns
- Develop public speaking skills
- Learn business skills through management of school and state chapters
- Learn cooperative decision-making, conflict resolution, and consensus building
- Connect with the nursing profession and learn about issues facing the profession
- Attend educational programs and career development workshops sponsored by NSNA
- Plan and implement a state association convention or workshop
- Mentor other students and connect with mentors in the profession
- Make connections and build professional networks
- Build a professional curriculum vitae (résumé)

reach consensus on how to meet the nursing needs of a complex society. Diversity in all aspects of humanity requires leaders who encourage and consider varied points of view and opinions The ability to find common ground so that one strong voice can be created from many requires sensitivity and an ability to articulate inclusiveness. Leaders of tomorrow must recognize that diversity multiplies the possibilities of human potential. Individuals need to be recognized for their uniqueness.

NURSING'S EARLY PRINCIPLES CONTINUE—HOLISM AND ETHICS

Future nursing leaders will embrace the concepts of holistic nursing practice—the care as well as the development of the total human being. Through an expanded world view, nurses will recognize the interdependence of individuals, families, communities, and the global environment on the health of human beings. A holistic framework will help leaders recognize and create new possibilities for addressing their own personal health needs as well as the needs of their clients.

Leaders who guide the human potential of others will advance leadership in the profession and ensure the preparation of future leaders. Leaders cultivate the development of leadership skills and sensibility and have a way of bringing new people into the fold. They empower people to take charge of their own lives and to have the courage and confidence to act.

Humanity faces complex moral and ethical issues surrounding advances in science and medical technology. Genetic engineering, for example, challenges fundamental beliefs and value systems. The principles of ethical and moral decision-making are shifting as individuals and professions reexamine their values and set new standards for social and medical responsibility. At every level of decision making, nurses confront ethical and moral dilemmas that cannot be ignored. Ethical principles will continue to guide the decision making of future nursing leaders.

As competition for human and material resources increases, leaders will understand how to connect people and organizations to accomplish collective goals. Networks of individuals associated with institutions and organizations will come to realize that greater things can be achieved through shared expertise and partnerships. The ability to recognize and act when synergistic opportunities occur will be one of the hallmarks of future leadership.

THE IMPORTANCE OF SELF-CARE AS A LEADER

To sustain creativity and insight, leaders must replenish their energy, center themselves, and reconnect with nature. Leaders in the future may become overwhelmed with work unless they find ways to enrich their own lives. Support from close colleagues, fellow NSNA members, family, and friends is essential to keep the meaning of one's life in focus. Observation and/or participation in the arts and humanities aids in the cultivation of new insights and sensibilities. Future leaders will recognize the value of living a well-balanced life.

SUMMARY

We discussed the history, attributes, essential elements, and vision for your nursing leadership development. NSNA is where your march along the critical path to leadership development begins. Nursing leaders of tomorrow will empower the profession to create and actualize a shared vision. In order for that vision to become reality, we must add our voices to those of our ancestors and current leaders who have recognized that for the profession "to advance—we must unite" (Draper, 1893). The critical path will take us beyond the shadows of the past and into the sunlight of the future march. But we can only arrive there by developing leaders to guide us—leaders like you. Your onward march along the critical path to leadership begins with a first step, and will be empowered through membership and active involvement in NSNA.

CRITICAL THINKING QUESTIONS

1. Reflect on a leadership experience you had or are currently having. How has that experience contributed to your growth potential? Consider the positive contributions as well as the challenges you have experienced. Discuss these with your mentor for feedback.

2. Select a leader (any leader) whom you admire. What leadership characteristics does this person demonstrate? Looking over the list in Table 11–1, which of these listed attributes do you identify in this leader?

3. What are your own leadership attributes? (Use the list in Table 11–1 for a reference.) How can you begin to develop those attitudes you still need? Keep a journal of your personal leadership development.

4. Why did you choose to enter the nursing field? Make a list. Next to each reason, determine the motivation for each (i.e., social, political, economic, spiritual, personal). Record this list in your journal and return to it when you feel discouraged, or when you discover new insights for wanting to be a nurse.

5. What are your technical abilities? What technical abilities do you need to acquire? Make a list of both, and compare it with a list of your interpersonal skills (such as empathetic listening) and those that you need to acquire. Revise and reflect on these lists from time to time to discover how you can keep the lists in balance (see Table 11–2). How can your involvement in NSNA help with these goals?

ACTIVITIES

1. Volunteer to participate in a school chapter activity or on a committee. Keep notes on how decisions are made and how participation is encouraged or discouraged. Identify how the leader (group facilitator) sees her or his role and the roles of others. Were the goals of the group accomplished? If not, why? If yes, what made it possible for the group to accomplish its goals? If you were the leader of this group, how would you have facilitated the group to plan and implement its goals?

2. Design and implement an independent study plan that will provide you with an opportunity to learn and practice leadership skills and self-governance.

3. Visit the NSNA home page on the World Wide Web (www.nsna.org) and send in your comments on what you like or how the site could be improved. If you have not yet established an e-mail address for yourself, set a goal to

establish one before the end of the semester. Visit the computer support center on your campus and obtain a list of computer classes. Set a goal of learning at least two new computer skills every semester.

4. Start your own home page on the World Wide Web.

REFERENCES

Carling, F. E. "The Possibility of Introducing Self-Government into Schools of Nursing." *AJN* XVII, no. 4 (January 1917): 302.

Draper, E. A. (1893). *The Necessity of an American Nurses Association*. Paper presented at the International Congress, Chicago, IL.

ADDITIONAL SUGGESTED READINGS

Astin, H. S., & Leland, C. (1991). *Women of Influence, Women of Vision—A Cross-Generational Study of Leaders and Social Change*. San Francisco, CA: Jossey-Bass Publishers.

Bartling, C. E. (1996, June). Leaders for the information age. *Association Management, 48* (6).

Below, P. J., Morrisey, G. L., & Acomb, B. L. (1987). *The Executive Guide to Strategic Planning*. San Francisco, CA: Jossey-Bass Publishers.

Bergquist, W., Betwee, J., & Meuel, D. (1995). *Building Strategic Relationships—How to Extend Your Organization's Reach Through Partnerships, Alliances, and Joint Ventures*. San Francisco, CA: Jossey-Bass Publishers.

Birnbach, N., & Lewenson, S. (eds.). (1991). *First Words: Selected Addresses from the National League for Nursing 1894–1933*. New York: National League for Nursing Press.

Bolman, L. G., & Deal, T. E. (1995). *Leading with Soul—An Uncommon Journey of Spirit*. San Francisco, CA: Jossey-Bass Publishers.

Botsford, J. (1997, August). President's message—We must empower our leaders to make a difference. *AORN Journal, 66* (2).

Brunner, N. A. (1997, July/August). From the president—Step into the future—The language of change. *Orthopaedic Nursing, 16* (4).

Collins, J. C., & Porras, J. I. (1996, September/October). Building your company's vision. *Harvard Business Review*.

Denning, P. (1997, July/August). A glimpse into the future. *Educom Review, 32* (4).

Feeg, V. D. (1997, July/August). From the editor. *Pediatric Nursing, 23* (4).

Gardner, H. (with the collaboration of Laskin, E.). (1995). *Leading Minds—An Anatomy of Leadership*. New York: Basic Books.

Garfield, P. (1995). *Creative Dreaming—Plan and Control Your Dreams to Develop Creativity, Overcome Fears, Solve Problems, and Create a Better Self*. New York: Fireside Books/Simon & Schuster.

Gouillart, F. J., & Kelly, J. N. (1995). *Transforming the Organization.* New York: McGraw-Hill, Inc.

Hesselbein, F. (1997, Summer). The power of civility. *Leader to Leader,* (5).

Hesselbein, F., Goldsmith, M., & Beckhard, R. (eds.). (1996). *The Drucker Foundation—The Leader of the Future.* San Francisco, CA: Jossey-Bass Publishers.

Kerfoot, K. (1997, Summer). On leadership—Glue: The essence of leadership. *NFSNO, 7* (1).

Klauer, P. T., Pozehl, B. J., & Mahaffey, T. L. (1997, May/June). Development of leadership within the university and beyond: Challenges to faculty and their development. *Journal of Professional Nursing, 13* (3).

Kristof, N. D. (1997, August 17). Where children rule. *The New York Times Magazine.*

Langer, E. J. (1997). *The Power of Mindful Learning.* New York: Addison-Wesley Publishing Company, Inc.

Larimer, L. V. (1997, January). Ethics—Evolutionary ethics. *Association Management.*

Levinson, H. (1996, July/August). When executives burn out. *Harvard Business Review.*

Mahoney, A. I., Senge, P., Covey, S., & Peters, T. (1997, January). Leadership lessons. *Association Management.*

Mahoney, A. I., & Romano, G. (1997, June). Exploring our toughest questions. *Association Management, 49* (6).

Mindell, P. (1995). *A Woman's Guide to the Language of Success—Communicating with Confidence and Power.* Englewood Cliffs, NJ: Prentice Hall.

Quigley, J. V. (1993). *Vision—How Leaders Develop It, Share It, and Sustain It.* New York: McGraw-Hill, Inc.

Redfield, J., & Adrienne, C. (1996). *The Tenth Insight—Holding the Vision (An Experimental Guide).* New York: Warner Books.

Senge, P. M. (1990, Fall). The leader's new work: Building learning organizations. *Sloan Management Review. Strategies for Success—Core Capabilities for Today's Managers.*

Skiba, D. J. (1997, May/June). Transforming nursing education to celebrate learning. *Nursing and Health Care Perspectives, 18* (3).

Temes, P. S. (ed.). (1996). *Teaching Leadership—Essays in Theory and Practice.* New York: Peter Lang Publishing, Inc.

Vance, C. (1997, July 14). Management perspectives—Transformative leadership. *The Nursing Spectrum, 9A* (14).

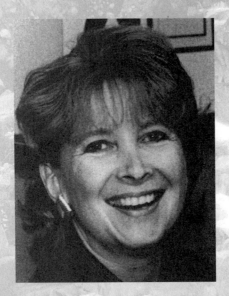

Virginia Trotter Betts,

MSN, JD, RN, FAAN

Virginia Trotter Betts is the immediate past president of the American Nurses Association, having served two terms 1992–1996, and has been involved in health care for over two decades as a clinician, administrator, educator, researcher, and policy activist. In 1998, she was appointed Senior Advisor on Nursing nd Policy to the Secretary and Assistant Secretary of Health at the US Department of Health and Human Services. She is also a founding partner and President of HealthFutures, a health consulting firm. A graduate of the University of Ten-

nessee, the Vanderbilt School of Nursing, and the Nashville School of Law, she is one of only 12 nurses to have been chosen for the prestigious Robert Wood Johnson Health Policy Fellowship. Virginia Trotter Betts has frequently represented the United States internationally on health issues. In May 1993, she was named Special White House Delegate to the 46th World Health Assembly; in September 1995, she was a member of the United States delegation to the Fourth World Conference on Women in Beijing; and in May 1996, she served as a delegate to the 49th World Health Assembly taking the lead in the World Health Organization Resolution on Nursing and Midwifery. At the conclusion of her term as ANA President, she served as Senior Health Advisor to the Clinton/ Gore Reelection Campaign.

From 1995–1997, she served as a Presidential appointee to the Military Health Care Advisory Committee. She is the author of scores of articles on nursing, health care, and health law and has given hundreds of presentations and speeches across the country to nursing, health, and community audiences. In 1997, Virginia Trotter Betts was inducted as a Fellow of the American Academy of Nursing. She is a native of Tennessee, and she and her husband, Steve, are the parents of two daughters, one of whom recently completed a nurse practitioner program.

CHAPTER 12

Political Action for Nurses–The Vision, the Path, and the Roles

INTRODUCTION

Nursing as a profession and nurses as health care professionals are dramatically affected both positively and negatively by the social context in which they exist. Public policy sets the direction, principles, and rules for health care practice, economics, innovation, and education. Thus, nurses must be vitally aware of and participate in health and social policy development.

In our society, one avenue for direct citizen policy participation is through political action. This chapter will highlight the need for professional nurses and nursing students to make shaping health policy through political action an essential part of their professional responsibilities both now and throughout their careers.

NURSES AND POLITICAL ACTION: WHY?

What are you concerned about in your life as a nurse?

1. Direct reimbursement for advanced practice nursing services
2. Sufficient numbers of RN colleagues to practice nursing safely in complex patient-care situations

3. Monies for upgrading your nursing credentials
4. Professional days off to obtain continuing education on the latest in nursing interventions
5. Being acknowledged as a primary care provider on managed care panels in your community and in your state's Medicaid waiver
6. Ensuring that your facility provide equipment and supplies that protect the staff from serious injury and illness

All these concerns (and many more!) are shaped by policy decisions in the public domain. These decisions that affect us are frequently made by the President—his administration and by Congress. They are also made by governors—their administrative structures, and the state legislature, and by mayors and city councils. These decisions are made in reasonably full public view, with the input of a variety of individuals and groups who contend that they are stakeholders in the issues.

Nursing and nurses are stakeholders in both nursing and health care issues and thus must be effective participants in the policy process. Policy is an overall direction or plan directed toward achievement of a certain goal. Public policy is that overall direction made by governments at many levels to reflect choices, priorities, and reactions to competing possibilities or addressing problems large and small. Policy is both a process and an identified outcome. The policy process has four steps that are distinct only in their description: problem identification, policy development, policy adoption, and policy evaluation. (This should sound very familiar!! **Think** the nursing process applied to a social context!) Nurses can and must become adept at participating in each of these policy activities.

One activity that is open to each and every nurse who has an interest in a particular policy outcome is politics. Politics embodies a variety of activities directed toward influencing the outcomes of public decisions about policy. Politics is the method (the how) to achieve the outcome (the what) nurses want from government on social, health, and nursing issues. Politics moves government officials (policy makers) to make authoritative decisions and allocate scarce resources such as dollars, time, access, and power in a focused manner. Thus, if nurses want particular policy outcomes, then political action directed toward those objectives is the route. Political action is required for successful completion of each step of the policy process.

HEALTH CARE POLICY

Just what does nursing want from health policy initiatives? Nursing has long spoken out for universal access to quality affordable health care services and wants primary care available in comfortable, convenient community sites for all regardless of ability to pay. Nursing wants viable programs in Medicare and Medicaid to assure access to and payment for comprehensive health services for our nation's elderly, disabled, and extremely poor. Nursing also wants to make health services for individuals, families, and communities more available and wants to make payment for services affordable for every citizen through public-private partnerships that truly have a safety net for changing personal circumstances. At different times and in varying jurisdictions, nursing has addressed these health policy goals at the federal, state, and local levels depending where the debate and action is.

HEALTH PROFESSIONS POLICY

In terms of health professions policy, nursing has a long history of policy initiatives that it both proposes and supports. The scope of nursing practice and the definition of nursing is one of the most critical policy issues affecting each individual nurse. The Nurse Practice Act (NPA) of each state controls nursing scope, requirements for credentialing and titling, and nurses' professional rights and responsibilities. Nurses have worked diligently for many years to bring their state's statutory definition and authority for practice up to modern day standards within the profession. Such policy initiatives have frequently been fraught with conflict, as both organized medicine and the hospital industry have inserted themselves as oppositional stakeholders to nursing's efforts to practice in modern, quality, and safe ways. After decades of serious and concerted policy/political effort, nurses now have the following: scopes of practice that include advanced practice nurses (APNs) in 49 states; independent practice in 26 states; mandatory title and scope protection in 49 states; and recognized autonomous functions in all states. Policy work to attain homogeneous initial credentials for professional nurses is the priority professional licensure issue of the next decade.

Just as nurses have long worked to shape professional definitional and licensure issues, nurses have also been very active in securing reimbursement for practice. Getting paid directly for one's clinical work has been a long term policy objective of the nursing community. Yet in payment plans such as Medicare, Medicaid, CHAMPUS, and Blue Cross/Blue Shield, direct nursing reimbursement resembles a patchwork, reflecting battles won and lost, rather than objective rational payment system policy. Nurses, especially APNs, want to be a part of all current payment systems for health service delivery such as fee for service, managed care panel fees, and staff model employee salaries. In the summer of 1997, APNs and nursing finally achieved direct Medicare reimbursement for nurse practitioner and clinical specialist services in all practice settings and geographical areas. This was a reimbursement victory that took nearly two decades of relentless political activity from nurses led by the American Nurses Association (ANA).

Monies for health professions education have long flowed from various governmental sources. For decades medical education has received billions of dollars annually to develop today's medical workforce with the predominant amount flowing through Graduate Medical Education (GME) funds for post medical school training. In 1996, GME funds directed to physician education totaled over $7 billion. Nursing has never received the same level of support for nursing education as medicine. Schools of nursing and nursing students have grown accustomed to some level of federal subsidy, which the nursing community has worked hard both to maintain and to grow. Nursing programs received $244 million through GME and $58.1 million from the Nursing Education Act (NEA) in 1996. A current grave concern of nursing organizations throughout the country is a 1997 proposal to cut the NEA as a part of an overall attempt to decrease federal spending and balance the federal budget in seven years. Nurses, as the primary stakeholders for the NEA, are urging all members of congress to protect the NEA and its appropriations level.

THE PATH TO POLITICAL ACTION

Nurses have strongly held beliefs and feelings about many of the contextual issues affecting nursing and health care as already mentioned herein (as well as countless others!). Yet no matter how strongly nurses care about an issue requiring policy intervention, we are left with the very real question of how to make an effective difference in its resolution. Certainly we know that our time, money, and energy will be required, but just how to focus, how to get started, and how to be successful remains a question.

PROFESSIONAL ORGANIZATION MEMBERSHIP

There are 2.5 million nurses in the United States. It is together that we can make our most significant impact on health policy. Nurses can best come together as professionals through membership in State Nurses Associations (SNAs) and the ANA. The ANA and the SNAs are the collective policy and political voice for all nurses, just as the National Student Nurses' Association is the voice for all nursing students. All professions have such a collective, and ANA is nursing's.

When the President or a member of Congress wants to know where nursing stands on a particular issue, nine times out of ten, the ANA is called upon to answer. At the state level, the same process occurs between the Governor, the Legislature, and the state nurses' association. Your voice with a policy idea, demand, or need is heard best when you are working toward an agenda in common with other nurses. Your policy effectiveness as an individual nurse begins with your SNA membership and is enhanced by your active participation with the ANA/SNA policy and political action committees.

The ANA/SNAs will be more effective as all nurses become members. They will bring manpower, fresh ideas, and sufficient resources to do the very necessary ongoing and future policy work for the profession. The ANA/SNAs provide solid expertise, an historical perspective, and a variety of in-place structures for nurses to engage in policy development and the political activity necessary to make policy happen.

To influence policy makers on matters of substance, the ANA/SNAs have set up one-on-one networking between nurses and elected officials. These nurse/official relationships are grown over time and usually are quite lasting. For example, every member of the United States Congress has an SNA nurse member from his or her state who serves as Congressional District Coordinator to communicate frequently, and in depth, with the Senator or Representative on a variety of issues important to nursing over time. To influence issues more narrowly but with great intensity, ANA developed in 1994 the Nurses Strategic Action Team (N-STAT) to serve as a grass-roots response vehicle. The SNA members of N-STAT have been able to turn out thousands of calls, letters, and faxes on a key policy initiative in less than 72 hours. N-STAT is a terrific example of nurses acting together making a visible difference in a policy outcome. While the CDC/SC Network and N-STAT focus on national and federal nursing concerns, some SNAs have used the CDC/SC and N-STAT models for their own state policy/political initiatives.

In addition to content driven influences, through the ANA and SNA political action committees (PACs), nurses also identify, endorse, support, and elect candidates who are health and nurse friendly. ANA/SNA endorsements are highly sought after by both federal and state candidates, and nurses have increasingly given generously of their time and dollars for campaigns of endorsed candidates through the nurse PACs. In 1994 and 1996, ANA PAC was the fourth largest federal health care PAC, distributing over $1,000,000 to federal candidates. SNA PACs follow a similar mode and have been very active and successful with state candidates.

AN HISTORIC MOMENT

A recent and an historic example of nurses, policy, and politics occurred between 1990 and 1994. During that time the profession of nursing, led by the ANA, engaged formally and significantly in the national debate on health care reform for the nation. In 1991, the ANA published nursing's in-depth, researched policy guide, Nursing's Agenda for Health Care Reform (see Appendix A) developed in collaboration with the National League for Nursing and the American Association of Colleges of Nursing, and receiving the endorsement of nearly all of organized nursing. The Agenda was nursing's simple, straight forward description of the health delivery problems of the nation in the areas of cost, quality and access, and the profession's equally simple but compelling policy recommendations for their solution. Through use of the ANA SC/CDC network, Nursing's Agenda was distributed to the 102nd Congress, and nurse members of the network participated in over 200 town meetings with fellow citizens and members of Congress in 1991 and 1992. The Agenda first and foremost focused nurses on their policy objectives for health care reform and was then used as a screening tool for political candidates in the 1992 elections.

Nursing's policy objective was clear—universal access to affordable health services of high quality delivered by a variety of health professionals, including registered nurses. Focused, dramatic political action was necessary in order to put policy makers in the Oval Office and in Congress who would then put health care reform on the front burner for action and whose policy ideals and values for health care matched nursing's. ANA PAC endorsed the Clinton/Gore ticket based upon these criteria as well as sustaining a 70 percent plus winners rate with members of Congress. Nursing then was included as friend (not foe) in the planning for what became the Health Security Act of 1993 (HSA). Nursing was also included in the complexity of congressional discussions from 1993 to 1994 as the HSA was debated. While the HSA was eventually withdrawn without passage, nursing as a policy and political force came out a big winner and continues as a real "player" in federal and state health policy and politics. Many of the elements of the HSA are still being debated and addressed in piece-meal fashion, and many of the nursing specific elements (such as direct Medicare reimbursement) have been enacted with strong bipartisan support. Having your policy and political "act together" pays off!!

NURSES' POLITICAL ROLES

Hopefully by now you are convinced that policy and politics are exciting, essential elements of nurses' lives. So, what roles are available to you? Which ones fit you now, and which will fit you in the future? Three roles for consideration are the nurse citizen, the nurse activist, and the nurse politician.

The nurse citizen role is a must for all nurses, and there is no excuse to not fulfill it. Nurses bring unique perspectives to their citizenship role, and the nation and the community are better for it. Nurses tend to vote for socially progressive candidates committed to better health care for all. A few examples of fulfilling the role of nurse citizen include: being a registered voter; voting in every election; knowing elected officials and candidates; and participating in public issue forums.

Nurse activists are nurse citizens with more of their energy focused on participating in policy or political concerns. Nurse activists are joiners and usually are members of their SNA, a political party, and one or more specialty organizations. They participate rather than just pay their dues. A few examples of fulfilling the role of nurse activist include: communicating with policy makers in order to influence health care/nursing policy; giving money to a PAC or a candidate; working in a political campaign; and providing leadership to other nurses in order to analyze or influence health legislation or regulation on behalf of ANA/SNA.

Nurse politicians are nurse activists who decide to move from influencer to decision maker, and we need more of them! We have only two nurses in Congress, but we are gaining numbers in state legislatures around the country. They all are making a real policy difference.

For example, our two nurse Congresswomen recently circulated among their colleagues a request for support for level funding for the Nursing Education Act—a federal appropriation of high priority at the ANA and throughout the nursing community. Being on the inside allows these nurse politicians to better articulate nursing's value and concerns while gaining support (and votes!) for our initiatives.

Nurses can fill the role of nurse politician through seeking an elected office; securing an appointed position; and becoming a key staff person to an elected official or health committee.

SUMMARY

Our nation needs better health care for all and a new paradigm for health care delivery.

Nurses have the ideas, commitment, and expertise to achieve these greatly needed goals. But, nurses must "live the necessity" of policy and political action in order to effect such change. At the national, state, or local levels, nurses need to come together; develop and push forward their policy plans; and then work within the variety of political roles just discussed to secure nursing's preferred future both for the profession and for health care. Nurse activists and nurse politicians are terrific in principle and too few in numbers. I hope YOU will change that—for the sake of nursing and the patients we serve!

CRITICAL THINKING QUESTIONS

1. How do policy and political activity differ?
2. How are policy and political activity interrelated?
3. What is a key health problem of concern to you? What health policy would you propose for its resolution?
4. What is your greatest nursing concern? What policy would you propose for its resolution?
5. How would you go about securing the adoption and implementation of your two policy proposals?
6. Are you a registered voter? Does your state hold, and have you attended a political party precinct caucus, or town hall meeting? What could you do to start a "get registered" and "get out the vote" campaign at your school?

ACTIVITIES

1. Attend the next meeting of your local District or State Nurses Association, an NSNA school chapter or state association meeting and find out the current health and policy concerns of your local colleagues.
2. Attend your State Nurses Association annual convention and go to the policy and political sessions. There is usually a discounted registration for nursing students.
3. Attend your SNA "Lobby Day" and offer to meet with your representative on a nursing issue.

4. Read your State Nurses Association and Board of Nursing newsletter/magazine.

5. Check out NursingWorld.org on the World Wide Web for the latest ANA policy and political materials.

6. Organize a voter registration campaign on your campus and in your community. Host a political debate for your campus between candidates, and ask them to talk about nursing and health care issues. Offer your assistance with the candidates you prefer. Encourage all candidates to talk to your State Nurses Association about health care/nursing issues.

ADDITIONAL SUGGESTED READINGS

Chitty, K. (ed.). (1997). *Professional Nursing: Concepts and Challenges* (2nd ed., chapters 3, 4, 13, 16, 21, 22). Philadelphia: WB Saunders Company.

Mason, D., Talbott, S., & Leavitt J. (eds.). (1998). *Policy and Politics for Nurses* (3rd ed.). Philadelphia: WB Saunders Company.

Trofino, J. (ed.). (1996, Spring). Politics, power, and practice. *Nursing Administration Quarterly: 20* (3).

The Stepping Stones of Mentoring and Networking

U N I T 4

In Unit Four, you will explore the interrelated stepping stones of mentoring and networking. Although separate concepts, they interact so frequently in our experiences as nurse leaders, we will address them together. Chapter 13 looks at the *student's perspective to mentoring and networking,* and includes some self-assessment and visioning exercises for you to complete as you make that important step towards acquiring a mentor. It also looks at how networking plays a valuable role in the process. Chapter 14 reviews the history and practice of *mentoring from a nurse leader's perspective.* Then in the next two chapters, you will look at the experiences, perspectives, and paths of three seasoned nurse leaders who have been mentored in their own careers, have mentored others, and experienced first hand the value of networking skills. Chapter 15 shares *one nurse's story of nursing as a launching pad for other options.* And in Chapter 16, two nurse leaders review a *variety of nurse's paths that have launched many important roles.*

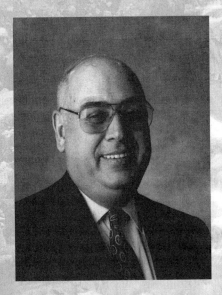

Dedicated to: Robert V. Piemonte,

RN, EdD, FAAN

Our first lesson in the student perspective to mentoring is that we should take opportunities to recognize the impact that mentors have made on our lives, and extend our gratitude.

Over the years, many NSNA Presidents, Boards of Directors, Committee members, Councils of State Presidents, and nursing student leaders on the school chapter, state association, and national level have all benefited from NSNA Executive Directors' and NSNA staff members' mentoring, creativity, encouragement, and vision. Too often we forget to thank these professionals—who are leaders themselves—for the difference they have made. Nursing leaders can often trace their growth to many such mentors over a lifetime.

For me, the majority of nurses that have had significant impact on my leadership development are contributing authors in this text. However, one mentor stands above the rest as a significant contributor to my leadership development and the leadership opportunities that I have been given. Dr. Robert V. Piemonte, served as Executive Director of the National Student Nurses' Association during my term as President. He retired in April, 1995, after over eleven years of exemplary service to the NSNA. Many nursing student leaders who experienced Dr. Piemonte's support, encouragement, and mentoring owe him a debt of gratitude. So on behalf of all of us, I take this opportunity for us to say Thank You. Both NSNA and nursing have benefited from your leadership and mentoring.

Chapter written by Carol A. Fetters Andersen, BSN, RN.

CHAPTER 13

Mentoring and Networking—The Student's Perspective

INTRODUCTION

A mentor can be defined as a wise and trusted counselor. In this dynamic era of reform in health care, the nursing leaders of tomorrow must learn from both the failures and successes of the past. The forces that are molding and shaping not only the profession of nursing, but the health and health care delivery system of our nation, are complex and ever changing. As a nursing student entering the profession, the best career move that you can make is to understand the mentor-protégé relationship. Then actively seek out an experienced professional to help you make the transition from nursing student to full-fledged registered nurse.

In this chapter, I challenge you to:

1. understand the student's perspective in the mentor-protégé relationship
2. begin to look within yourself to learn your current strengths and weaknesses
3. look at your networking potential
4. set goals for finding and acquiring a mentor to work with you as you begin your own career map

UNDERSTANDING THE MENTOR-PROTÉGÉ RELATIONSHIP

Perhaps the most critical piece to understanding the student's role in the mentor-protégé relationship is realizing that it is participatory. As with nursing education programs that have been accredited by the National League for Nursing (NLN) over the past few years, the student is expected to actively share in the responsibility of learning. The days of waiting as a vessel with outstretched arms to receive knowledge are being replaced by students sharing in the responsibility of teaching themselves. This is a big adjustment for students, especially older non-traditional students like I was. It is important that nursing students and faculty collaboratively work on curriculum committees to find the balance between 100 percent instructor taught and 100 percent student taught courses. For neither extreme will benefit the nursing leaders of tomorrow.

Transition to this education style will be critical for students who went through formal education that was almost entirely lecture-note taking instruction. This effective transition plan will help to decrease stress and help prevent burn-out and attrition. If you are a nursing student in this country, you understand how stressful nursing school is today! It's time for us to reduce that stress, whenever possible, so that the health we are promoting is also our own.

The good news for you as a student is that you don't have to take this learning journey alone. A mentor can help you develop the skills *you* need to succeed in nursing. However, remember that the process of learning is participatory. Your challenge is to maintain an autonomous position, building on your own strengths, while remaining open-minded enough to learn, consider suggestions, and accept some direction from an influential mentor whose care and patronage helps you to further your career in nursing. You will need to be assertive and trusting enough to share your own vision of the profession, and your strengths as well as your weaknesses.

ASSESSING YOUR STRENGTHS AND WEAKNESSES

Taking an inventory of your own strengths and weaknesses can be a challenging experience. To help you begin, I've made this chapter itself participatory. So keep a journal of your own as you discuss these topics in class or with a group of colleagues.

1. *What do you know about nursing's role in the health care delivery system in the United States? How does nursing fit into the bigger picture (past, present, future)?* List, discuss, and share with others your current knowledge.
   As a nursing student, what can you do to learn more about these issues? Where will you go to find out? Keep this list. Be committed to broadening your knowledge base regarding your profession. Begin to use the list!

2. *What do you know about nursing education, and nursing practice opportunities currently available in this country?* List, discuss, and share your current knowledge. This question will be valuable to look at again (in review) after you read this book. Where can you go to learn more?

   In past years, the National Student Nurses' Association at its fall Midyear Conference and National Convention in the spring has presented sessions called "Finding Your Niche in Nursing." Nursing leaders from various practice roles share with students about their careers in nursing. For more information call NSNA Headquarters, NY, NY, at (212) 581-2211.

   Also, you could put together your own program on various nursing roles to be held at your school. Often local nursing professionals are happy to come share with students about their careers free of charge.

3. *What leadership skills do you have?* Be courageous and share these with others. If you have a skill or strength, share why you believe it can be a benefit to nursing. Don't be shy—but be honest. This section also allows you to begin to learn what others in nursing view as strengths.

4. *What followership skills do you have?* List qualities you believe make you a good committee member, co-worker, and member of a group. Remember, the best leaders also know how to follow. Where can you get involved in group activities to practice and improve your followership skills? Your campus most likely has several committees for you to serve on. This is a good chance to develop an "Opportunities to be Involved" list to share with new students.

5. *Are you comfortable with public speaking?* As NSNA president, I spoke to groups as large as 10,000 people. But, I was not always comfortable doing that. First, I learned to speak about issues in small groups and in class. I studied the issues so that when I spoke I could do so articulately and knowledgeably. In larger groups, I forced myself to get up to the microphone at question time, introduce myself, and pose a well thought out (written out at first) question regarding the presentation as it related to the nursing profession as a whole. My fellow graduate students at the University of Iowa, College of Nursing, would laugh and say that's why I'm always looking for the "global perspective" on issues. I know this challenge to practice public speaking is not easy, but it is essential to nursing's future that you begin. The nursing leaders of tomorrow must be informed, articulate, and involved in the issues.

   Which groups you are involved with provide you opportunities to practice public speaking? Push yourself to keep interacting with larger and larger groups.

6. *When controversies occur are you part of the problem, or part of the solution?* Why do you feel so? The most effective nursing leaders that I have observed have developed the skill to help both sides of a controversy reach a solution that allows all parties involved to maintain their dignity. I call that finding a "win-win" solution. Nursing students and nursing leaders must remain com-

mitted to helping nursing's future leaders claim this skill as one of their strengths.

7. *What have you done beyond your basic nursing education to become an active part of the nursing profession?* List opportunities available to you as a nursing student. Often students are given very low registration rates at professional nursing programs. Remember, professional involvement does not replace the importance of nursing education and practice. Instead, it is the other half of your professional career. Become part of the big picture today. Both your education and practice will become more effective and alive for you.

8. *In two separate columns, list your strengths and your weaknesses.* Then take a minute to set three goals to help you work on your weaknesses for the next 30 days. Set a date to review your progress, reevaluate, and redesign as needed.

Now congratulate yourself! You've taken the first steps toward finding a mentor—you've gotten to know the protégé more.

LOOK AT YOUR NETWORKING POTENTIAL— A KEY TO ACQUIRING A MENTOR

You are entering a profession that is unique from others in one important way. The leaders of nursing are actively seeking to involve you in the issues, discussions, and solutions to our country's health care concerns. I will not tell you that all nurses who "eat their young" (so to speak) have disappeared. But, I can say that after meeting hundreds of nursing leaders professionally since graduation, through my role as NSNA President, and earlier as President of the Iowa Association of Nursing Students, I have never felt that my views were discounted in any way because I was a student. Instead, my thoughts were listened to respectfully and sought out on some occasions. Be assured that the current leaders in nursing are anxious to meet you.

In our society today, it's often said "it's not just what you know—but who you know." I don't believe that successful leaders can function with only one or the other exclusively. Decisions that affect our society should not be made in a vacuum or without knowledge of the whole issue. This is especially true of health care issues. As a future leader in nursing, you need both knowledge and collaborative connections. Networking focuses on developing who you know so that when you share what you have learned and experienced on an issue, you will be heard by someone who can make a difference. As a student, you can begin now to expand the networking potential that is available to you.

9. *List the influential leaders that you have met or could come in contact with.* Be sure to include all areas of nursing: education, practice, research, administrative, professional organizations, and other independent areas.

Now list other community leaders, political leaders (local, state, national), social leaders, and business leaders that you have met.

List friends and current nursing student leaders that you know.

Review these lists. What health care issues concern you the most? Who could you contact from your lists to let them know about your concerns? Volunteer to help them with efforts to learn about the issue and to seek solutions. Then when opportunities arise, people will know you are interested and consider you for involvement.

I would suggest that when you hear nursing leaders speak and are empowered by their message that you go up afterwards, introduce yourself, and ask for their business card. Then drop them a note to let them know how much you learned from their speech and enjoyed meeting them. It sounds like simple etiquette, however, in today's busy world the gesture is rarely done. It's always appreciated.

Nursing leaders are interested in student's leadership development and remember the students they meet much more often than you would expect. I'm reminded of when I met Dr. Lucille Joel, RN in Cedar Rapids, Iowa, at the joint convention between the Iowa Association of Nursing Students (IANS) and the Iowa Nurses Association (INA) in 1988. I was the IANS Membership Director then and went up and introduced myself to her. In the spring of 1991, in San Antonio, Texas, our paths crossed again as I was running for the office of NSNA President. I approached Dr. Joel again and said, "You probably don't remember that we've met. I'm Carol Fetters, a nursing student from Iowa." I was amazed when Dr. Joel said, "Yes, I do. We met a couple years ago in Cedar Rapids." That simple introduction in 1988 has lead to a professional colleague relationship, and her mentoring has been invaluable as I worked to move this book from my vision to reality. So, work on your networking potential. Don't underestimate the opportunities that you can have in the future when leaders know who you are, and know your leadership skills and interests. It often happens that while you are working on networking, you will meet your most significant mentors.

GOALS FOR FINDING AND ACQUIRING A MENTOR

Earlier in this chapter, you accomplished the first steps toward finding a mentor when you learned more about yourself. We talked about how the student perspective in the mentor-protégé relationship involves active participation. Your role balances autonomy with accepting the direction and critique of your mentor. I would like you to spend some time looking at your networking potential lists (Question 9), and your goals to improve your weaknesses (Question 8). Who on your networking potential list could best help you accomplish those goals?

If your first choice is unavailable, approach your second choice, and so on. You will have many mentors in your career. But this is an excellent place to begin.

SUMMARY

Finally, I ask you to join me in the commitment to mentor others as you have been mentored. Developing the protégé-mentor relationship will be worth your efforts. As nursing's future leaders, our strength will come when we embrace the concept that together in nursing we can accomplish even more than we've dreamed of alone.

CRITICAL THINKING QUESTIONS

1. Who has been the most significant mentor in your life (in general)? How has he or she helped you? Have you taken the opportunity to express your gratitude?

2. Why do you want to be a nurse? Define nursing here. How does your mentor or potential mentor define nursing?

3. Many national nursing organizations are opening up membership to nursing students. How did the autonomy/independence of nursing students voice come about? Should nursing students be members of NSNA first, before belonging to other professional associations? Compare and contrast collaboration and autonomy.

4. A new student has just entered your school's nursing program. You are interested in mentoring her or him. How would you do that?

5. How do you teach collaboration and conflict resolution? Who would be a good mentor to help you develop this skill?

6. Your mentor disagrees with your view or intended action on a nursing issue or decision. How would you handle this situation?

ACTIVITIES

1. Attend your State Nurses Association Convention and purchase a ticket to their award luncheon or dinner. Sit with a table of nurses that you don't know. Introduce yourself. Share that you are a nursing student interested in leadership development and that you would like to meet a nurse from the District Nurses Association where you live. Then follow-up with that person and attend a District Nurses meeting. Most of the time you can get a discount student ticket to state nursing functions, and often district meetings are free or have only a meal charge, if applicable.

2. Go back and answer the questions that you omitted in this chapter. Start discussing them with other nursing students, faculty, or nursing leaders. Your first steps in leadership development are up to you. *Carpe diem.*

REFERENCE

Microsoft Corporation [CD/ROM]. (1995). Microsoft Encarta '95 The Complete Interactive Multimedia Encyclopedia.

ADDITIONAL SUGGESTED READINGS

Brekke, M. E. (1993, July–August). Building on experiential learning in a leadership/management internship. *Nurse Educator, 18* (4), p. 5.

Klakovich, M. (1994, June). Connective leadership for the 21st century: A historical perspective and future directions. *Advances in Nursing Science, 16* (4), pp. 42–54.

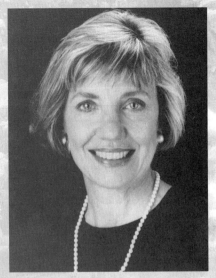

Connie Vance,

EdD, RN, FAAN

Dr. Connie Vance is Dean and Professor of Nursing at the College of New Rochelle School of Nursing in New York. Her research and writing have been in the areas of mentoring, leadership development, and the professionalization of nursing.

Dr. Vance has had many publications including one in *Image*, the publication of Sigma Theta Tau titled "Women Leaders: Modern-Day Heroines or Societal Deviants?" Besides writing, research, and education, Dr. Vance has a long history of leadership roles in professional nursing organizations. She is currently a member of the Board of Directors of the American Association of Colleges of Nursing and has served in many other roles, including: Chairperson of the Board of Trustees of the New York State Nurses Political Action Committee; member of the Board of Trustees of Our Lady of Mercy Medical Center, Bronx, NY; honorary member of the Association of Educators of Nursing and Pharmaceutical Schools and Colleges in Russia member of several committees of the Catholic Health Care Network in New York; and Congressional District Coordinator for the American Nurses Association.

Dr. Vance's commitment to mentorship and leadership development in nursing is evident in her many roles and is recognized and respected by the profession. She is a Distinguished Lecturer of Sigma Theta Tau International and enjoys mentoring nursing students. Her commitment to nursing leadership and education around the world is demonstrated by her service as a mentor to several Russian nursing leaders and professional associatons.

CHAPTER 14

Mentoring—The Nursing Leader and Mentor's Perspective

INTRODUCTION

In every career stage, from student to high-level leader, mentoring is an essential element of professional socialization. Indeed, the sustained involvement of various support persons, such as mentors, in the life and career path of every human being is a necessity. Anecdotal reports and research studies have demonstrated that support and guided assistance promote career commitment and a fully developed, satisfying career. Therefore, mentor relationships should not be an isolated phenomenon but should be integrated into one's daily professional life. Clearly, the complexity of a nursing career demands a substantial and consistent support system to ensure success and satisfaction in both personal and professional life.

The mentor connection is a developmental, empowering, and nurturing relationship extending over time in which mutual sharing, learning, and growth occur in an atmosphere of respect, collegiality, and affirmation (Vance & Olson, 1998). The mentor-protégé relationship can be viewed as a gift-exchange phenomenon (Gehrke, 1988), as it is characterized by mutual sharing and give-and-take. The reciprocity inherent in the relationship means that all who enter it, those who mentor and those being mentored, will receive the rewards of sharing and learning together. The mentor's gifts come from their life experiences, knowledge, and wisdom. The mentor guides, models, encourages, and inspires the protégé. The protégé receives the mentor's gifts and returns these gifts by her or his contributions to the profession and by eventually mentoring others. The traditional mentor relationship always occurred between an older, experienced professional and a younger neophyte in the discipline. Increasingly, however, peer-colleagues, friends, and family members are providing important mentoring functions, in addition to the classic mentor.

Nursing students are recognizing the value of mentor relationships. At the National Student Nurses' Association convention in 1996, the delegates passed a resolution in "support of the promotion, awareness, and development of mentorship programs" (NSNA, 1996). This resolution urged the establishment of mentor programs in schools and nursing organizations as well as dissemination about mentoring in publications. Through their collective action, student nurse leaders have communicated their desire for mentor support during their educational experience. Mentoring can promote students' progression and retention during the program of study, assist new graduates during their entry into professional practice, and encourage the leadership development of new professionals. Caring mentors can help with a broad range of professional and personal issues that confront the "new" nurse. These relationships contribute to the early success and satisfaction of being a young nurse and a potential leader. L. D. Beaulieu suggests that mentoring can bridge the gap between education and practice. It is a means to improve patient care by strengthening professional nursing practice (Beaulieu, 1988).

THE LEADER'S ROLE AS MENTOR

The empowerment and care of others are leadership tasks. The contemporary role of the leader is to develop others, to enable and empower people to grow. The "old" leadership paradigm was characterized by a bureaucratic, command-and-control, power-over-others style. Today, however, educational and clinical organizations need leaders who foster the development and empowerment of others through mentorship. Organizations exert considerable influence on people, either assisting or impeding the development of their potential. The "learning organization" described by P. Senge emphasizes support and sharing among all members, teacher and student, supervisor and subordinate, peer to peer (Senge, 1990). Today's leaders must establish climates in which people learn together—mentoring each other, so that each person and the organization realize their potential for growth and creativity.

Nursing leaders have both the obligation and privilege of serving as mentors. In his book, *The Paradox of Success,* O'Neil describes long-distance leaders or "success sustainers" who keep their pursuit of excellence in balance with their inner well-being. One of their characteristics is the seeking of opportunities to teach and serve as mentors (O'Neil, 1993). Nursing leaders are now challenging other nursing leaders to deliberately seek out students, new graduates, and novice nurses, facilitate their transition into the profession, and assist in their development (Joel, 1997; Schorr, 1978). Passing on wisdom to the next generation is inherent to being a good leader. This is the stage of "generativity" that Erikson speaks about, manifested by the human need to reach out to others to provide guidance and nurturance (Erikson, 1963). Inherent in generativity is the acceptance of responsibility for "passing the torch" to the next generation.

A key role of the mentor-leader is creating an environment that supports the development of both individual and collective mentor relationships. These relationships are particularly important during entry into the discipline and into specialty practice. A study of nurse managers reported that their most influential mentoring experiences occurred during the early years of their nursing careers. The most significant mentoring relationships occurred in superior-to-subordinate relations and colleague-to-colleague relationships (Boyle & James, 1990). It would appear that nursing leaders, therefore, have an important responsibility in shaping learning organizations in which nurturing relationships can easily occur among nurses at all levels. In particular, it is crucial that leaders link young nurses with mentors who will introduce them to the profession, serve as role models, and instill self-confidence.

In the learning organization, two types of mentor relationships are present: *informal* and *formal. Informal mentoring* consists of the traditional expert-to-novice relationship and peer-collegial relationship. This occurs when two people are drawn together through mutual attraction, shared interests and goals, a mutual desire to work with each other, and "chemistry." These relationships frequently develop in the educational and work settings and include the teacher-student, preceptor-student, superior-to-subordinate, or peer-to-peer relationships. *Formal or planned mentoring* is the organizational application of spontaneous informal mentoring. Many educational and clinical leaders understand that mentor relationships promote continuous learning, excellence in professional practice, and commitment to the organization and profession. These leaders are incorporating the concepts of mentoring into the value systems and relationships of schools and clinical settings. Formal mentor programs involve the matching of potential mentors and protégés with respect to commonalities of professional goals, specialty area, concerns, and needs. These formal programs require careful planning, orientation, training, support, and follow-up of the participants. Formalizing mentor programs gives mentoring heightened visibility, importance and durability, creates enhanced communication, motivation, and productivity (Duff & Cohen, 1993; Murray & Owen, 1991).

In the educational setting, a growing number of formal mentor programs for undergraduate nursing students are occurring (Olson & Vance, 1998). These programs report various benefits to students: improved communication, technical and organizational skills; enhanced academic performance; increased self-confidence and motivation; leadership development; and facilitation of the entry into professional practice (Alvarez & Abriam-Yago, 1993; Baldwin & Wold, 1993; Gonzalez, 1994; Wold, 1993). Through active mentoring, students gain self-assurance, experience reduced anxiety, and feel "cared about" as they progress toward their educational and professional goals. Mentors serve as important role models and help students gain insight into the realities of the nursing world.

In clinical settings, the mentoring of new graduates increases their self-confidence in skill performance, work satisfaction, professional commitment, and retention. System-wide mentor programs promote cultures where professional development, open communication, and conflict resolution can occur more easily. It is believed that quality patient care is delivered more consistently by nurses who have been mentored, as they tend to possess a career commitment and are satisfied with their work. Several research studies provide information about the many positive outcomes of mentor programs for the novice nurse (Butts & Wither, 1992; Carey & Campbell, 1994; Hamilton et al., 1989; Martin et al., 1995; Nayak, 1991).

THE MENTOR RELATIONSHIP

Since the mentor relationship is reciprocal, both mentor and protégé have the responsibility for initiating the relationship and maintaining it. The leader is frequently instrumental in the selection process. The leader must possess an attitude of openness and willingness to serve as a mentor. This entails being on the lookout for promising persons who could benefit from the experience, knowledge, and connections of a mentor. Likewise, the protégé must possess an attitude of willingness to receive help. This involves being on the lookout for experienced persons who could provide guidance and support. In addition, opportunities should be sought for networking and interacting with leaders. The protégé must present herself or himself as someone worthy of the mentor's time and investment (Vance, 1990). Practically speaking, this means being serious, passionate, and dedicated to one's career and ongoing growth and development. Maintaining the mentor relationship requires the same nurturing and care as any other human relationship. There must be mutual trust and regard and a commitment to each other. Some degree of "chemistry" is helpful, but respect is as essential as liking the person. Regular communication is necessary in strengthening the relationship.

One myth about mentoring says that anyone who wants a mentor can find one. This is not always the case; mentors still remain in short supply for many people. For the most part, senior people need to make mentoring happen. "It is not bad people or abusive people who derail or ruin careers. It is the indifference of people who become so involved in their own work that they forget the junior people" (Hoffman, 1995, p. 43). The first investigation of mentoring activity among national nursing leaders demonstrated that they did indeed have mentors and that they were actively mentoring others (Vance, 1977, 1982). This finding has been consistent in many nursing studies (Vance & Olson, 1991; Olson & Vance, 1993). Anecdotally, however, there are mixed reports of mentoring involvement from clinical and academic leaders, particularly for nursing students and young nurses. Factors that contribute to the lack of widespread mentoring include leaders who don't mentor ("queen-beeism"); the presence of oppressed group behavior; work environments that isolate and alienate; and the absence of mentor programs in academic and clinical settings. The types of help that leaders can provide to their protégés is best summarized in three categories: *guidance, role modeling,* and *advocacy.*

Guidance

The mentor-guide is a teacher and counselor who provides expert advice and guidance about the career and profession. The guide shows the way, pointing to opportunities and pitfalls. The mentor provides information that may prevent mistakes along the career path. Coaching occurs through dialogue and clarifying career options and educational routes.

Role Modeling

The mentor-model provides an exemplar of professional commitment and serves as an inspiration to the neophyte. Future possibilities are articulated and modeled for the protégé. Knowledge and wisdom are shared that gives the protégé a larger world view.

Advocacy

Protégés are empowered by the mentors' belief in them and the high expectations set by the mentor-advocate. The protégés' gifts and dreams are championed and supported. The mentor motivates and opens doors for the neophyte. Through the networks and sponsorship of the mentor, opportunities and new learning experiences are created for the protégé.

A leader-mentor speaks about her role: "My entire professional career has been involved with mentoring. I see my protégés as family, like nieces and nephews. I hold them in high expectation with deep affection. It is my hope that when they get older they will become mentors to others. I enjoy the mentor role and feel that as nurses we need to mentor our students. We can all learn from each other" (Thomas, 1998).

BENEFITS OF THE MENTOR RELATIONSHIP

The two major developmental outcomes of mentor relations are professional and personal success and satisfaction. These benefits accrue to mentors and protégés, to the workplace, and the profession. Studies, anecdotal accounts, and self-reports suggest the following benefits of the mentor connection (Vance, 1982):

- promotion of career success and advancement
- increased work satisfaction
- enhancement of self-esteem and self-confidence
- preparation for leadership roles and succession
- strengthening of the profession

Mentoring is particularly important during the transition from student to new professional. Mentor relationships make a significant difference in career development. Students achieve easier and faster with the support of active, involved mentors. An investigation of staff nurses reported that 95 percent of their mentors were both manager-leaders and peers. These nurses perceived mentoring to be a large factor in their successful career development, particularly in the early career stage (Angelini, 1995). In another study of staff nurses, there was a significant difference between the professionalism scores of mentored and non-mentored nurses, with mentored nurses achieving higher scores (Just, 1989). A study of beginning nurses' diagnostic reasoning behaviors showed a high level of beginner uncertainty and problems with independent diagnostic reasoning. The need for carefully planned mentoring of the novice nurse was demonstrated (Haffer, 1990).

Mentors believe that their own clinical and teaching skills are refined and that their professional and personal learning is stimulated through their mentoring of students and beginning nurses (Atkins & Williams, 1995). Mentoring is an investment in the future. By influencing new people in the discipline, mentors leave a legacy. Through their protégés, their voice and values are extended into the future. It is clear that those who are mentored will mentor others. Nurses who are mentored internalize that mentoring experience as an important dimension of their own professional practice and leadership style. They carry forward the traditions and values of the profession through the extension of their mentor connections.

A nursing leader believes that the gifts they give to protégés contain these benefits: their knowing that I cared about them as individuals; wanting them to succeed in their nursing program; assisting them in establishing their nursing career; and sharing professional insights that could further their development (Opitz, 1997). The reciprocal and dynamic nature of the mentor connection among mentors and protégés is illustrated through analysis of interviews of the participants in a school of nursing mentor program consisting of over 65 mentor-protégé dyads. The themes of these interviews suggest the following benefits of the mentor connection to both leader-mentor and student-protégé: teaching and learning, guidance and support, and reflection and insight. "The protégé brings an openness that is not empty but full of life experiences, curiosities, naiveté, hunger, ideas, questions, insecurities, and enthusiasm, as well as a wish to seek the wisdom of someone who has been there" (Bamford, Hullstrung, & Niedzwiecki, 1997, p. 137). Faculty, advisers, and other mentors struggle with these issues along with students. They know that resolution of them is beyond the traditional modes of teaching and socialization. Mentor connections can be a motivating framework for the reciprocal growth of both mentors and protégés.

MENTORING FOR THE FUTURE

Leader-mentors will increasingly view themselves as learning partners rather than patriarchs (Kaye & Jacobson, 1995). They will join with students and novice nurses as partners in mentoring. This collaboration will require mentor relationships in every stage of professional life. This means that leader-mentors must seek opportunities to mentor neophytes, involving themselves as collaborative partners in learning. Mentoring means that caring involvement is kept as a core value in our work, not only with clients but with each other. In relationship, leaders help students and new nurses tap into their unique strengths. Through reciprocal involvement, both mentors and protégés are empowered in their personal and professional lives.

In order to be successful as mentors and protégés, various qualities are required. A good leader-mentor should be: (1) generous of their time and energy—mentoring is going above and beyond the usual commitment; (2) self-confident—mentors cannot be oppressed and self-absorbed; (3) a wise expert—competency and experience provide security in sharing one's knowledge; and (4) open to mutual growth—mentors must be respectful of their own and others' need for lifelong learning and development. Likewise, a good student-protégé should be: (1) open to learning and receiving help—asking for advice and guidance is essential; (2) possess a career commitment—the protégé must be serious and motivated; (3) a self-starter—it is important to take the initiative in making oneself known to potential mentors; and (4) respectful of self—the protégé should identify with and model the mentor while still maintaining her or his own unique identity. These qualities will promote a healthy mentor relationship characterized by mutual respect and admiration. Full reciprocity can occur in these relationships. Mentors and protégés should expect to ask and receive help many times over the course of their careers. There are appropriately different mentors for different reasons; a variety of both expert and peer mentors is very beneficial.

An encouraging phenomenon is that fine mentoring seems to beget fine mentoring (Hardcastle, 1988). These mentor connections strengthen nursing's role and contributions and assure leadership succession. Since a major issue facing all organizations and professions is preparation for assumption of leadership, current leaders, through mentoring, ensure this succession (Holloran, 1993). Many schools and clinical organizations are incorporating mentoring into their everyday value systems and working relationships. It is understood that mentoring and learning are interconnected. In these learning organizations, mentors and protégés together expand their capacity to grow, learn, and create.

SUMMARY

Nursing's collective power and future success depends to a large extent on the mentoring relationships among leaders and the developing persons in our profession—students and novice nurses—our protégés. Mentors and protégés give gifts to each other, which are in turn passed on to future generations of mentors and protégés. Mentoring is an investment in the future. It entails a belief in the potential and promise of each nurse and the profession. Building mentor connections creates bridges to nursing's future.

CRITICAL THINKING QUESTIONS

1. What are the characteristics of the two types of mentoring: (1) informal, (2) formal or planned?

2. What are the unique benefits of the mentor relationship?

3. Are there potential problems in the mentor relationship? If so, what are these? What are the responsibilities of the mentor and the protégé?

4. What factors contribute to the lack of widespread mentor relationships? Describe how these factors contribute.

5. How does a mentor select a protégé? How does a protégé find a mentor?

ACTIVITIES

1. Talk to three nurse leaders and explore with them their experiences as a mentor.

2. Talk to three nursing student leaders and explore who their mentors are or have been. Explore with them their experiences as a protégé.

3. Make a commitment to nursing's future. As you have been mentored, begin to mentor others.

REFERENCES

Alvarez, A., & Abriam-Yago, K. (1993). Mentoring undergraduate ethnic-minority students: A strategy for retention. *Journal of Nursing Education, 32* (5), 230–232.

Angelini, D. J. (1995). Mentoring in the career development of hospital staff nurses: Models and strategies. *Journal of Professional Nursing, 11* (2), 89–97.

Atkins, S., & Williams, A. (1995). Registered nurses' experiences of mentoring undergraduate nursing students. *Journal of Advanced Nursing, 21,* 1006–1015.

Baldwin, D., & Wold, J. (1993). Students from disadvantaged backgrounds: Satisfaction with a mentor-protégé relationship. *Journal of Nursing Education, 32* (5), 225–226.

Bamford, P., Hullstrung, R., & Niedzwiecki, E. (1997). Developing caring connections: Nursing students, alumni, faculty. In International Mentoring Association, *Diversity in mentoring* (pp. 134–140). Kalamazoo, MI: Western Michigan University.

Beaulieu, L. P. (1988). Preceptorship and mentorship: Bridging the gap between nursing education and nursing practice. *Imprint, 35* (2), 111, 113, 115.

Boyle, C., & James, S. K. (1990). Nursing leaders as mentors: How are we doing? *Nursing Administration Quarterly, 15* (1), 44–48.

Butts, B. J., & Wither, D. M. (1992). New graduates: What does my manager expect? *Nursing Management, 23* (8), 46–48.

Carey, S. J., & Campbell, S. T. (1994). Preceptor, mentor, and sponsor roles: Creative strategies for nurse retention. *Journal of Nursing Administration, 24* (12), 39–48.

Duff, C. S., & Cohen, B. (1993). *When Women Work Together: Using Our Strengths to Overcome Our Challenges.* Berkeley, CA: Conari Press.

Erikson, E. (1963). *Childhood and Society* (3rd ed.). New York: Norton.

Gehrke, N. (1988). Toward a definition of mentoring. *Theory into Practice, 27* (3), 190–194.

Gonzalez, L. (1994). Faculty mentors for minority undergraduate students. *Journal of Cultural Diversity, 1* (4), 90–94.

Haffer, A. G. (1990). Beginning nurses' diagnostic reasoning behaviors derived from observation and verbal protocol analysis (Doctoral dissertation, University of San Francisco, 1990). *Dissertation Abstracts International, 52,* 160B.

Hamilton, E. M., Murray, M. K., Linkholm, L. H., & Myers, R. E. (1989). Effects of mentoring on job satisfaction, leadership behaviors, and job retention of new graduate nurses. *Journal of Nursing Staff Development, 5* (4), 159–165.

Hardcastle, B. (1988). Spiritual connections: Protégés' reflections on significant mentorships. *Theory Into Practice, 27* (3), 2–208.

Hoffman, B. C. (1995). Mentoring of women and minority faculty and students. In E. Rubin (Ed.), Building the workforce for a diverse society. *Proceedings of the 3rd Congress of Health Profession Educators* (pp. 41–47). Washington, DC: Association of Academic Health Centers.

Holloran, S. D. (1993). Mentoring: The experience of nursing service executives. *Journal of Nursing Administration, 23* (2), 49–54.

Joel, L. A. (1997). Charged to mentor. *American Journal of Nursing, 97* (2), 7.

Just, G. (1989). Mentors and self-reports of professionalism in hospital staff nurses. (Doctoral dissertation, New York University, 1989). *Dissertation Abstracts International, 51,* 664B.

Kaye, B., & Jacobson, B. (1995). Mentoring: A group guide. *Training & Development,* 23–27.

Martin, M. L., Tolleson, J., Lakey, K. I., & Moeller, E. (1995). VALOR students: A creative type of preceptorship. *Federal Practitioner, 12* (4), 47–50.

Murray, M., & Owen, M. (1991). *Beyond the myths and magic of mentoring.* San Francisco, CA: Jossey-Bass.

National Student Nurses' Association. (1996). *Resolution: In Support of the Promotion, Awareness, and Development of Mentorship Programs.* New Orleans, LA: National Student Nurses' Association, House of Delegates.

Nayak, S. (1991). Strategies to support the new nurse in practice. *Journal of Nursing Staff Development, 7* (3), 64–66.

Olson, R. K., & Vance, C. (1998). Mentorship in nursing education. In K. A. Stevens (Ed.), *Review of Research in Nursing Education, 8,* New York: National League for Nursing.

Olson, R. K., & Vance, C. (1993). *Mentorship in Nursing.* Houston, TX: University of Texas Printing Services.

O'Neil, J. R. (1993). *The Paradox of Success: A Book of Renewal for Leaders.* New York: G. P. Putnam's Sons.

Opitz, M. (1997). *Mentoring Mementos.* Unpublished manuscript.

Schorr, T. (1978). The lost art of mentorship. *American Journal of Nursing, 78,* 1873.

Senge, P. M. (1990). *The Fifth Discipline: The Art and Practice of the Learning Organization.* New York: Currency Doubleday.

Thomas, V. (1998). My role as mentor. In C. Vance & R. K. Olson, *The Mentor Connection in Nursing.* New York: Springer Publishing Company.

Vance, C. (1990). Is there a mentor in your career future? *Imprint, 36* (5), 41–42.

Vance, C. (1982). The mentor connection. *Journal of Nursing Administration, 12,* (4) 7–13.

Vance, C. (1977). A group profile of contemporary influentials in American nursing. *Dissertation Abstracts International, 38,* 4734-B.

Vance, C., & Olson, R. K. (1991). Mentorship. In J. J. Fitzpatrick, R. L. Taunton, & A. K. Jacox (Eds.), *Annual Review of Nursing Research, 9* (pp. 175–200). New York: Springer Publishing Company.

Vance, C., & Olson, R. (1998). *The Mentor Connection in Nursing.* New York: Springer Publishing Company.

Wold, J. (1993). *The Effectiveness of a Mentor Program on Student Satisfaction and Retention in a Baccalaureate Nursing Program.* Unpublished doctoral dissertation, Georgia State University, Atlanta.

ADDITIONAL SUGGESTED READINGS

Benner, P. (1984). *From Novice to Expert: Excellence and Power in Clinical Nursing Practice.* Menlo Park, CA: Addison-Wesley.

Cahill, M. F., & Kelly, J. J. (1989). A mentor program for nursing majors. *Journal of Nursing Education, 28* (1), 40–44.

DeMarco, R. (1993). Mentorship: A feminist critique of current research. *Journal of Advanced Nursing, 18,* 1242–1250.

Huang, C. A., & Lynch, J. (1995). *Mentoring: The Tao of Giving and Receiving Wisdom.* New York: Harper San Francisco.

Jeruchim, J., & Shapiro, P. (1992). *Women, Mentors, and Success.* New York: Fawcett Columbine.

Johnsrud, L. K. (1991). Mentoring between academic women: The capacity for interdependence. *Initiatives, 54* (3), 7–17.

Jowers, L. T., & Herr, K. (1990). A review of literature on mentor-protégé relationships. In G. M. Clayton, & P. A. Baj (Eds.), *Review of Research in Nursing Education* (Vol. 2, pp. 49–77). New York: National League for Nursing.

Larson, B. A. (1986). Job satisfaction of nursing leaders with mentor relationships. *Nursing Administration Quarterly, 11* (1), 53–60.

Nelson, L. (1995). Mentoring toward a longed for life. In P. Munhall, & V. Fitzsimmon (Eds.), *The Emergence of Women into the 21st Century* (pp. 361–375). New York: National League for Nursing.

Orth, C., Wilkinson, H., & Benfari, R. (1990). The manager's role as coach and mentor. *Journal of Nursing Administration, 29* (9), 11–15.

Pilette, P. C. (1980). Mentoring: An encounter of the leadership kind. *Nursing Leadership, 3* (2), 22–26.

Policinski, H., & Davidhizar, R. (1985, May–June). Mentoring the novice. *Nurse Educator, 3,* 3.

Prestholdt, C. (1990). Modern mentoring: Strategies for developing contemporary nursing leadership. *Nursing Administration Quarterly, 15* (1), 14–28.

Pyles, S. H., & Stern, P. (1983). Discovery of nursing gestalt in critical care nursing: The importance of the gray gorilla syndrome. *Image: Journal of Nursing Scholarship, 15* (2), 51–57.

Ramsey, D. R., Thompson, J. C., & Brathwaite, H. (1994). Mentoring: A professional commitment. *Journal of the National Black Nurses' Association, 7* (1), 68–76.

Rogers, J. L. (1988). New paradigm leadership: Integrating the female ethos. *Initiatives, 51* (4), 1–8.

Strachura, L. M., & Hoff, J. (1990). Toward achievement of mentoring for nurses. *Nursing Administration Quarterly, 15* (1), 56–62.

Taylor, L. J. (1992). A survey of mentor relationships in academe. *Journal of Professional Nursing, 8* (1), 48–55.

Vance, C. (1995). The teacher as mentor. *International Nurse, News and Views, 8* (2), 6.

Vance, C. (1979). Women leaders: Modern day heroines or societal deviants? *Journal of Nursing Scholarship, 11* (2), 37–41.

Vance, C., & Olson, R. (1997). A new paradigm for mentorship. In International Mentoring Association, *Diversity in Mentoring* (pp. 249–259). Kalamazoo, MI: Western Michigan University.

Yoder, L. H. (1990). Mentoring: A concept analysis. *Nursing Administration Quarterly, 15* (1), 9–19.

Yoder, L. H. (1995). Staff nurses' career development relationships and self-reports of professionalism, job satisfaction, and intent to stay. *Nursing Research, 44* (5), 290–297.

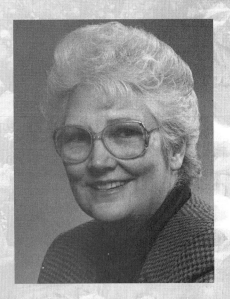

Mary Mallison,

BSN, RN

Mary Mallison was born and grew up in rural Iowa. She graduated from Iowa Methodist Hospital School of Nursing in Des Moines, and received her BSN with honors from the University of Iowa (U of I) in Iowa City. At the U of I, she was elected to the Gamma chapter of Sigma Theta Tau.

Mary's extensive nursing experience has included work in obstetrics, family psychiatry, community health, and in acute medical surgical nursing. Most of her career, however, has been spent in nursing journalism. Mary joined the *American Journal of Nursing* in New York City as a young assistant—associate editor beginning at the age of 28. Later, during her 12-year tenure as Editor, she piloted *AJN's* redesign and refocus of content. During those years, *AJN* was a finalist four times for the National Magazine Award for general excellence. (The American Society of Magazine Editors gives this award, considered the Oscar or Emmy of the magazine industry.) Mary's editorials also won media awards from ANA's Academy of Nursing, from Sigma Theta Tau, and from the New York Business Press Editors. Mary is perhaps best known for her attempts to teach nurses how to tell their own "hero stories"—celebrate heroic acts of creative caring.

From 1994–1996, Mary was Executive Director of the Georgia Nurses Association in Atlanta. You may reach her by e-mail: mmallison@aol.com.

CHAPTER 15

Nursing as a Launching Pad for Other Options— One Nurse's Story

INTRODUCTION

OK, I admit it. I'm a listener and a learner who's most at ease when invisible, intensely attending to the lives of others. So what have I gotten myself into, agreeing to talk about my own life instead of someone else's?

I agreed only because the intended reader is you, a nursing student, and because nurse colleagues and friends have been there for me when I was in need. The question I've been asked to answer is "How did you get where you got in your career?"

My story demonstrates that nursing is a lifelong profession that nourishes the ongoing process of one's self-development. Suprisingly diverse leadership positions available to nurses are outgrowths of nursing concerns. Those leadership roles are extensions of one's career as a nurse—not an abandonment of nursing. My career was shaped by a drive to find, develop, and use the talents I'd been given. Such a quest is both joyful and painful. It is never free of risk.

MY STORY BEGINS

Like many who've later become nurses, I was first impressed by nurses because of my experience of being seriously ill as a child. As a six-year-old, I was astonished by the nuns in the rural Iowa hospital where I lay recovering from pneumonia. They made a pallet on the floor so my mother could sleep in the room (long before parent-friendly visiting policies). They put up my hair in exotic French braids so it stayed off my hot face. Most of all, they moved with a quiet kindness, confidence, and surety that I could later call professionalism. I was permanently awestruck. They had once been little girls like me. Could I become someone like them?

Unlike many who claim they'd always wanted to be nurses, however, I claim no such thing. I loved reading most of all (still do) and fortunately had a mother who actively nurtured it. Even before I could read words, I struggled to decipher the political cartoons on the front page of the *Des Moines Register*. In that pre-TV era, I believe they ignited my interest in the uses of visual communication.

My first attempt at writing arose (as writing often does) from frustration. Bored with playing cowboy with my younger brother and his friends, I wrote a fairy tale princess story, with starring parts for the neighbor girls. (Even then, it seems, I preferred writing and directing to performing.) My brother's cooperation was assured by our father's alarmed discovery that our cowboy game included a saloon we'd constructed of boards at the top of a corncrib. We were banned from playing any more bar scenes copied from movies, even though we'd never considered tossing down shots of anything but Kool-Aid.

High school teachers encouraged my writing, and I was editor of the yearbook. Superintendent Swanson asked if he could place my school newspaper essay on the shrinking schoolyard in the town paper, since it might help pass a bond issue for a new school. When the bond issue was voted in, he credited my essay. Years later, of course, I realized he was probably just being a generous teacher.

So why didn't I major in journalism? Or English? It never occurred to me that one could earn a living in journalism (it's always been difficult) and attempting to teach Shakespeare to high schoolers seemed a fate worse than death. Moreover, I had learned a caregiver role: My father, a farmer, had lost an arm in a cornpicker accident, then developed laryngeal cancer and was saved with a permanent but messy trach; my mother retreated into what was probably paranoid depression. Nursing offered the hope of learning how to cope with these horrifying illnesses. It was also the most affordable and practical choice.

My teachers were disappointed. The home ec teacher was the most outspoken: "Nursing is just glorified first aid!" I wanted to ask her what home economics was but didn't want to cast aspersions on her career.

MY NURSING EDUCATION

A scholarship from the Iowa Cancer Society, plus the determination of my Methodist minister, enabled me to jump from a town of 600 where I was the class valedictorian, nicknamed "The Brain," to Iowa Methodist School of Nursing in Des Moines where I was one of scores of talented valedictorians in a nursing class of nearly 100. Up through the 1950s and 1960s at least, diploma schools like Iowa Methodist were able to choose from the top five or ten percent of high school graduate women. I breathed in the equality and camaraderie, free of competition: We were not pitted against one another but instead against an ideal. Our highest clinical praise was "Shows the capacity to become a good (operating room, obstetric, pediatric, you-name-it) nurse." It was (rightly) assumed that almost everyone who survived the three years would pass Boards.

The predictability and structure was also a welcome relief, at first, then (predictably) gave me something I could rebel against. At first I wrote parodies of nursing procedures and made fun of pretentious terms like "pediculosis" for lice.

Then my rebellion flowered in religious zeal. Though I couldn't have explained it this way at the time, I'd found the ideal target: Challenging a school founded by a church to be unafraid of dormitory Bible studies and religious conversions. The director of the school was definitely displeased. Her unspoken concern seemed to be: What if we should suddenly lose all common sense and turn bedbaths into baptisms? Of course we hadn't and we didn't. Thus I learned by age 21 that administrators get fierce when money (offending patients and losing admissions) is even peripherally at stake.

The "we" included my roommate Marilyn Bower, who went on to a career as a missionary in Crete. Upon graduation from Iowa Methodist, we had both applied to the University of Iowa's BSN completion program. Despite equally high grades, I got a "come now" letter and she got a "not yet" letter. Seeing this clearly as God's will, Marilyn went on to the University of Nebraska and the Navigators where she met her husband and her future.

I was thrilled for my dear friend but puzzled about my own future. Like most late teens-early twenties people I was awash in hormones, but unlike most, I avoided—even ran from—marriage. I had seen my three elder stepbrothers choose early marriage instead of higher education. And I had my mother's and grandmother's injunctions ringing in my brain: "Wait to marry! Marriage is a trap!" From childhood I'd wondered: What is the purpose of getting married to have children who then get married to have children? Who will contribute to the world beyond the family circle? Please remember that in those days women—at least, the women I knew—who had children stopped working outside the home.

I had also determined not to return home to fulfill what I later realized was the script the rest of the family had written: As the only daughter, I was to remain our parents' main caregiver. A nursing education would have been fine as long as I used it to return home. But I was certain I had to flee from my mother's desperate, clinging dependence. When I did, I became an unpredictable oddity.

I delighted in the broad sweep and scope of the liberal arts as taught at the University of Iowa. I've never quite understood nurses who say, "How will I ever use (this or that college course) in my work?" I've used every scrap, every ounce of my education and experience in one way or another in my work as a nurse. Readings from the Holocaust helped me relate to elderly European refugees who'd lived through it. Community sociology taught me to look at communities and organizations in new ways. They underpinned my lifelong interest in how to get things done. A class in modern American drama helped me understand the beginnings of the union movement, and also provided a colorful taste of the times during which my older patients grew up. Of course I scooped up an abnormal psychology course like a kid eating ice cream.

The nursing courses themselves also opened new doors because the faculty encouraged investigation into what Faye Abdellah called nursing problems. A faculty member pointed me toward Melzak's beginning studies of pain; another encouraged my interest in community/home care nursing.

A painful love affair led to my own private library investigation into the characteristics of the feminine ideal in history—some early feminism before I knew such explorations were going on elsewhere. College did for me what it purports to do: I learned how to learn. I glimpsed the riches behind doors that I could enter and explore if I chose. The knowledge that doors exist, even if one doesn't know their names, seems to me the overarching benefit.

Evenings and nights in obstetrics and a semester as a dorm nurse easily paid my way through school. The security of being able to earn a living as a nurse was an incredible relief. The question, though, of what I was intended to accomplish with my life hung permanently over me. You can see that I felt I needed to justify my desire to escape from my family's dutiful daughter script. So, partway through college, when I met a psychiatrist in private practice who was seeking to break new ground in what would now be called family therapy and behavior modification, I jumped at the chance to work with him.

MY FIRST MENTOR

We bonded like Superglue, and he became my first mentor. Psychiatry had been my first choice for a nursing career, but I saw as a nursing student that the graduate nurses in the state hospital supervised techs and gave meds; it appeared to me that their direct therapeutic activity with patients was small. Now I had a chance to work one-on-one with patients, families, and an intense, brilliant therapist. We worked together off and on for nearly five years. During that time I marshalled my family and committed my mother to a state hospital (having learned how to go about it); completed my BSN; and helped the psychiatrist get published. By then the Superglue had badly loosened. Professionally, we worked together seamlessly, but personally we were inimical. In *Passages,* Gail Sheehy describes how career women outgrow their first mentors, usually men, and the profile fit.

A MOVE TO NEW YORK
AND COMMUNITY HEALTH

So I arranged a job as a visiting nurse in New York City, fastening my idealism to the life of Lillian Wald. Once in New York, I pored over the public library's collection of Lillian Wald's handwritten letters. I was awed by her amazing clearsightedness and persistence in obtaining resources for the poor immigrants of New York's lower east side. Later that year, I contrasted my experiences with hers in writing. It never occurred to me to show the results to anyone.

I loved caring for patients at home and was well-equipped to do it. I marveled at their diverse backgrounds, cultures, and language excesses, compared to the (external) homogeneity and taciturnity of Midwesterners. To some of these New Yorkers, I was the corn-fed kid from—Ireland? Idaho? Perhaps because of that appearance, I was assigned the regular beat of the rich and famous: Park Avenue and Sutton Place. So I divided up my hours and spent them with people who needed attention more than they needed simple injections of Vitamin B_{12}. That got me in trouble with a supervisor who'd gotten stuck in her wartime military belief that nurses should be faceless interchangeable parts. She thought I must be doing something wrong since the patients called to request me by name. After I attempted to explain, I'd be sent off many mornings with "There she goes, off to give psychological care." The tone sounded gruffly good-humored, but it felt more like a form of hazing, an attempt to extrude an unwanted growth. I didn't feel I could talk over the situation with the next level of administration, since that person was my supervisor's best friend.

My reality shock set in further as I learned the reimbursement rules. Only three visits to a multiple-problem family? "Did you refer to the appropriate agencies?" Yes, of course. But was that any substitute for the caring involvement Lillian Wald would have offered?

As I've looked back on these early years in nursing, I've seen so many ways I might have communicated better and sought common ground with peers. I'm a strong believer in the local nurses association in part because that's where one can put outriggers on one's canoe to keep it from tipping over. The "outriggers" are nurses outside one's own unit and place of employment who can offer safe commiseration and suggestions. But until I was in my mid-thirties, I didn't access the local association's strengths; I kept my idealistic anguish to myself. I hope you, reading this, will be different.

With hindsight it would have made sense to return to school, but in the 1960s even a BSN was sometimes a barrier to bedside nursing, which I wanted to continue. I believed then (as now) that the greatest art takes place in the nurse-patient relationship, and in those days, I felt that a master's degree would have separated me from the learning I wanted most.

So in the depths of what Marlene Kramer later called reality shock, I resigned as a visiting nurse and immediately succumbed to measles meningitis. I recovered slowly at the home of a kind nurse friend. In catching up on reading and writing, I realized that I really wanted to combine my nursing with writing. That meant working for the *American Journal of Nursing*.

It didn't happen right away, of course; as I regained my strength, I worked as a private duty nurse at a major teaching hospital in New York. At a friend's suggestion, I attempted to continue learning about patient care by writing a three-column evaluation of the care given the previous shift, the care I gave, and the care I *might* have given had I thought of it soon enough. This self-audit led to some memorable encounters with patients, families, and other nurses (since some of the nurses gave better care than I did, and I admired their work). It also reinforced a long-term interest in the appropriate uses of touch in patient care.

MY FIRST ROLE WITH THE *AMERICAN JOURNAL OF NURSING (AJN)*

To my amazement and delight, *AJN* hired me as an assistant editor at the ripe old age of 28. All those years of reading and asking questions, plus a proofreader's eye and a habit of writing, and a genuine admiration of other nurses' accomplishments meant that I'd finally found my niche. I found my second mentor, too: Thelma Schorr, RN, who was then senior editor.

Each editor was assigned certain areas of practice. Mine was the emerging area of med-surg that would soon be called critical care. Chief editor Barbara Schutt, RN, was convinced that *AJN* articles should be written by nurses, not physicians. So it was my (often unsuccessful) job to find these nurses and persuade them to write. The nurses, in turn, were busy opening coronary care units and frantically hurrying to teach other nurses how to read ECGs. I traveled to Los Angeles County's CCU to put into print its nurses' revolutionary new responsibility: Following a protocol, not waiting for an MD's agreement, to give lidocaine based on the nurse's interpretation of the arrhythmia. That was almost exactly 30 years ago.

I asked various trailblazers what sort of education and experience they thought nurses in these new units should have. Too often, they described backgrounds exactly like their own. On one hand, such responses were myopic since all backgrounds differ. On the other, one could understand that they thought *all* their own previous experiences were essential in meeting these new challenges. See what I mean about using everything, every scrap of education and experience in one's life as a nurse?

Such I'm-the-template responses permanently warned me off prescribing career moves for nursing students and new graduates. Who knows where *your* particular combination of life skills and education might lead? Yes, two years of med-surg is great generic advice. But will it fit you? My experience warns: Find the person you can best learn from and work there if you possibly can—even if it's peds and you wanted geriatrics. I realized, too, that I sought out OB and psychiatry first because those were the specialties of the nurse faculty I admired most (plus, I was more apt in psychiatry because I'd practiced it defensively years before I became a nurse).

Speaking of the influence of nurse faculty brings up the delightful long-distance teaching I received from Chicago's Myra Estrin Levine. I met her as her editor then learned to save money for her occasional NY visits, because she would run through bookstores with me, piling my arms with books I must read on cultural anthropology and science. Her uncompromising intellect, like Thelma Schorr's, pulled me forward with loving intensity.

Coverage of med-surg meant attendance at lots of medical specialty meetings because most of today's nursing specialty organizations had not yet emerged. Many medical papers, I learned, offered weak science or fuzzy reasoning; I was often astonished at the stories my colleagues, newspaper science reporters, spun from what looked like straw. One can understand the public's hunger for Amazing Breakthrough stories, but one can also understand the public's increasing cynicism over the years. Too many false hopes were raised from reports from dog labs, Petri dishes, or one or two transplant patients. Meanwhile, I played "Search Out the Nurse" (*Cherchez l'Infirmiere?*) in the hospital units of the physicians whose work I admired.

A LUNCH MEETING WITH GEORGE MALLISON

The operating room nurses—AORN—held a particularly memorable national meeting for me. Like the newspaper science reporters, I had to come home with news stories, as well as manuscripts solicited. The Center for Disease Control's expert on disinfection and sterilization, a sanitary engineer named George Mallison, was a final speaker on a morning panel. Suddenly a light bulb went on in my head. I could gather together at lunch the 8 or 10 nurses asking him questions and figure out their current concerns on these topics. I was thoroughly humiliated by the OR nurses' responses: "I had only one question; I'm headed to the exhibits; I'm meeting someone else." The speaker was quick to let me take him to lunch—alone. Stinging from my humiliation, I stared down at my notebook as I plied him with questions. He slid around my questions until I thought I had him pinned down: "Really, what disinfectant would you use on thermometers?" His flippant reply, "It doesn't matter what kind of sheep dip you use," finally startled this former Iowa farm girl enough to look up into his dancing blue eyes, and I fell right in. (George decided his epitaph for me would be: *She's great—if you can just get her attention.*)

Two years later we were married. This was one of the toughest decisions of my life, because I knew I was in the right job; I was partway through graduate school; and I loved my mentor, her family, and my colleagues at *AJN*. Yet George was plunged deeply into his career—plus he had three pre-teen children—in Atlanta.

A MOVE TO ATLANTA AND BACK TO STAFF NURSING

So I reentered staff nursing in Atlanta, but getting hired wasn't so easy. In addition to med-surg, I'd covered economic and general welfare—nurses' union issues—for *AJN,* and the rumor spread that I was perhaps an undercover union organizer, especially since I sought a staff nurse job. Fears were high because the Georgia Nurses Association, with ANA help, had just led a mass resignation at a major hospital.

Fortunately, Mary Woody was the director of nursing at Grady Memorial Hospital, Atlanta's huge city-county teaching hospital. She simply asked me directly about the rumor. Startled, I answered "Would I get married and move 900 miles just to start a local unit?" She shared my enthusiasm for bedside nursing, so she understood my desire to return to it, though she later explained that she knew she wanted me to work with her directly. She extracted my promise that if I saw a need to organize nurses, I'd at least talk with her first.

Mary Woody became my third mentor, this time in nursing management. The above exchange took place when she was 42 and I was 32. Her great talent as a leader-administrator was based on just such direct, clear, careful communication. She never assumed. She asked and verified. Nor was she directive; she asked questions to lead people in problem-solving. As long as you focused on the best interests of patients, she was gentle, tuned in, and enthusiastic—whether you were an aide or an MD. If not, she became cool and disengaged.

MY ENTRANCE INTO NURSING MANAGEMENT

I found my clinical footing on the hemodialysis unit where I kept saying "let me do that," so I could get needed practice. I also listened constantly to patients and families. In five months the head nurse resigned and I took her position. I decided to work all four 12-hour shifts each week instead of the requisite three because the unit was so troubled. I'd already made a habit of staying late cleaning up each evening because the attending MD would drop by to talk. These long talks, mostly about patients and families, taught me a lot but also changed the behavior of the MD, who'd been accustomed to exploding in stormy tantrums when problems caught him unaware.

A major source of trouble was the phenomenon I've called "tech takeover" (Mallison, 1988, p. 787). The blue-collar values of narrowly trained technicians swamped the white-collar professional ethics and clinical strategies of the RNs. Some blue-collar examples: Get-'em-on and off dialysis as fast as possible (even if you're terrifying the patients and changing their blood volume too fast); treat every patient the same (even though some are sturdy and some are fragile); acting heroically in an emergency is more fun than keeping the emergency from occurring. Using Patricia Benner's formulations, these are stances of uninvolved task performance compared to involved, caring task performance (Benner, 1989). Of course the lines can't be neatly drawn by education or profession. Some techs are very caring, thoughtful people and some RNs and MDs aren't.

It's easy to summarize this clash of values but difficult to live through, especially if you don't understand what's going on—it took me a while. Behaviors are justified by beliefs, so both have to change over time. Meanwhile, I went home every night to my new husband and either burst into tears or fell asleep on the sofa. Then I'd weep afresh as I worried whether our new marriage could withstand my distress. Fortunately, George was amused and supportive: "It's your first job as a manager! I had to deal with fistfights in mine!"

I knew the tide had turned when two earnest young RNs came to talk: "Mary, we know your way is the right one, but we want to go back to the way it was." Astonished, I asked, "Would you repeat to yourself what you just said?" They simply said, "Oh!" and the dominance of tech values was ended.

Who could foresee that such clinical and political experiences would someday translate into magazine editorials?

EDITOR OF THE FIFTH DISTRICT NEWSLETTER

Meanwhile, the executive director of the Georgia Nurses Association, Katherine Pope, RN, asked for help with the association newspaper. So on my midweek off day, I'd often work for GNA. Katherine asked then-Governor Jimmy Carter to underwrite a statewide master planning committee and later, a conference and report on nursing in Georgia. So through Katherine and Mary Woody (both staunch GNA/ANA supporters even when many nurse administrators boycotted it), I was involved with the writing and editing of this work. In the process I got to know many nurses.

It was from watching another Grady staff nurse, Mary Long, that I learned what could happen with a local (District) nurses association. I attended the lackluster District meetings but didn't know how to turn them around. Mary did. She ran for nominations chair, then she and her committee persuaded Atlanta's bright young movers and shakers to run for office. The first new president was Mary Lou Keener who later got a law degree and now heads up the national legal department of the Veterans Administration. (Mary Long later became state president, then an ANA board member. She became vice-president for legislation for the National Arthritis Foundation.) I started a District newsletter and reported what was going on locally. Clare LaBar, who later went on to a research staff position at ANA, contributed her analytic skills to a comparison of Atlanta's cost of living and lagging salaries and benefits *vs.* other parts of the United States. In the midst of a nursing shortage, those fact sheets were hot potatoes. If you look back at *AJN* in the 80s and early 90s, you'll see that we continued the comparisons nationwide.

We did many other things to influence public thinking about nurses. A surgeon's RN wife helped us create a flyer, "Dear Doctor: Are You a Part of the Nursing Shortage?"

that listed 10 escalating ways surgeons drive off nurses. A District group dressed up in power suits and, smiling sweetly, handed it out at the American College of Surgeons' national meeting in Atlanta. (I've always thought it a bit craven to picket/leaflet at meetings where people are likely to agree with you—like, say, the American Public Health Association. Why not beard the lion in its den?) Use of the flyer was reported nationwide. I loved the call from *NBC News:* "Are you the editor of the *Fifth District Newsletter?*" I always valued that call higher than "Are you the editor of *AJN?*" because it was so much less likely.

We also began publishing the nursing-related voting records of our district's state legislators. We knew we'd made an impact when one called insisting that we run a correction: He'd voted our way and wanted to be sure the nurses knew it.

At my paying job, I had taken emergency leave from the dialysis unit to intervene with our troubled teenager. Easier for me than for the parents, especially since I'd done such work years before. Mary Woody kept me going as a part-time assistant to her, and the dialysis unit brought me back as a part-time researcher of hepatitis B, which meant I got to visit dialysis families at home. Once our family crisis resolved, Mary Woody brought me on full-time as assistant director of nursing for special projects—meaning, no line supervision, but whatever the director of nursing needed help with at the time. This was terrific experience because it was like a graduate residency in nursing administration. I helped with the move to the problem-oriented record, with patient education, quality assurance, infection control; with hospital marketing and recruitment; with nursing support services and budget; with the support of nurse practitioners, nurse midwives and clinical specialists, as well as with students and refresher nurses—whatever needed organizational development, analysis, writing and backstage support, but not "ownership."

EXPLORING THE MENTOR-PROTÉGÉ RELATIONSHIP

Another door opened when Mary introduced me to the work of Peter Drucker and other management writers. They were a revelation to me because most textbooks I'd seen on management were too often rigidly prescriptive or overly cautious in principles without the necessary case material. I began a love affair with business books.

I hope this gives you a picture of what a true mentor does in one's career. It is definitely a two-way street; each must select the other, and the learner must adapt to the mentor's pace, hours of work, shifting priorities, and assignments. When Mary Woody stepped outside her office asking, "What are you doing right now?" I knew the right answer was, "Nothing that can't wait."

If you haven't already had the experience of a would-be mentor selecting you and you feel uneasy about it, let me warn you it might happen. Some people want you to become a moon to their sun, reflecting their glory as a prisoner in their orbit, totally dependent upon them for light and warmth. One tipoff is the excessive use of "I." Another tipoff is an attempted bribe, such as, "I can get this (scholarship, position, appointment) for you." An attempted bribe disturbs your ethical sense and should disturb common sense, as well. If the Sun thinks you can get whatever it is, aren't others likely to think so, too? The most important tipoff: A Sun has little interest in ideas or achievements that fall outside its own orbit. To avoid an angry backlash, take care how you say no to a Sun. Often the "no" can be covert; you simply become busy elsewhere.

ANOTHER ROLE AT *AJN*

Through these years, I'd done occasional writing for *AJN,* including coverage of nursing news in Georgia. I talked fairly often with Thelma Schorr, who'd been editor for 10 years. When she said she was moving up to CEO/publisher, I couldn't imagine who might step into her shoes. A mutual friend told me Thelma said I was a potential candidate, but she thought I had put down roots and was unlikely to leave Atlanta. Shocked—I'd never considered the possibility—I talked first with my husband, who said gallantly, "You moved for me the first time, and I'll move for you this time."

Timing and a combination of circumstances led to the decision to "go for it." As you can, I hope, see from the previous events, I'd taken several huge leaps into the unknown. All were difficult, filled with pain as well as joy. Much of that pain comes from pulling away from close contacts, which causes them pain, too, which adds to one's own.

My biggest fear was for my husband. If he'd be unhappy, I'd feel miserably guilty. Instead, he adapted beautifully to his part-time consulting and full-time hobbies. At the time, I was enormously buoyed by his level-headed good cheer. Hindsight shows he was relieved. Three years later at 56, he started showing signs of the familial Alzheimer's that had caused his mother's death at the age of 57.

I focused intently on *AJN's* immediate needs, while getting to know the perspectives of its staff and varied stakeholders. My Grady experience had prepared me in countless ways; the staff and budget of a magazine are small compared to those of a major hospital. My nursing organization experience was crucial. One of my cousins, an agricultural engineer, reflected that all his good career moves had been outgrowths of his activism in his professional organization. I agree wholeheartedly.

Thelma showed enormous self-discipline and support by giving me a free hand. Each new leader builds on the platform of the previous one; each has new problems to attack, standing on that platform. Early in her tenure as editor, Thelma had brought into being the vision of Barbara Schutt: *AJN* articles were nurse authored. Early in my tenure, I set up a peer review system that built on Thelma's work. I also measured editors' performances partly by the yardstick of how many pages each contributed monthly, and set quotas for clinical articles that reflected the most common reasons for hospitalization. In the 11 years I'd been in Atlanta, *Nursing* had started up and risen like a rocket. Dozens of nursing specialty organizations had started, each with its own journal. No longer could one monthly journal attempt to reflect all the details of nursing practice. Nor would advertisers support so many nursing journal pages, especially since many of them still believed their target market was MDs. (Think about this: The United States has half as many MDs as RNs, yet 10 times as many medical as nursing journals—advertising money.) My job, then, was to refocus and redesign the content of *AJN,* but do it in fewer pages and with less money. I also wanted to reflect the awesome power that nurses exert in daily patient care. In Atlanta, a staff nurse had remarked in a district planning meeting that nurses didn't know—and therefore didn't appreciate—what other nurses do. I was sure she was onto something; Tom Peters' book *In Search of Excellence* helped me figure out how to call attention to everyday nursing excellence by focusing on hero stories. Patricia Benner was able to place much of this excellence in understandable context. Her article "From Novice to Expert" appeared in the March, 1982, *AJN,* and her "Dialogues with Excellence" became a regular feature.

We also planned one or two major surveys a year, in addition to salary and wage comparisons. Thus, we examined nurses' consensus on what they considered to be non-nursing functions; nurses' job satisfaction and reasons for leaving their jobs or staying; the kind of patient-care assignments in use and what the daily load looked like; and so forth. Editors and freelancers also rounded up nurses' experiences, research, and opinions for articles on issues such as workplace safety and healthcare reform.

You can see that full-time editors don't just sit and wait for manuscripts to appear, then select those they want. Good editors do, of course, rejoice at the occasional unexpected treat that appears in the mail or over the phone. So don't get the impression that it's hopeless to send in something unbidden; it's certainly not. Editors just can't afford to hang around hoping. Nor do editors while away their days slowly spinning editorials. As I recall, Barbara Schutt spent about a week on hers; Thelma Schorr, probably much less; I took about three work days, not counting nights and weekends. Time and talents are all relative: Conservative political columnist William F. Buckley once confessed he spent all of 20 minutes writing a column (on writing) for the *New York Times Book Review.* Ouch!

Nor are most editors pedants who enjoy identifying careless language usage. That would be like saying nurses enjoy seeing disease. No; editors enjoy finding nuggets of exciting content, just as nurses scan for signs of healing.

It seemed to me from the outset that, if I were lucky, I'd get to remain *AJN* editor for 10 years. I left after twelve. I'd had my say, and it was time for someone else. I was also physically exhausted from the years of 60- or 80-hour weeks, then taking over the weekend care of my husband, who'd passed through the wandering, paranoid, and combative episodes of his Alzheimer's disease process. I'd hired Dorothy, a sensitive, sensible caregiver who stuck with him through thick and thin. It seemed to me less stressful to care for him at home than to worry over what might be happening elsewhere. We also had great support from New York University's aging and dementia research program, which had followed us as research subjects from the onset of George's short-term memory loss. Of course, I became fascinated by the stories of caregivers in my support group, by the changes wrought by the disease, and especially by George's heart-melting grace and good humor. If you'd told me when I was 25 that someday I'd become interested in people with Alzheimer's, I'd have said, "No way!"

MY RETURN TO ATLANTA AND THE GEORGIA NURSES ASSOCIATION

So we moved back to Atlanta—George, Dorothy and I—where our three grown children still lived, and where I was offered the position of Executive Director of the Georgia Nurses Association (GNA). I stayed in the position for two years, then left and cared for George full-time until his death in October, 1996.

I was intensely interested in taking the GNA position because I wanted to examine, and try to assist, districts in identifying their unique work. *Megatrends* and *The Third Wave* and lots of management literature talk about bottom-up, not top-down, organizations. ANA had reorganized itself in the mid-1980s to give each state much greater flexibility and autonomy. How were the states, in turn, helping their districts? I wanted to see what tools districts needed to flourish instead of wither; it's largely at the district level that members are won or lost. So I sent "insider" information to District Presidents in our weekly mailings and, with student help, created district-specific orientation materials.

It was also nursing students who immediately gave me crucial staff nurse views of hospital employment conditions (nurses stretched too far). So, we quickly published a survey of nurse:patient ratios and held forums around the state. GNA assisted nurses in one small hospital in their attempt to organize for collective bargaining; the effort was fought off by the hospital's corporate owners, and we lost by two votes. We also disseminated information nurses could use to help themselves if working conditions were unfair or unsafe. We also worked closely with a coalition of nursing specialty organizations, and assisted advanced practice nurses in their attempt to gain less restrictive prescriptive privileges.

SUMMARY

That's where this story ends, for now. Isabella Rosselini called her autobiography *Some of Me.* A truthful title for this chapter would be *Some of Me With the Aid of Lots of Other People.* Because I've named only a few (lists are boring to read), please understand that my work exists only within a huge supportive matrix. What you are examining in this chapter is one cell in a larger organism—just one nurse's story.

Another truthful title would be *How God Uses You Despite Your Flaws and Stumbling.* As a farm girl, I learned about sheep, as well as sheep dip. So I know when the Bible likens us to sheep, it is hinting at God's incredible patience—and sense of humor.

CRITICAL THINKING QUESTIONS

1. What is your own childhood memory of nurses? Did that memory influence your career choice?

2. Did you discuss a potential nursing career with teachers or counselors? If so, did their perceptions of nursing fit with what you now know about it? If their perceptions need correcting, can you arrange to talk with them?

3. Which of your college courses do you think will be most useful in your career as a nurse? Which do you think will be least useful? Write the answers, then look at them at significant dates in the future: your birthday, five years, and ten years from now.

4. What are two attributes of mentors and two ways to spot would-be mentors who don't have your best interests at heart?

5. Have you identified someone you want to learn from, perhaps as a mentor, once you graduate? If you plan to apply for a position where you don't know anyone, how could you use your networking skills to identify positive, helpful nurses at the intended workplace?

ACTIVITIES

1. Interview two staff nurses to see if they experienced reality shock in their first years out of school. Had they been armed by the activities suggested in Marlene Kramer's book? Did they seek support in their workplace or elsewhere? Or did they withdraw?

2. Explore the following:

   Are you aware of a "script" your family expects you to fulfill? If so, is the script in your own best interests or does it serve the interests of others? Do you agree with the script or do you plan to take another path?

REFERENCES

Benner, P. (1982, March). From novice to expert. *American Journal of Nursing, 82,* 402.

Benner, P., & Wrubel, J. (1989). *The Primacy of Caring.* Menlo Park, CA: Addison-Wesley.

Mallison, M. (1988, June). Of tasks, techs, and control. *American Journal of Nursing, 88,* 787, (tech values).

Peters, T. J., & Waterman, R. H. (1982). *In Search of Excellence.* NY: Harper & Row.

Sheehy, G. (1977). *Passages.* NY: Bantam Books.

ADDITIONAL SUGGESTED READINGS

Kramer, M., & Schmalenberg, C. (1974). *Reality Shock: Why Nurses Leave Nursing.* St. Louis, MO: C. V. Mosby.

Mallison, M. (1981, October). Our eyes are on results. *American Journal of Nursing, 81,* 1813.

Mallison, M. (1982, August). Nursing's third wave? *American Journal of Nursing, 82,* 1207.

Mallison, M. (1984, May). The shoes of the clinician. *American Journal of Nursing, 84,* 587.

Mallison, M. (1986, May). Letter to a high school counselor. *American Journal of Nursing, 86,* 517.

Mallison, M. (1986, September). Wring-'em dry mismanagement. *American Journal of Nursing, 86,* 989.

Mallison, M. (1987, April). How can you bear to be a nurse? *American Journal of Nursing, 87,* 419.

Mallison, M. (1987, September). Are you ready for Oprah Winfrey? (introduces Dial c Excel) *American Journal of Nursing, 87,* 1127.

Mallison, M. (1987, November). Two million a day is not chicken feed. *American Journal of Nursing, 87,* 1401.

Mallison, M. (1988, May). Exactly like a nurse. (metaphors for what nurses do) *American Journal of Nursing, 88,* 629.

Mallison, M. (1988, September). The (Health Care) reckoning. (Halberstam & allied health) *American Journal of Nursing, 88,* 1165.

Mallison, M. (1988, October). Unsinkable nurses. (hero stories) *American Journal of Nursing, 88,* 1317.

Mallison, M. (1989, May). Lives that sing. *American Journal of Nursing, 89,* 637.

Mallison, M. (1990, May). Guts, brains, and heart. *American Journal of Nursing, 90,* 7.

Mallison, M. (1990, October). Ninety years through nursing's lens. *American Journal of Nursing, 90,* 15.

Mallison, M. (1991, May). An occasional walk in magic moccasins. *American Journal of Nursing, 91,* 7.

Mallison, M. (1992, August). Welcome to postgraduate year two. *American Journal of Nursing, 92,* 8.

Mallison, M. (1993, May). My name is *nurse. American Journal of Nursing, 93,* 7.

Mallison, M. (1993, June). Remnant of a great vision. (Lillian Wald) *American Journal of Nursing, 93,* 7.

Starr, P. (1983). *The Social Transformation of American Medicine.* NY: Basic Books, Inc.

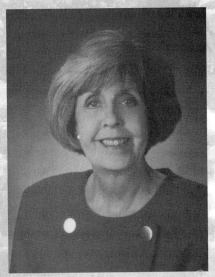

Carole A. Anderson,

PhD, RN, FAAN

Dr. Carole Anderson serves as Dean of the Ohio State University College of Nursing and Assistant Vice-President for Health Sciences. In addition, she holds an academic appointment in the department of Psychiatry, College of Medicine. She came to Ohio State in 1986 from the University of Rochester where she served as Associate Dean in the School of Nursing.

Dr. Anderson received her BS in Nursing, her MS in Psychiatric Nursing, and her PhD in Sociology from the University of Colorado. Her career has included roles as a staff nurse, clinical specialist, and psychotherapist. Currently, Dr. Anderson maintains a clinical practice with the Aids Clinical Trials Unit (ACTU), Division of Infectious Diseases, College of Medicine at Ohio State.

During her career, Dr. Anderson has played an active role in changing and shaping baccalaureate and graduate nursing education with particular emphasis on the desired linkages between nursing education and nursing practice. She served as President of the American Association of Colleges of Nursing (AACN) from 1996–1998.

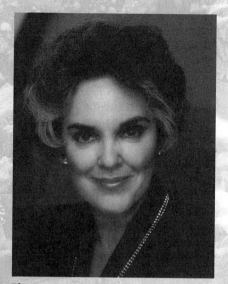

Photo courtesy of Glamour Shots®

Geraldine Bednash,

PhD, RN, FAAN

Dr. Geraldine Polly Bednash was appointed Executive Director of the American Association of Colleges of Nursing (AACN) in December, 1989. In her role, Dr. Bednash oversees the educational, research, government affairs, databank, publications, and other programs of the only national organization dedicated exclusively to furthering nursing education in America's universities and four-year colleges.

Dr. Bednash received her Bachelor of Science in Nursing from Texas Woman's University, Master of Science in Nursing from the Catholic University of America, and PhD in Higher Education Policy and Law from the University of Maryland. She has experienced many roles in her nursing career including: work on the development of resource policy for the Geriatric Research, Evaluation, and Clinical Centers of the Veteran's Administration; serving as nurse practitioner and consultant to the family practice residency program at DeWitt Army Hospital at Fort Belvoir, Virginia; and service as an Army Nurse Corps staff nurse in Vung Tau, Vietnam.

Prior to her appointment as AACN Executive Director, Dr. Bednash headed the association's legislative and regulatory advocacy programs as Director of Government Affairs. Dr. Bednash has directed AACN's efforts to secure strong federal support for nursing education and nursing research, coordinated new initiatives with federal agencies and major foundations, and co-authored AACN's landmark study of the financial costs to students and clinical agencies of baccalaureate and graduate nursing education.

CHAPTER 16

Nursing as a Launching Pad for Other Options— A Variety of Nurses' Paths to Important Roles

INTRODUCTION

As each of the authors of this chapter finished their nursing education, neither envisioned the options that would become available to them during the course of their careers in nursing. Beginning as a staff nurse, at a young age, the world seemed clearly defined by practice as a nurse, in an acute care setting, and providing direct patient care. Patient care has always remained central to the careers that the authors have had in nursing, but the ways in which each has practiced nursing to affect patient care have been varied. Moreover, the skills and knowledge gained in their nursing education programs provided the authors with the ability to participate in multiple and different types of organizations.

Graduation from nursing school provides the graduate nurse with a beginning view of the possibilities available for a professional career. Experience and additional graduate education provides a means to expand the rich diversity of options available. Nursing is a launching pad for a number of opportunities.

NURSING PRACTICE: A BROAD DEFINITION

Nursing is a unique discipline characterized by skills and knowledge related to human behavior, as well as physiological responses. Nursing is practiced in hospitals, homes, offices, corporations, schools, universities and colleges, and in associations. The growing emphasis on community-based health care has brought greater awareness of the need for the unique skills of nurses to assess, design, and implement programs and interventions that will improve or enhance the health of groups of individuals and the community. Although care for individual patients is still a major goal of nursing clinicians, health care providers and policy makers are increasingly aware of the need to have access to professionals who can design broad community-based interventions to improve health for populations.

The ability of nurses to function at both the individual and the community level is a major reason why nurses have a wide variety of options available to them during their career. Clinical practice for nurses has historically begun in hospitals. New graduates have often sought the security of practice in an acute care facility for the entry level practice experience, believing that will sharpen and refine the skills acquired in school. Increasingly, however, that option is not the first available employment opportunity. Employment in nursing homes, home health care agencies, visiting nurse agencies, or managed care organizations has created a demand for nurses that have the ability to function in less structured, more autonomous ways. In these newly emerging entry level employment sites, employers seek clinicians that have the ability to assess complex and diverse individual or group needs, set priorities, design interventions, and implement them in more autonomous ways. For professional nurses, the ability to function as a member of an interdisciplinary team and the ability to function in ambiguous environments also creates a growing need for nurses to have the best education possible, and to continue their education so that they maintain a high degree of competence despite rapid and continuous changes in the world of health care delivery.

Many of the career options available to nurses are directly tied to the educational experience and credentials that the nurse has acquired over his or her career. There is a growing focus on differentiation of nursing roles in the design of care delivery systems. This differentiation designs roles that are specific to educational preparation of nurses. Consequently, nurses will have limited options available to them unless they acquire additional education. In health care organizations as well as the full market of employment in today's society, education and educational credentials are increasingly recognized as evidence that the individual being employed has not remained static and has sought additional knowledge or skills that are an asset to organizations.

The rapid expansion of knowledge and the growing dependence upon the use of complex technologies—for both information management and patient care delivery—demands that the nurse not assume that the education and skills gained in their initial basic academic program will suffice for a whole career. Rather, a variety of learning experiences both formal and informal, as well as additional work to expand the nurse's credentials, will be central to a career that is challenging, varied, and rewarding.

EDUCATION AS A MEANS TO EXPANDED CLINICAL PRACTICE OPTIONS

The sign of a professional is a commitment to lifelong learning. The variety of options available for a nurse are directly related to the learning that the nurse does throughout his or her career. The changes in clinical practice will require that the competent professional continue to learn about new treatments, nursing interventions, and technologies. However, learning must extend beyond the knowledge base that is directly relevant to nursing. This learning can occur through credit granting course work, continuing education programs, reading of the professional literature related to nursing and health care, and participation in the community of nursing and health as a member of organizations focused on these interests. Formal and informal learning about the system in which nursing is practiced, the policies and organizations that frame the delivery of health care, and the economics of health care delivery will provide the nurse clinician with a broader understanding of the world in which nursing is practiced and will also give the nurse a greater potential to move into unique or influential new career paths.

For instance, the changes that have occurred in health care delivery have resulted in a dramatic increase in the demand for nurses to serve in roles as advanced practice nurses (APNs). Practice as an APN allows a nurse greater autonomy, expands the employment sites that are available for practice, and also brings greater financial reward. APNs have acquired a graduate education to function in roles such as nurse practitioners, clinical nurse specialists, nurse anesthetists, or nurse midwives.

APNs are assuming greater importance in the world of health care delivery because of the enhanced clinical decision-making and management skills that they bring to health care. However, APNs are also sought because of their ability to deliver care to groups of patients with complex health care needs and to assist these patients to maintain an optimal level of health. Research on the effectiveness of care by APNs provides good evidence that these clinicians provide high quality care, achieve clinical care outcomes as good as and sometimes better than those achieved by physicians, and are also able to provide patients with a greater sense of satisfaction about the quality of that care.

Nurses in advanced practice roles report tremendous satisfaction in their work. This satisfaction is evidenced by their long-term commitment to clinical practice. However, other nurses with advanced degrees also serve important roles in the health care delivery system. For instance, nurses with graduate level education in administration of nursing and health care systems are an important resource in today's sophisticated and often complex health care organizations. These nurses assume roles as executives in a health care organization managing a complex array of interdisciplinary clinicians, and often have responsibility for oversight and expenditures of large budgets. These nurses are shaping the way care is organized, making decisions about the kinds of clinicians that are necessary to provide good nursing care, and improving the organizational structures that are designed to support care delivery.

Nurse executives in these leadership roles often have advanced degrees in nursing that have given them education related to principles of management, economics, and policies of health care systems, leadership, quality improvement, clinical outcome assessment, and personnel. With this enhanced level of knowledge, these nurses are changing the face of health care delivery and are able to respond and grow in the evolving world of health care.

NURSING EXPERTISE AS ENTRÉE FOR OTHER ROLES

Although the majority of nurses in the United States have continued as clinicians in direct care or in the oversight and administration of health care systems and organizations, nurses have more recently been sought as important advisors on policies related to the health care system. These nurses have served as legislators, legislative advisors, policy analysts, or administrators of governmental bureaucracies. For instance, Marilyn Goldwater, RN, served as a representative in the state of Maryland and also filled an important role as policy advisor to the governor of Maryland on issues related to health care. In addition, Rep. Bernice Johnson (D-Texas) was elected to the United States House of Representatives in 1993 because of her experience as a nurse, and her understanding of health care and the issues that are confronting her constituents. She has served in important roles as a member of a variety of Congressional committees dealing with legislation. In turn, her experience as a legislator has brought new understanding to policy makers of the contributions that nurses make to the care of individuals, families, and communities.

Sheila Burke, RN, serves as the Executive Dean of the Harvard University John F. Kennedy School of Government. Ms. Burke began her career as a staff nurse and then served as a staff member in the National Student Nurses' Association (NSNA). During her work at NSNA, she gained a greater understanding of the importance of federal policies to the lives of individuals needing good health care. Sheila Burke worked in a number of policy roles and eventually moved to a position as Chief of Staff for Senator Robert Dole (R-KS). Policy makers recognized the expertise that she brought to her understanding of the complex issues surrounding health care policies. Her advice and counsel were instrumental in shaping many of the country's current policies related to Medicare, Medicaid, and health care reimbursement.

Mary Wakefield, PhD, RN, serves as Director of the Center for Health Policy at the College of Nursing and Health Science, George Mason University, Fairfax, VA.

Dr. Wakefield began her role as a nurse in the rural state of North Dakota and was active in her state nurses association. During her career she moved through a variety of clinical and educational positions. Her knowledge and understanding of the needs of rural Americans resulted in her eventual employment as Chief of Staff for both Senators Quentin Burdick (D-ND) and Kent Conrad (D-ND). Both of these senators understood that their rural constituents had unique health care needs, and they sought the expertise of this nurse to assist them in developing policies that would address these needs. Dr. Wakefield now directs a major health policy institute that focuses upon leadership development in health professionals, development of health policies for rural populations, and development of policy expertise in health professionals.

Carolyn Davis, PhD, RN, serves as a National Health Care Advisor for Ernst & Young. She began her nursing career as a clinician giving patient care. But, over the span of her career developed new skills, acquired additional education, and eventually moved into a role as a chief academic administrator of a nursing program. In her various roles including that of Dean of a School of Nursing, Dr. Davis understood the need to use her nursing expertise to shape the political process and change policies related to health care. She worked as a strong participant in the policy process and was eventually appointed by President Ronald Reagan as head of the Health Care Financing Administration. This federal agency is the largest organization in health care with an annual budget that exceeds $360 billion. HCFA has responsibility for the oversight of both the systems of Medicare (which insures health care for the nation's elderly) and Medicaid (which provides health care to the nation's poor and disabled). The policies and initiatives set by HCFA serve as a driving force and model for the policies of the remainder of the health care market. Dr. Davis' experience and expertise as a nurse were instrumental in moving her to that position.

Each of these nurses have achieved success because they defined the practice of nursing very broadly and also knew that the unique perspectives they had developed as nursing professionals provided them with the ability to make positive contributions in arenas outside traditional nursing practice. Yet, each was, and is, a practicing nurse as they work to influence the way health care is delivered, paid for, or conceptualized.

ASSOCIATIONS AND ORGANIZATIONS AS A MEANS TO NEW OPTIONS

Much of the early work of nurses in important leadership positions, as policy makers or in other roles, was formed and shaped by their experience with nursing and higher education associations. Nonprofit associations are organizations that serve the public by working to improve quality of life, or influence the social environment in which education, health care, or practice occur. Because of the important work they do to enhance the social fabric of our society, the federal government has made these organizations tax exempt. In nursing, a wide array of nursing organizations exist to address specialized or profession-specific issues. For instance, the American Association of

Colleges of Nursing serves the public in many important ways. This organization, formed approximately 30 years ago, was developed to enhance public awareness of baccalaureate and graduate nursing education for improving the public's health.

Through work in the array of associations, many nurses learn what the issues are that will shape health care or education, identify ways and means to influence the policies that will address these issues, and then work to implement these policy solutions. Participation in a professional association is an important way to contribute to the profession. The most direct and simple means of participation is to simply join an association. However, the most influential means of participation is serving on committees, boards, or as officers, to do the work of the organization. For example, Dr. Carolyn Davis' work in a political campaign, through her professional nursing organization, was the path that led President Reagan to choose her for that important federal role as the chief administrator of HCFA.

Many associations have public policy initiatives directed at influencing federal or local governmental policies for health. Professionals have a responsibility to know about the policies that shape their professional careers and also have a right to intervene in shaping these. The professional association gives that opportunity. More importantly, however, through active participation in a nursing association, the nurse is able to expand his or her awareness of the ways that change can be made and the variety of other career options that are available for nursing practice.

THE AUTHORS' EXPERIENCES

Each of the authors of this chapter have had numerous twists and turns in their professional careers. One of us started her educational life in a diploma program. After graduation from that program, there was a clear understanding that a true career in nursing required continued study and more formal education.

The first author, Dr. Carole Anderson, RN, FAAN, graduated from a diploma school, which at the time was the most common type of nursing education. Sometime during her senior year, the realization came that the educational program had been focused exclusively on nursing. What was missing was more general knowledge about the world, our country, social organizations, and human behavior. Consequently, enrollment in a baccalaureate degree completion program came immediately following graduation. Sometime during her senior year of that baccalaureate program, Dr. Anderson decided to continue on into graduate school and obtain a masters degree in psychiatric nursing. That program prepared individuals for advanced practice in a specialty area. Following completion of her graduate program, she began her nursing career dedicated to advanced practice, teaching, and academic administration (Department Chair, Associate Dean, and Dean). Throughout Dr. Anderson's career, those three activities (advanced practice, teaching, and academic administration) have been ongoing, and eventually were expanded to include being named the Assistant Vice-President for Health Sciences at a major academic health center.

Throughout her nursing career, involvement in professional organizations at the local, regional, and national level was deemed essential. With time, election to national office became a reality. She served as secretary of the American Academy of Nursing and then President of the American Association of Colleges of Nursing.

Dr. Anderson's background in nursing also led her to seek volunteer roles in her community as a member of a group of women who founded a shelter for battered women and their children, member of the Board of Director's of a community mental health center, and serving as a member of the city Board of Health. In these roles, the nursing perspective has been brought to bear as policies are developed to serve the needs of the agency's clients.

The second author, Dr. Geraldine Polly Bednash, RN, FAAN, graduated from a baccalaureate program as the first level of education. The variety of nursing experiences by this author have included active military service in the Army, including a tour of duty in Vietnam, work as a staff nurse in an intensive care unit, and work in a public health department. Along the way, graduate degrees were acquired in nursing, with a masters degree in adult medical surgical nursing, and a doctoral degree in education policy and law. In addition, a fellowship experience from a major foundation allowed this author to develop advanced practice skills for a role as a nurse practitioner with eventual practice in an ambulatory family practice clinic, and a role as a consultant to a family medical practice residency program. She has also enjoyed a volunteer role in a homeless shelter providing primary care services to the homeless.

Dr. Bednash served as an educator in diploma, associate degree, baccalaureate degree, master's and doctoral degree programs over the span of her career. Service and leadership in the state nurses association were a routine and ongoing interest with various roles including chair of the Political Advocacy Committee of the State Nursing Association. From this blended mix of clinical practice and service as an educator, her career advanced toward doctoral studies in education policy and law. As a result of this combination of practice and education roles, Dr. Bednash served as the lobbyist for the AACN for three years and eventually assumed the role of Executive Director at the AACN.

SUMMARY

Nursing has been a wonderful career with many options that were never envisioned as each of us entered our careers as nurses. Nursing has allowed us to touch lives in ways that have improved the lives of our patients by giving expert nursing care to overcome illness, educating patients about ways that they can be healthier and more proactive in maintaining their health, and by supporting them through difficult times. Nursing has never limited us, but has instead provided options that have changed as our professional expertise and interest has changed. Moreover, the roles that we have each assumed at this point in our careers are enhanced by the skills we bring from nursing. The unique and central interest of nursing in the interpersonal component of care delivery allows nursing professionals to facilitate change in a supportive and effective fashion.

The options available to the nursing student or the nursing professional are directly related to the commitment and interest that the individual brings to the profession. Nursing allows the individual to grow and change with the assurance that his or her career will grow and change too. Nursing practice and nursing leadership skills will never be irrelevant. The impact that nurses have on lives and organizations are directly related to the skills and knowledge that are core to the practice of nursing. As each of us has changed our careers and practiced nursing in various roles, we have never stopped being nurses. Instead we have practiced nursing in different ways—educating students, patients, consumers, policy makers, and other professionals about the health care issues that must be addressed and the kinds of solutions that nursing has to offer.

Never be limited in your view of nursing. Instead, consider your own interests, unique skills, knowledge, and recognize that there are a myriad of opportunities to blend these with your professional knowledge to shape nursing. The future of the health care system and its ability to deliver effective, efficient, and high quality care to the consumers of that care is directly dependent upon the leadership that will be exhibited by clinicians. Nurses are one of the most important groups in assuring that these goals are met. If you, as a future nursing professional, continue your education, hone your skills, participate in the life of professional organizations, and expand your view of how practice can best be implemented, you will have more options than can be chosen in one lifetime in the leadership profession called *Nursing*.

CRITICAL THINKING QUESTIONS

1. What skills, knowledge, and expertise in nursing prepare nurses for practice in nontraditional roles?

2. What are the unique capabilities that you bring to the discipline of nursing? How will the various practice opportunities available in nursing allow you to use these capabilities?

3. What are the leadership roles that nurses assume? How will a nursing background allow the nurse to succeed in these roles?

4. What health care system changes are most likely to be influenced by the skills and capabilities of the professional nurse? How can the nursing professional assume a leadership role in addressing these changes?

5. What career path do you expect? How can you assume a leadership role in this career path?

ACTIVITIES

1. Select five various nursing journals such as *Nursing Outlook, Journal of Nursing Education, Journal of Nursing Administration, Nursing Economics, American Journal of Nursing, RN Magazine, The American Nurse* or many other excellent examples that your school nursing library should carry. Look for editorials or articles that make predictions about nursing education and nursing practice in the next century. Think critically about what they are saying. In order to understand their predictions of impacts to your future practice and the lives of the patients you will serve, make a list of the major categories that their predictions fall under. Do you agree with what they are saying? If not, what are your own predictions?

   Ask your Dean to address your leadership or issues class about these categories, and predictions. Ascertain from that discussion, how nursing education at your school or university is striving to meet future predictions, and how nursing education groups (AACN, NLN, etc.) that your Dean is involved with are striving to meet those predictions.

ADDITIONAL SUGGESTED READINGS

Anderson, C. A. (1995, March–April). What do our numbers look like? *Nursing Outlook, 43,* (2), 55–56.

Nornhold, P. (1990, January). Predictions for the 90s. *Nursing 90,* 34–41.

Tanner, C. A. (1995, February). Living in the midst of a paradigm shift. *Journal of Nursing Education, 34,* (2), 51–52.

Empowerment for Your Path to Leadership Development

We have explored the stepping stones of *Education, Nursing Practice, Professional Nursing Involvement, Mentoring, and Networking.* It is our goal as the writers of this text to leave you empowered for travel along your own path to leadership development. There are four remaining areas that we want to discuss together. The first two involve the growing use of computers in nursing, health care, and society. In Chapter 17, we'll look at a *key tool for empowerment in the twenty-first century: Informatics literacy.* Chapter 18 explores the *nursing challenges, roles, and opportunities in a World Wide Web environment.* This chapter is a valuable guide for nursing students still developing in the information age. We have tried to help you find sites on the internet that may prove beneficial to you as a nursing student. However, remember directions and paths to sites change. Our goal is to provide you with enough street signs to allow you to surf a little, but still find your way. One of the most valued steps you will take is to graduate and enter practice. In Chapter 19, a recent nursing student leader shares *the privilege and the challenge of entering the profession in today's world.* Included are some valuable insights into practice and interviewing for nursing positions. Finally in Chapter 20, one of today's most influential nurse leaders provides information about the value and process of *career mapping:* a process that can empower you as a future nurse leader.

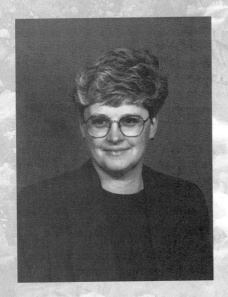

Connie White Delaney,

PhD, RN

Dr. Connie Delaney is an Associate Professor at the University of Iowa (U of I), College of Nursing in Iowa City. She also holds an Affiliate faculty position in the U of I Center for Health Services Research, and maintains an Adjunct Clinical appointment in nursing informatics at the University Hospitals & Clinics.

Following completion of her undergraduate studies in nursing and mathematics at Viterbo College in LaCrosse, Wisconsin, Connie worked as a staff nurse in ICU. She earned her Master's Degree at the U of I in 1978 and accepted her first faculty appointment at Luther College in

Decorah, IA later that year. At that time Connie and a colleague founded a nursing education and consulting business. Later in 1984, she continued her commitment to lifelong learning and pursued doctoral studies in educational administration and computers. With the recent arrival of the microcomputer, these studies proved to be quite interesting. Thus she began her commitment to an area called "informatics," although the term was used very limitedly in nursing at that time. Perhaps her early studies in mathematics helped develop her "fit" with this specialty. With her PhD completed in 1986, at the U of I, she continued teaching there and still teaches nursing informatics and health informatics classes.

Dr. Delaney's research focuses on knowledge representation in the computer-based patient record and on large database research using the Nursing Minimum Data Set (NMDS). She is working towards the refinement of the North American Nursing Diagnosis Association (NANDA) Taxonomy and the development and testing of the Nursing Management Minimum Data Set (NMMDS). Dr. Delaney serves as Vice-Chair of the ANA Nursing Information & Data Set Evaluation Center (NIDSEC) Advisory Committee, and Third Vice-President of the Iowa Nurses Association. Connie Delaney was named Outstanding Faculty Member for Iowa by the Iowa Association of Nursing Students in 1993. She views this as her most treasured award.

CHAPTER 17

Informatics Literacy— A Key Tool for Empowerment in the Twenty-First Century

INTRODUCTION

Yes, we are living and practicing within a health care system that is in crisis. Our professional discussions and readings are permeated with descriptions of:

1. changing patient/client characteristics
2. a need for budget driven policy
3. demand from all consumers for quality care and proven effectiveness
4. an explosion in the use of biotechnology and information technology
5. an increasingly complex health care delivery system

Simultaneously, the paradigm shift contains elements of reshaping the environment, preserving the human focus, orientation toward health and wellness, and a radical change in values. Autry (1991) asserts that the new values for the twenty-first century include spontaneity, connectedness, vulnerability, self-knowledge, wisdom, authenticity, truth, communication, and focusing on potential versus permanence. Nurses have long known, and society recognizes, that nursing embodies those very values, in fact the twenty-first century values, appropriate for meeting such complexities. The nurse's role as information manager and processor, knowledge worker in decision support is unequivocal.

Purpose

The emergence of nursing informatics as a specialty arose out of such demands, crises, and technological developments. The purpose of this chapter is to support your transition to nurse leader by examining the contribution of nursing informatics to your practice, the profession, and health care in the twenty-first century. This chapter will explore information resources/technologies within the human and social context, describe the emergence of nursing informatics, address the power of nursing informatics to serve nursing practice, suggest strategies to increase your involvement in nursing informatics, and propose a vision for the future.

INFORMATION TECHNOLOGIES WITHIN THE HUMAN AND SOCIAL CONTEXT

You have begun to experience the sights, sounds, tastes, smells, and touches of nursing care. These experiences are occurring within a United States health care system, possibly an international system, and within the nursing profession during perhaps the most wonderful, stimulating, chaotic, and transformational period that history will ever record. You have read essays from prominent nursing leaders in *Nursing Student to Nursing Leader: The Critical Path to Leadership Development*. Now, I ask you to pause and reflect.

Consider a specific information technology or resource. Focus your attention on electronic communication, the Internet, computerized care planning, on-line documentation, imaging, video-conferencing, bibliographic databases, clinical datasets, standardized vocabularies, automated decision support, the computer-based patient record, and others. Ask yourself the following questions:

1. How has this technology changed my nursing practice?
2. Are these changes visible or invisible to me?
3. Are these changes visible or invisible to the people I serve?
4. Are these changes visible or invisible to the profession?

You have undoubtedly discovered that the use of any information technology or resource changes what you do and how you do it. It also changes your values, the values of care recipients, the nursing profession, health care in general, and even society. You may also have discovered that many of these changes become invisible. There are characteristics of all technologies that provide greater insights into your discoveries.

McGinn (1990) noted that all technologies, including information technologies, share several characteristics. They are concerned with material, involve purpose, expand human possibilities directly or indirectly, require resources for development and use, are knowledge, and involve method. Most important to our discussion is the fact that all technologies grow out of an enabling socio-cultural-environmental context, and in turn they generate context. Moreover, every technology has a profound relationship to the practitioner's mental set—the practitioners who developed the technology as well as the practitioners who use the technology. Technology is indeed value laden. McGinn goes on to assert that all technology confers benefit to someone or something. It has become so institutionalized that the products and values the technology serves are no longer determined by the practitioner's values. Rather, products and values that specific technologies serve are determined by institutions. All technologies convey certain individual preferences, tastes, and world views. These characteristics of all technologies demand your critical analysis.

Although it is clear that technology is needed to support nursing practice, it is equally certain that those technologies must be wisely selected and critically used. Clinician knowledge and skill that go beyond computer literacy and the use of computer applications are needed. Are you prepared to wisely select and critically use the appropriate information technologies to support your practice?

EMERGENCE OF NURSING INFORMATICS

Developments in information science, information theory, cognitive science, psychology, electrical engineering, biomedical engineering, medical computing, and computer science supported the formal identification of "informatics" as a discipline in the late 1960's. It is readily apparent that informatics has been, and is, an interdisciplinary specialty. The nursing profession came on board and transitioned from a focus on computer applications to nursing informatics in the mid-1980's. This transition was supported by early work of nursing leaders in the recognition and development of standardized language and the efforts of nurse pioneers in implementing computerized hospital and nursing information systems.

The Study of Nursing Informatics

The study of informatics focuses primarily on the data, information, and knowledge needed to support patient care; it is secondarily focused on the computer as a vehicle to meet these information needs. That is, nursing informatics is about coalescing data (facts), information (interpretation of facts with a value added), and knowledge (a set of rules, formulas, or heuristics used to create new information and ideas).

The study of nursing informatics focuses on:

1. Providing better health care access, quality, and cost-effective care
2. Supporting patient care, research, and education
3. Use of data, information, and knowledge
4. Appropriate use of the technology to complement human skills
5. Communication within health care
6. Identifying the capabilities and limitations of technology

THE POWER OF NURSING INFORMATICS TO SERVE NURSING PRACTICE

The impact of the information paradigm shift is beyond measure. James Bailey in *After Thought* succinctly notes that "This is truly an electronic computing revolution; its intellectual impact will be greater than anything since the Renaissance, possibly greater than anything since the invention of language" (Bailey, 1996, p. 6). The force of this shift, more aptly described as an "information revolution," is indisputable throughout all sectors of the health care delivery system. The demand from consumers and payers alike for quality and effectiveness verification is based on the assumption that data and information about such aspects of health care as cost, quality, satisfaction, and outcomes, are available. The reliance of policy makers on existing large computerized data banks is a case in point.

Reliance on Information Accessibility— Where Is Nursing?

The Agency for Health Care Policy and Research (AHCPR, 1991) clearly outlined the existence and use of computerized administrative, clinical, federal medical and health services research databases, death and disease registries, and many other computerized state and private resources for health care policy development. It is particularly noteworthy that these federal, state, and private databases often contain millions of patient records and data about medical diagnoses, treatments, related charges, and in some cases, dental care. Most disturbing, however, is that no nursing data are present in these hundreds of health care databases and millions of patient records represented within these databases.

And we, in nursing, wonder why the patients' responses to health are not visible. We wonder why the health care system is not more health oriented. It is indeed quite unlikely that these perspectives will emerge from electronic databases that focus on all but health promotion, illness prevention, and the patients' responses to birth, health, illness, and death. As nurses, we have a responsibility to be active partners in this electronic world of computerized databases. You are invited to engage in this transforming revolution, support the visibility of our patients, clients, families, and communities, and expand the comprehensibility of the nursing profession within the broader health care context of our society.

EFFORTS TOWARD NURSING'S VISIBILITY IN COMPUTERIZED DATABASES

For several years, nursing has focused on the data and information needs of the profession to support a presence in computerized databases. This work has been driven by the underlying principle of atomic-level patient data being collected once, and then used many times. That is, individual patient data documented while providing care serves as the foundation for agency-wide, community/region-wide, nation-wide, and world-wide uses and decisions. The following discussion will highlight several of these major accomplishments of nursing, particularly in support of capturing patient specific data and the relationship of these accomplishments to fostering the information power of the profession.

Nursing Minimum Data Set

Without doubt, one of nursing's first major attempts to identify a standardized collection of essential nursing data was lead by Werley and Lang (1988). Following an invitational conference and follow up discussions, the Nursing Minimum Data Set (NMDS), composed of 16 key data elements, was identified. The sixteen elements were organized into three categories: service, demographics, and nursing care. The service elements include unique facility number, unique health record number, unique number of principal registered nurse provider, episode admission and discharge dates, disposition of patient, and expected payer of the bill. Demographic elements include personal identification, date of birth, sex, race and ethnicity, and residence. Although 10 of the 12 elements comprising the service and demographic categories have been consistently collected since 1975, two elements of "unique registered nurse provider number" and "personal identification" are still not accessible. Nationwide efforts are underway to outline a strategy to collect these data.

The third category, nursing care, is comprised of four defined elements: nursing diagnosis, nursing intervention, nursing outcomes, and nursing intensity. Capturing the nursing care elements of the NMDS is the linchpin to nursing's survival in an electronic information society. Retrieval of all elements of the NMDS will support establishing comparability of nursing data across clinical populations, settings, geographic areas, and time. Access to these data will also support nursing's ability to describe nursing care of patients and their families in institutional and non-institutional settings, and nursing's ability to project trends in care, stimulate research, and provide the essential data needed to influence clinical, administrative, and health policy decision making. Realizing the benefits of the NMDS, however, requires a common standardized nursing language.

Standardized Nursing Language

Clear evidence of nursing's commitment to standardized language is the development of numerous languages to describe nursing's work. Actual implementation of these languages, however, was clearly facilitated by the American Nurses Association (ANA) when they assumed a major leadership role in developing a mechanism for recognizing standardized languages through the ANA Steering Committee on Databases to Support Clinical Nursing Practice. To date, five classifications have been recognized: the North American Nursing Diagnosis Association (NANDA) (1996) Taxonomy, the Nursing Interventions Classification (NIC) (1995), the Omaha System (OS) (Martin & Scheets, 1992), the Home Health Care Classification System (HHCCS) (1991), and the Nursing Outcomes Classification (Iowa Outcomes Classification, 1997).

Nursing is becoming empowered to participate in the electronic world. First, the essential nursing data were identified in the NMDS, and second, languages necessary to actually capture the NMDS data have been developed and share common quality criteria. However, these activities alone will not accomplish the goals of the NMDS. The languages need to be actually implemented with computerized information systems.

Computerized Information Systems

Clearly, significant progress has been made toward the development of languages to communicate nursing's contribution to health care. Realizing this visibility, however, is dependent upon implementing these languages in computerized nursing information systems. Again, the ANA has provided significant leadership to support the implementation of the recognized languages. For example, the NEXT Generation Nursing Information Systems (Zielstorff, 1993) describes the essential characteristics of nursing information systems for professional practice. This product describes functional requirements; it is a guide to nurses who are involved in the development and/or selection of a nursing information system.

To further the adoption of standardized nursing language and the essential characteristics of nursing information systems, ANA has established the Nursing Information & Data Set Evaluation Center (NIDSEC) (ANA, 1997). Specific standards and scoring criteria have been created to evaluate data sets, both those marketed by vendors and those custom designed. This recognition mechanism is designed to encourage vendors to design products that truly support nursing practice, including the use of standardized nursing languages.

Using the Data

Nursing leaders involved in the development of the NMDS clearly saw its potential to describe nursing practice and influence health care policy. ANA has consistently supported the NMDS trajectory. Saba and McCormick (1986, 1996) further clarified the research power of computers and computerized databases to define nursing science through articulating a taxonomy of nursing research foci.

This taxonomy has three components:

1. Nursing science in patient care
2. Efficacy of nursing strategies in solving problems
3. Nursing care organization and delivery

The following queries illustrate some of the power to provide answers when nursing data are retrievable from computerized information systems: What is the frequency of nursing diagnoses, signs and symptoms, interventions, or medications administered for a selected patient population? What are the predictions of nursing data for prevention, deterioration, and stabilization of patients? Is there a correlation between nursing data and medical data? How does nursing care compare to the care provided by allied health professionals? What nursing interventions are effective with which patients? Is there a correlation between nursing interventions and the data representing the organization and delivery system? What are the expected and actual outcomes of patient care? What are the benefits of nursing care on physical outcomes and emotional outcomes? What is the frequency of error reporting/safety/incidents? What is the clinical decision-making process of nurses?

Nursing has actually moved toward using computerized nursing data. Evidence distinctly demonstrates that nursing data are being used and some of the research potential of these data elements is being realized. For example, ANA has taken a lead role in implementing nursing's first report card (ANA, 1997). This study is one of the first longitudinal studies of RN staffing, length of stay, and patient outcomes conducted across three states. Moreover, Ryan and Delaney (1995) have reported the actual use of the NMDS to define nursing practice.

Power of the NMDS. The power of the NMDS is extended by the identification and implementation of the Nursing Management Minimum Data Set (NMMDS) (Delaney & Huber, 1996). Designed to capture the context within which nurses provide care, the NMMDS will facilitate across site and setting comparisons of financial and personnel resource expenditures and quality measures.

International Strategies

Efforts to build on the commonalties of the nursing classifications to establish a unified nursing language system (UNLS) continue in the United States. ANA is also an active participant in the development of an International Classification of Nursing Practice (ICNP). Imagine the power of the NMDS and other data sets when nursing data can be communicated throughout the world. Nursing's continued progress in the world of large database methodologies to profile our practice is up to you and others.

STRATEGIES TO INCREASE YOUR INVOLVEMENT IN NURSING INFORMATICS

First, become knowledgeable in one of the newest specialties in nursing, nursing informatics. Excellent resources include *The Scope of Practice for Nursing Informatics* (ANA, 1994) and *Standards of Practice for Nursing Informatics* (ANA, 1995b). Such knowledge is imperative regardless of your nursing role and practice setting. Moreover, many of you may decide to become nursing informaticists. There are several excellent nursing informatics programs to explore.

Second, recognize the power of the NMDS, standardized languages, and the NMMDS for describing what nurses do, how good they do it, and with whom. Accept individual professional responsibility for learning each classification. Through understanding the classification, the patient information that you record will be more accurate. Fully use the classifications to document all of the health care problems, interventions, and outcomes of each patient you serve. This is, indeed, a significant responsibility. At the same time that you must care for expanding numbers and increasingly sicker patients, the number of staff is often being decreased. The pressure is on you to do more with less. And, now, you are being asked to COMPLETELY document the care you deliver. It may help to remember that every time you choose to take a short cut—only document the more important nursing diagnoses in the patient, only the key interventions that are reimbursed, or only one outcome of care—YOU are making nursing, nursing care, and most importantly, the human experiences of health and wellness, invisible. Celebrate the inter-relatedness of your individual practice to the profile of nursing practice described regionally, nationally, and internationally. Accept the responsibility and accountability for complete documentation of your practice.

Participate in computerized nursing information system selection, implementation, and evaluation. Nurses are the experts in knowing what information systems must provide. Welcome opportunities to understand system capabilities and limitations. Foster your ability to communicate these needs with non-nursing personnel. The resources identified in this chapter will be invaluable.

Be involved. ANA welcomes input on the issues and strategies outlined in this chapter. Likewise, if nursing is to develop a common international language, nurses must work together, dialogue, and critique methods. The International Council of Nurses welcomes your interest.

The use of electronic communication technologies can greatly expedite this work. Internet resources, electronic mail, listservs, etc. are waiting for your contribution. Celebrate the power of representation that is afforded those that participate.

Commit to working together to create something that will outlast you and will outlast today. Every nursing diagnosis, nursing intervention, and nursing outcome that you document in a computerized information systems that meets the quality criteria supported by the ANA can become a part of a database that describes patient/client care in your delivery setting, in your health care delivery system, your state, national, and even ultimately, become a part of international databases of nursing care.

A VISION FOR THE FUTURE

The most important view of our shared vision of the future is that the electronic technologies we adopt support nursing's social contract. It is our shared responsibility to ensure that information systems support the accurate delivery, documentation, and knowledge development in the areas identified in our Social Policy Statement (ANA, 1995a, p. 8). Pause and reflect. How can you help ensure that the information systems and the knowledge resources you use support:

1. Care and self-processes
2. Physiological and pathophysiological processes
3. Physical and emotional comfort, discomfort, pain
4. Emotions related to experiences of birth, health, illness, death
5. Meanings ascribed to health and illness
6. Decision and choice-making
7. Perceptual orientations
8. Relationships, roles, and change
9. Social policies

Do our information systems provide the flexibility to document individual preferences in self-care? Do our systems provide the versatility to document physiological processes through pictures and graphics? Do they provide a mechanism for you to document, I mean record, your patient's voice of pain or discomfort or the first birthing cry? Do our systems provide a way for you to capture the meaning of an illness or the relationship of the individual's meaning of illness to adherence to prescribed interventions? Does the information system support individual decision making? Does it support equal access of patient/client and health care provider to the health information? Does the information system support family caregiving and family documentation of caregiving? Does it support documentation of the relationship of energy fields, vitamin therapy, or spirituality on health? Does the information system uphold advanced nursing practice? Does it sustain integrated interdisciplinary health care practices? Does the information system nurture collaboration among health care providers? Does it support socially responsible financial accountability for health care?

My vision of the interrelationship between my practice and computerized information systems is that both individually and as a professional group we will use electronic resources with integrity. That is, as Scott Peck (1993) has aptly described, we will use computerized information technologies as a "means to achieve wholeness." Maintaining integrity means that you and I are cognizant of the "meaning of technology" and the human and social context of electronic resources we choose to use. Maintaining integrity means that you and I foster a sense of responsibility within ourselves and in others to determine which technologies should be used, the strengths and limitations of these technologies, and the short-term and long-term implications of their use. Maintaining integrity means that you and I consider our advocacy role and its relationship to the use of common languages, information systems, and shared databases.

SUMMARY

Alan Drengson (1990) describes the evolution in our relationship with technology. The attitudes and values toward technology exist on a continuum from technological anarchy, technophilia, and technophobia to appropriate technology. He asserts that people can move from viewing technology simply as a way to preserve wealth, power, and tame nature to being enamored with their own mechanical cleverness, techniques, tricks, and technical devices and processes. Further, people can continue to grow toward recognizing that only human and humane values can curb the threats of technology out of control, reject technological control, and assert human autonomy.

Consider your future contributions as a nurse leader, and the balance that you must responsibly maintain between your talents and emerging technologies. Strive to live a philosophy of appropriate technology which Drengson describes as a maturing of our relationships among technology, people, and the world (Drengson, 1990, p. 31–32). Drengson describes this view of technology as one that:

1. Preserves diversity
2. Promotes balanced interactions between people, technology, and the environment
3. Conserves energy
4. Balances all costs
5. Promotes human development through use

You are invited to come together with your colleagues in nursing. You are invited to see, have the courage to change, and possess the strength to do. You have been invited to see technologies within a human and social context. You can develop the courage to move into the future by celebrating the strengths that the nursing informatics specialty brings to nursing. Acknowledging, accepting, and using the power of nursing information supports your courage to practice confidently in the twenty-first century. Now, do it!

Suggestions have been offered to you to begin your involvement in the informatics contribution to our profession. It is now your decision to accept the invitation to work toward our common goals: strong, consistent communication; a sense of direction; and a common spirit of unity.

CRITICAL THINKING QUESTIONS

1. What is the function of nursing informatics in the twenty-first century?
2. Can the profession create knowledge without large databases?
3. How do we give meaning to words or actions in computerized information systems?
4. What are our responsibilities to the patient as a consumer in terms of electronic access? electronic care? electronic resources?
5. Are electronic technologies and resources adjuncts to care or are they *THE* care?
6. Can machines create and/or record intelligence?
7. How is computer information different from verbal information or written information?
8. What will happen to our oral culture?
9. Are we becoming more vulnerable to the total destruction of all knowledge?
10. Do electronic resources create a poverty of attention? How does one conserve attention?
11. What determines the limit on what we do? Is it "time"?
12. How will virtual reality change the way nurses practice? What is the meaning of "space" in a virtual world of health care? What is the meaning of "reality" in a virtual world of health care?
13. Do you think our five senses will be all of the senses that will serve us in the twenty-first century? Do you think the human race will develop additional senses in the information age?

ACTIVITIES

1. Search Internet. What informatics organizations did you find? What listservs related to informatics did you find?
2. Search Medline US. Search Medline European. What did you discover? Is there a difference? Is scholarly information controlled?
3. Visit the home page of the American Medical Informatics Association at **http://www.amia.org**

4. Visit a comprehensive www forum for health care professionals at **http://www.healthcareforums.com**

5. Visit the Government Accounting Office www for up-to-date information on legislation related to the computer-based patient record and advocacy at **http://www.gao.gov**

6. Visit the National Library of Medicine at **http://www.nlm.gov**

7. Visit the home page for the development of the computer-based patient record at **http://www.cpr.org**

REFERENCES

Agency for Health Care Policy & Research. (1991). *Report to Congress: The Feasibility of Linking Research-related Databases to Federal and Non-federal Medical Administrative Databases* (AHCPR Pub. No. 91-003). Washington, DC: Government Printing Office.

American Nurses Association. (1994). *The Scope of Practice for Nursing Informatics*. Washington, DC: ANA.

American Nurses Association. (1995a). *Nursing's Social Policy Statement*. Washington, DC: ANA.

American Nurses Association. (1995b). *Standards of Practice for Nursing Informatics*. Washington, DC: ANA.

American Nurses Association. (1997). *Implementing Nursing's Report Card*. Washington, DC: ANA.

American Nurses Association. (1997). *Nursing Information & Data Set Evaluation Center: Standards & Scoring Criteria*. Washington, DC: ANA.

Autry, J. (1991). *Love & Profit: The Art of Caring Leadership*. New York: William & Morrow & Company, Inc.

Bailey, J. (1996). *After Thought*. New York: HarperCollins Publishers.

Delaney, C., & Huber, D. (1996). *A Nursing Management Minimum Data Set (NMMDS): A Report of an Invitational Conference*. Chicago, IL: AONE

Drengson, A. (1990).Toward a philosophy of technology. In L. Hickman, *Technology As a Human Affair*. New York: McGraw-Hill Publishing Company.

Iowa Outcomes Project. M. Johnson & M. Maas (Eds.). (1997). *Nursing Outcomes Classification (NOC)*. St. Louis, MO: C.V. Mosby.

Martin, K., & Scheets, N. (1992). *The Omaha System: Applications for Community Health Nursing*. Philadelphia: W.B. Saunders.

McCloskey, J.C. & Bulechek, G.M. (1995). *Nursing Interventions Classification* (2nd ed.). St. Louis, MO: Mosby-Year Book, Inc.

McGinn, R. (1990). What is technology? In L. Hickman, *Technology As a Human Affair*. New York: McGraw-Hill Publishing Company.

North American Nursing Diagnosis Association. (1996). *North American Nursing Diagnosis Association: Taxonomy I: 1996–1997.* St. Louis, MO: NANDA.

Peck, S. (1993). *Further Along the Road Less Traveled.* New York: Simon & Schuster.

Ryan, P. & Delaney, C. (1995). *The Nursing Minimum Data Set: Research findings and future directions.* In Annual Review of Nursing Research Vol. 13, Springer Publishing New York, NY.

Saba, V., O' Hare, P., Zuckerman, A., Boondas, J., Levine, E., & Oatway, D. (1986). A nursing intervention taxonomy for home health care. *Nursing & Health Care, 12,* (6), 296–299.

Saba, V., & McCormick, K. (1986). *Essentials of Computers for Nurses.* New York, NY: J. B. Lippincott.

Saba, V., & McCormick, K. (1996). *Essentials of Computers for Nurses.* (2nd Edition). New York, NY: J. B. Lippincott, 596.

Werley, H., & Lang, N. (1988). *Identification of the Nursing Minimum Data Set (NMDS).* New York: Springer.

Zielstorff, R., Hudgings, C., & Grobe, S. (1993). *NEXT-Generation Nursing Information Systems.* Washington, DC: ANA.

ADDITIONAL SUGGESTED READINGS

Anderson, B. (1992). Nursing informatics: Career opportunities inside and out. *Computers in Nursing, 10* (4), 165–170.

Andrew, W. F. (1994). New technologies mean a cable-free future for point-of-care. *Health-Care Informatics, 11* (5), 33–34, 36–44.

Ball, M., & Collen, M. (Eds.). (1992). *Aspects of the Computer-based Patient Record.* New York: Springer-Verlag.

Barnsteiner, J. H. (1993, Spring). The on-line journal of knowledge synthesis for nursing. *Reflections, 8.*

Blois, M. (1987). What is it that computers compute? *Clinical Computing, 4* (3), 31–33, 56.

Brunner, B. K. (1993). Health care-oriented telecommunications: The wave of the future. *Topics in Health Information Management, 14* (1), 54–61.

Cassey, M. Z., Kane, W. P., & Sutton, L. S. (1993). On-line access to nursing literature. *Computers in Nursing, 11* (5), 230–235.

Dick, R., & Steen, E. (Eds.). (1991). *The Computer-based Patient Record.* Washington, DC: National Academy Press.

Graves, J., & Corcoran, S. (1989). The study of nursing informatics. *Image, 21* (4), 227–231.

Heller, B., Damrosch, S., Romano, C., and McCarthy, M. (1989). Graduate specialization in nursing informatics. *Computers in Nursing, 7* (2), 68–76.

Kuhn, T. (1970). *The Structure of Scientific Revolutions.* Chicago, IL: The University of Chicago Press.

Lange, L. L., & Jacox, A. (1993). Using large databases in nursing and health policy research. *Journal of Professional Nursing, 9* (4), 204–211.

Maher, M. P. (1994). The CNS and nursing informatics. *Clinical Nurse Specialist, 8* (2), 103–108.

Meyrowitz, J. (1995). *No Sense of Place—The Impact of Electronic Media on Social Behavior.* New York: Oxford University Press.

Millholland, D. K. (1994). Privacy and confidentiality of patient information. *Journal of Nursing Administration, 24* (2), 19–24.

Mills, M., Romano, C., & Heller, B. (Eds.). (1996). *Information Management in Nursing and Health Care.* Springhouse, PA: Springhouse Corporation.

Moritz, P. (1990). Information technology: A priority for nursing research. *Computers in Nursing, 8* (3), 111–115.

Nicoll, L. H. (1994). An introduction to the internet part I: History, structure, and access. *Journal of Nursing Administration, 24* (3), 9–11.

Nicoll, L. H. (1994). An introduction to the internet part II: Addresses and resources. *Journal of Nursing Administration, 24* (5), 11–13, 59.

Nicoll, L. H. (1994). An introduction to the internet part III: The internet and other on-line services. *Journal of Nursing Administration, 24* (7/8), 15–17.

Nicoll, L. H. (1994). Modern day pirates: Software users and abusers. *Journal of Nursing Administration, 24* (1), 18–20.

Ozbolt, J., & Grave, J. R. (1993). Clinical nursing informatics, developing tools for knowledge workers. *Advances in Clinical Nursing Research,* 409–429.

Simpson, R. (1991). Electronic patient charts: Beware the hype. *Nursing Management, 22* (4), 13–14.

Simpson, R. L. (1994). Ensuring patient data, privacy, confidentiality and security. *Nursing Management, 25* (7), 18–20.

Simpson, R. L. (1994). How technology can encourage collaborative practice. *Nursing Administration Quarterly, 18* (4), 79–83.

Simpson, R. L. (1995). Ethics in the information age. *Nursing Management, 26* (11), 20–21.

Simpson, R. L. (1995). How will state-level reforms affect your information systems? *Nursing Management, 26* (5), 20–21.

Sparks, S. (1993). Electronic networking for nurses. *IMAGE: Journal of Nursing Scholarship, 25* (3), 245–248.

Staggers, N., & Mills, M. E. (1994). Nurse-computer interaction: Staff performance outcomes. *Nursing Research, 43* (3), 144–150.

Stone, A. (1995). *The War of Desire and Technology at the Close of the Mechanical Age.* Cambridge, MA: MIT.

Talob, R. (1994). Copyright, legal, and ethical issues in the internet environment. *Tech Trends, 39* (2), 11–14.

Trofino, J. (1993). Voice-activated nursing documentation: On the cutting edge. *Nursing Management, 24* (7)28–33.

Tufle, E. (1974). *Data Analysis for Politic and Policy.* Englewood Cliffs, NJ: Prentice-Hall.

Valiant, S., & Rosenberg, R. (1993). Evolving private networks in Europe. *Telecommunications, 27* (2), 28–33.

Waldrop, M. M. (1994). Software agents prepare to sift the riches of cyberspace. *Science, 265*, 882–883.

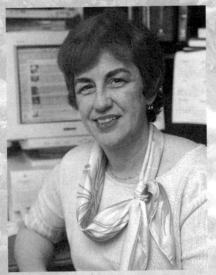

Photo courtesy of Stephan Hopkins

Florence L. Huey,

RN, MA

Florence L. Huey, RN, MA, has spent her professional life straddling patient care and nursing journalism/health care communications. Since 1996, she has served as Managing Editor of the first solely on-line, full-text clinical journal for primary care clinicians providing health care to women—*Medscape Women's Health*. The Medscape Web site grew in registered members from 15,000 in its first year to nearly 500,000 by its third year.

Huey began her journey into nursing leadership and communications in her first year in nursing school with her election first to Recording Secretary, then President of the Louisiana Association of Nursing Students. In 1968 during her junior year, Florence Huey was elected President of the 65,000 member National Student Nurses' Association (NSNA). That same year NSNA debuted its national publication, *Imprint*. To assist with the publications content, Huey wrote a column that examined the key issues of the time.

Florence Huey's vast experiences include several positions with the American Journal of Nursing (AJN), eventually serving as the editor of AJN. Over the years, Huey has been active on committees of the American Nurses Association, New York State Nurses Association, New York State Nurses Foundation, and Sigma Theta Tau.

Of all the honors in nursing and journalism that Florence has received, the two she cherishes most are the LSU Honorary Distinguished Alumnus Award and the NSNA Honorary Membership bestowed on her by the NSNA House of Delegates.

Carolyn —
Best wishes meeting the
challenges in nursing.
Florence L. Huey

CHAPTER 18

Nursing Challenges, Roles, and Opportunities in a World Wide Web Environment

INTRODUCTION

Not since Guttenberg invented the printing press has there been such a revolution in the dissemination of information as that provided by the Internet, which includes the World Wide Web (WWW). Just as the printing press made possible the multiple copies of books and the birth of periodicals, the Internet brings more information directly into the homes of millions than could be found in the largest single library.

At the dawn of the Information Age, people applauded the explosion of information gained from research while they lamented the difficulty in its dissemination. It could take five years, and often longer, for research findings to be disseminated widely enough to change practice. For instance, more than a decade after portable capillary glucose testing devices became widely available and research had clearly proved that measuring urine glucose levels (especially in elders with glomerula filtration changes) was a meaningless waste of time and money, urine glucose tests continued to be the routine practice for monitoring diabetes. Similarly, it took years for clinicians to stop doing pre-op shaves the night before surgery, to stop icing injectates for cardiac output measures, and the list goes on. Now, information has become so widely available, that often if health care providers don't know what is the latest in acceptable practice or therapy—their patients will tell them.

Opportunities to use the Internet to link people and resources has captured the imagination of millions worldwide. Health care providers routinely use the Internet for several activities including:

1. answering client questions, monitoring health status, and providing patient education
2. seeking consultation or making referrals to colleagues
3. promoting a private practice by creating a Web page to notify colleagues and potential clients of services
4. reviewing clinical practice guidelines, finding career opportunities, clinical books, and professional supplies
5. obtaining and providing continuing education

Stories of patients who have discovered their own cures, or at least major leads to innovations in treatment, have become so common that health care providers realize they need to be "on the Net"—that is connected to information resources on the Internet—to keep up with health care consumers. Stories of nurses who are using the network of computers to network with professional colleagues are demonstrating the value and necessity of mastering Internet-access skills. Consider, for example, a few of the many ways nurses are using the Internet to communicate and retrieve information.

EXPANDING ROLES: EXAMPLES OF NURSES ON THE NET

1. In Minnesota, a nurse in the Medical Policy Department of an insurance company is responsible for gathering information on new procedures and devices in order to propose policy for utilization and reimbursement approvals. As quickly as new procedures are introduced, she needs to find and evaluate whatever reports are available on their effectiveness, on what types of providers should be permitted to perform the procedures, and on what patients, under what conditions. Searching for information on the WWW and using Internet discussion groups to consult colleagues saves countless hours searching for resources and at the same time gives her more current information than she could find in a library (Glasgow, 1996).

2. An experienced obstetrics nurse enrolled in a nurse midwifery program with the Frontier Nursing Service in Kentucky, sits in New Jersey, boots up her computer, and logs on to the Internet to download class lectures, upload homework assignments, and participate in group discussions. Kentucky's Frontier Nursing Service and the University of Kansas Primary Care Nurse Practitioner Program are among the pioneers in a growing list of nursing education programs that are offering advanced-practice and graduate-level courses via the WWW. Besides virtually opening university doors to students not geographically near the schools they want to attend, these on-line classes

offer scheduling flexibility. Students need not juggle days off to attend class; instead, they can access course work and submit homework via electronic mail at any time. Some say students in these Internet classes get more 1 to 1 personal attention than they would sitting in a classroom.

3. In Alaska, a nurse practitioner checks his e-mail and responds to questions and requests for prescription renewals from his patients. One message is from a homebound diabetic patient who reports fluctuations in her blood glucose that makes the NP decide to add an ultra lente insulin to the woman's treatment regimen. Via e-mail, the NP advises the patient of his plan and then sends a message to the bush pilot about to leave on the mail run to bring the insulin to the woman.

4. In Russia, a nurse whose husband is being transferred from his US government position in Moscow to Houston, Texas, logs on to the Internet and visits a few job bank sites on the WWW to check out positions advertised. Then as she is reading the messages from colleagues in a nursing discussion group she regularly participates in, she decides to post her questions about job opportunities and specific facilities in Houston and asks nurses to respond to her privately via her personal e-mail address.

5. In Florida, a nurse is completing the form to renew her RN license when she realizes she is short the mandated number of CE credits. She boots up her computer and begins searching professional health care information sites for CE-credit-bearing articles in her clinical area.

6. To accommodate family caregivers unable to attend support group meetings, a nurse forms a "virtual support group" by collecting e-mail addresses and copying all group members on messages and responses.

7. In a rural clinic, a nurse practitioner having trouble treating a wound, photographs the wound with a video camera and transmits the image to a vascular clinical specialist who examines the wound and recommends treatment.

8. A nurse seeking to establish an independent practice as a geriatric case manager specializing in the care of elders whose families are in other parts of the country creates a Web page to promote her services.

9. In New York, a visiting nurse travels from home to home carrying a laptop computer in her bag. When she arrives at the home of a client, she plugs the computer into a phone line to access the client's record located on a server at the agency. She downloads the client's record so she can compare her current findings with those recorded on the last visit and check for any changes in the medical plan. Then, she uploads the documentation of her findings, interventions, and treatment plan changes from this visit to the agency's main computer.

10. In Hays, Kansas, a rural community with a population of 16,000 and about 200 miles from the nearest large city, an interactive home health nurse uses telehealth equipment to monitor patients in their homes—checking blood pressure, following up on health teaching, answering health care questions—

as she sits in her office at the Hays Medical Center. The time she might otherwise spend sitting in her car traveling from home to home she spends in direct patient contact. The telemedicine position doesn't replace F to F [face to face] home care visits, but it supplements them in a way that has averted unnecessary hospitalizations (Canavan, 1996).

Telehealth care, like the programs in Hays, KS, offers the promise of bringing a higher level of health care resources to a larger number of people in a shorter time. In 1996, the National Library of Medicine (NLM) embarked on a major initiative, awarding $42 million for 19 multiyear telemedicine demonstration projects in 13 states. One grant to the University of Southern California, for example, proposed to bring health care services to underserved center-city elders in North Hollywood and to isolated islanders off the coast of Catalina; another funded the University of Washington's creation of a telemedicine network permitting collaboration among clinicians in Washington, Wyoming, Alaska, Montana, and Idaho; a $1.8 telemedicine grant to the University of Iowa National Laboratory for the Study of Rural Telemedicine funded a project to measure the effectiveness of video consultation for patients with special needs (National Library of Medicine, 1997).

The Internet offers nurses the opportunity to locate resources for managing personal and patient-care problems, continuing their education and staying current, increasing continuity of care by linking patients with providers and with support groups, and shaping the political health care agenda.

NURSE PIONEERS/EXPLORERS ON THE NET

The Nightingale listserv—an electronic discussion group maintained at the University of Tennessee—was one of the early settlers on the Net and very quickly proved a global link for Net nurses worldwide. Now, countless nurses are involved in designing and maintaining Web sites, including their own home pages on the Web, as well as maintaining mailing lists to exchange information on such topics as nursing research [NURSERES <listserv@kentvm.kent.edu>], nursing issues [NURSENET <jnorris@oise.on.ca>], and countless other topics.

So many "ordinary nurses" now have Web sites for promoting their services, offering patient education, providing nursing resources to colleagues, and collaborating in research and entrepreneurial ventures with other nurses that a who's who of nurses on the Web would become incomplete as it was being written.

The corps of nurses who were early Internet explorers includes Susan Sparks, RN, PhD, FAAN, who was tracking patient and nurse chat groups even before many discovered the existence of the Internet. From her position in the Division of Extramural Programs at the NLM, Dr. Sparks was named to direct four of the NLM's telemedicine contracts. There is Mary Anne Rizzolo, RN, EdD, FAAN, who as Director of Interactive Technologies for the American Journal of Nursing Company created a national computer network to deliver information and continuing education to nurses in remote rural areas. At Langara College in Vancouver, Canada, there is Jack Yensen, RN, PhD, who maintains the Virtual Nursing College home page, an early Web settlement first established in June, 1993. The site is rich in resources to help nurses learn how to search and find the information they want on the Web. There is Leslie Nicoll, RN, PhD, editor-in-chief of *Computers in Nursing,* who launched the Hospice and Palliative Care Education Network for Internet support of cancer patients. There is Judy Norris, RN, who has long had a home on the Web at the University of Alberta's site and has been active in developing and maintaining listservs for nurses. Robert T. Smithing, RN, MSN, FNP, whose early activity promoting an electronic forum for nurse practitioners, is well known to many advanced practice nurses. There is the team of RNs, Mark and Mary Carraway, Ron Phelps, and Linda Anderson, associated with three different nursing sites—Nursing Net, Virtual Nurse, and Whole Nurse—who collaborated to create a mentor matching program **<http://virtualnurse.com/mentor/Mentor.html>.** This on-line mentoring program matches nursing students and novice nurses with experienced nurses who are willing to serve as mentors via the Internet.

The growing Net activity of nurses led the 1996 ANA House to adopt a resolution directing the association to develop model guidelines and policies for professional nurses' participation in telenursing and telehealth that address complex practice, education and legal issues; ethical concerns raised by telehealth and telenursing practice; and reimbursement issues.

NUTS AND BOLTS OF NETWORKING

Keep in mind that the Internet—commonly called The Net—is not the same as the World Wide Web (WWW). The Internet is the global network of computer connections that permit the home care nurses remote access to the agency's computer, and the NP in the rural clinic to transfer the video image file. The WWW is just one part of the Internet—the flashy part with pictures, sound, videos, animated text, links from one page to another. The other part of the Internet is electronically delivered messages, or e-mail.

Internet

The Internet emerged in 1968, but it had been more than a decade in planning. In the 1950s, at the height of the Cold War, the U.S. Department of Defense set out to design a computer network of networks that, like the mythological Hydra, would function despite severed heads. No matter how many computer centers were disabled, the Department of Defense would continue to have access to vital defense information

Given this beginning, not surprisingly, a checklist of the benefits of the Net for nurses sounds like the benefits of communication:

1. Talking with colleagues on a daily basis
2. Quick access to information to avoid reinventing the wheel
3. Resource sharing: news, job leads, and client referrals
4. Collaborative research projects
5. Political action
6. Collegial support
7. Professional socialization—lurk & learn what colleagues are discussing

Web

The World Wide Web is a 1990s phenomenon. The first "point and click" software for accessing the sights and sounds of the Web was called Mosaic. When Mosaic was released in 1993, there were only 50 hypertext Web servers or sites. Just 4 years later in 1997, there were more than 250,000 Web sites and more than a dozen software programs for accessing the Web.

The WWW of today is a multimedia environment that offers a vast array of audio-visuals—pictures, sound, video, animated text. It opens up a new world of educational and collaborative possibilities. For example, you can view images like PET scans, see histology tissue changes on a slide, or examine photos of pressure ulcers at various stages. On the WWW, you can visit a mental health site that allows you to listen to a patient's responses during a mental status exam, a cardiology site where you can hear heart sounds, and an oncology information site that features an animation of the pathway of cancer metastasis. What you find on the WWW can advance your own education as well as that of patients.

A key feature of information on the WWW is the speed in disseminating information. When the Agency for Health Care Policy and Research (AHCPR) first began to produce and distribute research-based clinical practice guidelines on conditions ranging from pain management to controlling and correcting urinary incontinence, it could take six weeks or longer to receive a copy after the document was requested from the Government Printing office. Now it can be obtained as soon as it is published by opening the document on the WWW and printing a copy.

E-Mail

The workhorse e-mail is straight text—no bells and whistles or flashing lights and images there. But it can keep you connected to colleagues and patients. In 1997 more than 50 million people in 160 countries had an e-mail address. E-mail permits you, at any time of the day or night, to send instructions or a reminder to a patient, to respond to a patient's question, or to contact colleagues for an answer to a question of your own. E-mail is sent according to the sender's schedule and received when the recipient is ready to log on and read mail. Listservs turn individual e-mail into group electronic discussions. Most often, e-mail communications of listservs members are asynchronous—that is, individuals pose questions and make comments; then, several hours later the answers, comments, and questions of others arrive via e-mail.

E-MAIL ESSENTIALS

Establishing an E-mail Address

Setting up an e-mail address to send and receive messages is a good first step in connecting to the Net. When you set up an e-mail address, you can select any sequence of letters and numbers as long as no one else has registered the same address. Because it is easier to remember words than numbers, most people register either their given or a nick name as their e-mail address. In an academic, government, association, or commercial site, often the e-mail address will be a full name or initials plus the last name.

Listserv Basics

There are thousands of mailing lists, listservs, e-forums, or discussion groups. For a sample of nursing listservs, see Table 18–1. To be on the mailing, you must send an e-mail message to whomever is maintaining the list. Then, anytime a comment is submitted, the message is delivered to all who have registered. For basic net etiquette rules on listerv communication, see Table 18–2.

There are 6 critical commands for Listserv:

   1 & 2—subscribe and unsubscribe, or join and leave list
   3 & 4—receive and cancel the digest form of list postings
   5 & 6—temporarily suspend and resume list mail

The commands must be executed exactly according to instructions, and current general guidelines (at the time of this writing) are included here for your convenience.

To subscribe. The typical protocol is to send a one-word message, "Subscribe," and conclude with the name you want to appear on the list.

Save the receipt. After you send the subscribe message, you will get an acknowledgment and, most important, the commands needed to get off the mailing list, suspend participation, and request the digest form of list messages. Save this.

Digest the information. An active list can generate a lot of e-mail. If you pay for your e-mail service by the number of messages, you can save money by asking for the digest form of the list messages.

Table 18–1: Nursing Listerv Sampler

Below is a sample of the growing number of electronic discussion groups that focus on aspects of nursing. After the name of each list is the address for subscribing plus a brief description of the nurse participants or discussion focus. Two nurse managed sites maintain an extensive list of nursing lists: NurseNet
<http://www.ualberta.ca/~jrnorris/nursenet/>
and Rod Ward's Home page
<http://www.shef.ac.uk/~nhcon/nulist.htm>
(Rizzolo 1997).

- ITNA (International TeleNurses Association) <listserv@listserv.bcm.tmc.edu>: telenursing
- NURSENET <listserv@listserv.utoronto.ca>: nursing issues
- NRSING-L <listproc@lists.umass.edu>: nursing informatics
- NURSERES <listserv@kentvm.kent.edu>: nursing research
- RN-JOBS <majordomo@npl.com>: professional nursing employment
- RNPHDC-L <listserv@mizzou1.missouri.edu>: doctoral nursing students
- SNURSE-L <listserv@ubvm.cc.buffalo.edu>: nursing students
- RNMGR <rnmgr-request@cue.com>: nurse managers
- CARENETL <carenetl@humber.bitnet>: nurse faculty
- NRSINGED <listserv@ulkyvm.louisville.edu>: nursing education

Specialty Clinical Areas
- ADDCTNSG <listproc@list.ab.umd.edu>: addictions nursing
- CLForNsg <listserv@ulkyvm.louisville.edu>: forensic nursing
- EYENURSE <maiser@mailgw.ornet.med.umich.edu>: ophthalmologic nursing
- GERO-NURSE <gero-nurse-request@list.uiowa.edu>: geriatric nursing
- HCARENURS <listserv@listserv.medec.com>: hospice and home care nursing
- IVTHERAPY-L <listserv@netcom.com>: IV therapy nursing
- NEPHRO-RN <majordomo@majordomo.srv.ualberta.ca>: nephrology nursing
- MIDWIFE <midwife-request@csv.warwick.ac.uk>: midwifery
- OHN-LIST <listerv@oise.utoronto.ca>: occupational health nursing
- PERIOP <listproc@uwashington.edu>: perioperative and OR nursing
- PNATALRN <pnaatalrn@ubvm.bitnet>: perinatal nursing
- NP Info <npinfo@npl.com>: advanced practice
- PNN-L <majordomo@interaccess.com>: advanced practice
- PSYCHIATRIC NURSING <mailbase@mailbase.ac.uk>: psychiatric nursing
- SCHLRN-L <schlrn-l@ubvm.bitnet>: school nursing

Table 18-2: Netiquette

Here are a few tips on Net etiquette, or proper Internet behavior (Jamieson, 1995).

1. **Don't be a stranger.** Get in the habit of signing your name at the end of every e-mail message you send because not every mail program passes along the header information. While those who frequently use e-mail quickly learn to decipher the "return address" to figure out the source of the message, it is best to identify yourself.

2. **Open and answer your mail.** Things happen quickly. Once you begin communicating by e-mail, you need to be prepared to act quickly both in responding and posting messages. You may get a response within minutes or at the very least within hours. It is only polite to be prepared to respond with relatively equal speed.

3. **Do Not Shout.** Typing in a word all in capital letters is considered shouting. While it is fine to emphasize a single word by putting it in caps, a message in all caps is hard to read and best avoided.

4. **"Smile" Discretely.** Smileys, or emoticons, are the graphics used to convey feelings from happiness [:-)] to displeasure [:-(]. Tilt your head to the left to see the faces. An occasional, well placed emoticon can be useful as long as not overused.

5. **Do Not Parrot.** If you want to respond to a posting on a chat-line or listserv, it is considered a waste of reader time and e-mail space to re-post an entire message. It is preferable that you copy only the portion to which you are responding and post it with a > at the left margin of every line.

6. **Lurk Before You Leap.** When you first subscribe to a chat-line or listserv, follow the discussion for a while to get a sense of what people are talking about and what the tone of the discussions are before jumping in with your opinions.

7. **Know Your FAQs.** Conference groups generally have a FAQ, a frequently-asked-questions list, that newcomers can use to find out the subjects discussed. The FAQ can spare you from asking dumb questions that waste members' time.

8. **Think Twice, Speak Once.** A thoughtless comment can be very painful, and the written word on screen has more staying power than a slip of the lip.[Time]

9. **Don't Be Too Forward.** When you want to share one message with several others, most mail programs permit forwarding the message, but that is not always a good idea. Unless you want the person who originally sent the message to be included in the general discussion, it is better to copy the message and send it on. Otherwise, at any point that someone decides to "respond to all" the originator of the message will be sent a copy of the discussion.

Table 18-2: Netiquette *(continued)*

10. Net Acronyms
  ROTFL—rolling on the floor laughing
  LOL—laughing out loud
  IMO—in my opinion
  IMHO—in my humble opinion
  IMNSHO—in my not-so-humble opinion
  BTW—by the way
  FAQ—frequently asked questions

Electronic Publications

Electronic newsletters are distributed via e-mail like messages from a listserv. But unlike a list, electronic newsletters don't invite a response. For example, Health Infocom Newsletter **<listserv@asuacad>** is a weekly newsletter of medical information. To subscribe, send message "Subscribe Mednews. <your name>" to listserv@asuacad/.

FINDING YOUR WAY ON THE WEB: SEARCHING

You can browse sites for information, or search for it—basically it's the difference between thumbing through journals and books versus looking at the contents page or an index. While browsing can be interesting and stimulating, the volume of information on the Internet can be overwhelming if you don't know how to search out what you're looking for. Imagine trying to find a book in a library with books arranged in no particular order and without a card catalogue.

There are 3 basic ways to find information on the Internet:

1. *Surfing* or wandering from site to site by clicking on hyperlinks can be useful when looking deeply into a specific topic.

2. *Browsing* or looking at directories, much like scanning books in a section of a library, is a more direct way to find information than just wandering around.

3. *Searching* or using one of more than about 60 individual and metasearch search engine sites, however, can be the most direct and efficient way to get the exact information you need (Wootton, 1997).

It has been said that the most frequently accessed site on the WWW is Yet Another Hierarchical Officious Oracle, better known as YAHOO, an Internet search engine. Search engines—aka spiders, crawlers, wanderers, robots—scurry around the millions of sites to index information. They tend to list documents tagged according to probability of relevance based on such factors as how many times key words appear in the document and how close they are to the top of the document. Search engines generally achieve volume, not subtlety. To increase the precision of your search, use Boolean syntax [and, not, or].

When you're searching for the information you want on one or more of the WWW's more than sixty million web pages, your success will be related to the breadth of the search engine's database and to your ability to describe your search. Now the use of metasearch engines allows users to greatly expand their searches by using several individual search engines at once. Please see Appendix C for a summary of nursing bookmarks for the Internet.

SUMMARY

Thanks to the remarkable strides in access to information via the Internet, the turn of the Twentieth Century could well mark the time when nurses generally consider a computer with Internet access as essential a piece of equipment as a stethoscope. As computers shrink in size to no more than the dimensions of a paperback book, nurses can carry their own electronic notebooks as they now carry their own stethoscopes.

Distance learning will continue to expand while the number of classrooms on campuses will shrink. Students will log in and download lectures, but will also participate in real time seminar chats on-line. Aside from breaking the geographical boundaries for students, the World Wide Web also will increasingly break geographical boundaries for faculty who need not even be in the same country much less the same room with the students in class.

Telemedicine will dramatically revise where and how patients receive health care services. Patients in the most remote rural communities will have access to health care without needing to travel great distances. Indeed, health care providers with finely honed specialty skills will not need to be in highly populated urban centers. Nurses already have a prominent presence on telemedicine networks. Health maintenance organizations rely on a national cadre of nurses to provide health education and answer patient inquiries to reduce the unnecessary use of more expensive health care services. In the "Ask-A Nurse" programs that have developed in the '90s, the patient posing the question could be in Oregon while the nurse answering it could be at a computer console in Tennessee. One emerging issue a national approach to delivery of health care is raising is: Is the Tennessee nurse counseling the Oregon patient practicing nursing without a license in Oregon?

Telemedicine technology will dramatically change clinical rotations for nursing students. Instead of faculty being actually present on selected patient visits during a home care clinical rotation, faculty can be virtually present with every student on every home care visit.

Nurses, like almost everyone else, will increasingly use the Web to disseminate professional, political, and patient education information. In fact, nurses maintaining home pages for patient education, colleague collaboration, and to promote entrepreneurial services isn't the future, it is the present. The population of nurses on the Web can only be expected to increase. According to a survey by the New York State Nurses Association, 39 percent of nurses in the state had access to the World Wide Web in 1996. Given the way use of the Web has grown exponentially, it isn't unrealistic to expect that percent to reach 90 percent or more by the turn of the century.

Perhaps the greatest challenge in the future will be what has always been the challenge of information—how to ensure that information is available to those who need it without violating confidentiality. How shall we restrict access without creating barriers? Who should pay for the maintenance of information on the Web?—those who access it? or those who want to reach those who access it? That is, user or advertiser?

As experience with the Web increases, so too will the challenges and the questions. But the bright side is that the opportunities can be expected to grow in equal measure.

CRITICAL THINKING QUESTIONS

1. Where would you find the latest immunization recommendations for young children? travelers? Hepatitis B?
   Where would you find patient education material on herpes?
   Where would you find a support group for lupus patients?

2. How comfortable are you with communication via the computer and the Internet? In what ways do you foresee that computer technology will affect your nursing practice in the next five years? How can you prepare yourself as a future nurse leader to be part of the leadership that will bring quality changes about in this area?

3. Using examples of how nurses could use electronic communications, how would you explain the difference between the Internet and the World Wide Web?

4. In a search for information on US Congressional support for graduate nursing education, on treatment guidelines on hepatitis D, and on state regulations governing advanced practice nursing, how would you compare the quality and quantity of the hits using three different engines?

5. How would you evaluate the usefulness of the following Web sites in terms of the following criteria: ease of access, original material versus links to other sites, frequency of updating content and links, use of such unique features of the Web as interactivity and audiovisual transmission?

American Nurses Association (ANA) **<http:nursingworld.org>**
Medscape **<http://www.medscape.com>**
NursingNet **<http://www.nursingnet.org>**

Nursing.Net <**http://www.nursing.net**>

National Student Nurses' Association (NSNA) <**http://www.nsna.org**>

NursingCenter <**http://www.nursingcenter.com**>

ACTIVITIES

1. Using one of the on-line job banks, make a list of 12 different nursing positions available in a state at least 500 miles away from where you live.

2. Using only the resources on the Internet, generate a list of 10 articles published within the past two years on nursing and the Internet.

3. Find on the WWW, a nurse's home page—a site on nursing. Find and print a nursing history photo from two different sites.

4. Prepare a bookmark for each of the following sites: nursing association, nursing journal, government, university, medical center, job bank, and on-line CE.

5. How would you explain the following joke? *Paul Revere Virus: Revolutionary virus that does not horse around. It warns you of impending hard disk attack: Once if by LAN; twice if by C.*

REFERENCES

Cailliau, R. (1995). A little history of the world wide web [on-line] W3C, 1995; **http: www.w3.org/History.html/**

Canavan, K. (1996, November–December). New technologies propel nursing profession forward. *American Nurse, 28* (8), 1–3.

Glasgow, V. (1996, July–August). Grateful med is a hit with managed care companies in Minnesota. *Gratefully Yours,* 1.

Jamieson, E. L., & Seaman, B. (Eds). (1995, Spring). Welcome to cyberspace: guide to the ways and words of cyberspace. *Time 145* (12), 42–48.

NA. (1996). What is the world wide web [on-line] MdGateway Internet Learning Center. **http://www.mdgateway.com/mdgatwaytrain/whatweb.html/**

NA. (1997). Choosing an ISP [on-line]. *Currents.* **http://www.currents.net/resources/netprov/inyquest.html/**

National Library of Medicine. (1997). NLM national telemedicine initiative [on-line] National Library of Medicine. **http://www.nlm.nih.gov/research/telemedinit.html/**

Nicoll, L. H., & Ouellette, T. H. (1997). *Computers in Nursing's Nurses' Guide to the Internet.* Philadelphia, PA: Lippincott-Raven Publishers.

Rizzolo, M. A., Sparks, S., & Norris, J: (May 29, 1997). Nursing lists. Handout at ICN'97 Nursing and the Internet, June 1997.

Scoville, R. (1996). Find it on the net. *PC World Online.* **http://www.pcworld.com/software/internet_www/articles/jan96/jan9635.html/**

Seiter, C. (1996). NetSmart. *Macworld On-line* [on-line]. **http: //www.macworld.com pages/december.96/Column.2893.html/**

Sparks, S. (1997). WWW search tools: let the spiders do your crawling [on-line]. **http://www.interactive-healthcare.com/97Sum4.htm#www Search/**

Wolf, G. (1994). The (second phase of the) revolution has begun [on-line]. Wired. **http://nswt.tuwien.ac.at:8000/cs/papers/mosaic-revol.html/**

Wootton, J. C. (1997). Search engines. *J Women's Health,* 6 (3), 345–347.

ADDITIONAL SUGGESTED READINGS

Bair, A. H., Brown, L. P., Pugh, L. C., Borucki, L. C., Spatz, D. L. (1996, July–August). Taking a bite out of CRISP. Strategies on using and conducting searches in the Computer Retrieval of Information on Scientific Project's database. *Computers in Nursing,* 14 (4), pp. 218–24, quiz pp. 225–226.

Bergren, M. D. (1995, February). Electronic communication. Part III. *Journal of Scholastic Nursing,* 11 (1), pp. 7–9.

Bichoff, W. R. (1997, March). The internet and the world wide web. *Advances for Nurse Practitioners* 5 (3), pp. 65–67.

Carlton, K. H. (1997, January–February). Redefining continuing education delivery. *Computers in Nursing,* 15 (1), pp. 17–18, 22.

Fawcett, J., Buhle, E. L. Jr. (1995, November–December). Using the Internet for data collection. An innovative electronic strategy. *Computers in Nursing,* 13 (6), 273–279.

Griffith, H. (1996, January–February). Internet magic. *Journal of Professional Nursing,* 12 (1), 3.

Hostetter, T. A. (1996, March–April). Ophthalmology's interaction with the Internet (you say, "Internet what?"). *Journal Ophthalmic Nursing Technology,* 15 (2), 57–59.

ILC glossary of internet terms (on-line). (1997). Internet Literacy. **http://www.matisse.net/files/glossary.html/**

Lybecker, C. J.(1997, June). A nurse explores the internet. *American Journal of Nursing* (6), 42–50.

McCormick, K. A, Cohen, E., Reed, M., Sparks, S., Wasem, C. (1996, November–December). Funding nursing informatics activities. Internet access to announcements of government funding. *Computers in Nursing,* 14 (6), 315–322.

Milholland, D. K. (1996). New information technologies suggest new roles for nurses. *American Nurse* 28 (6), 2–3.

Murphy, S. C; Start, N. E; Widzinski, L. J.(1996). Nursing sites on the world wide web. *Journal of NY State Nurses Association,* 27 (1), 19–21.

Nicoll, L. H. (1994, March). An introduction to the Internet. Part I: History, structure, and access. *Journal of Nursing Adminstration,* 14 (6), 9–11.

Nicoll, L. H. (1994, May). An intro to the Internet. Part II: Addresses and resources. *Journal of Nursing Administration,* 14 (6), 11–13, 59.

Nicoll, L. H. (1994, July–August). An intro to the Internet, Part III: The Internet and other on-line services. *Journal of Nursing Administration,* 24 (7–8), 15–17.

Prohaska, J. L., Chang, B. L. (1996, June). Using the Internet to enhance nursing knowledge and practice. *Western Journal of Nursing Research,* 14 (6), 365–370.

Rogers, G. (1995, April). Nurses and the Internet. *Journal of Emergency Nursing,* 21 (2), pp. 60–62.

Shearer, B. S. What's Up on the internet (on-line). (1997). *Medical Practice Communicator* 4 (3), 7; **http://www.medscape.com/HMI/MPCommunicator/1997/v04.n03/mpc0403.05. html/**

Shellenbarger, T., Thomas, S. (1996, July–August). Creating a nursing home page on the World Wide Web. *Computers in Nursing,* 14 (4), pp. 239–245.

Simpson, R. L. (1995, July). "Surfing" the internet. *Nursing Management,* 24 (7), 18–19.

Simpson, R. L. (1996, February). Will the Internet supplant community health networks? *Nursing Management,* 27 (2), 20, 23.

Simpson, R. L. (1996, November). Wireless communications: a new frontier in technology. *Nursing Management,* 11 (11), 20–21.

Sparks, S. M. (1997, March). Using the Internet for nursing administration. *Nursing Administration,* 27 (3), 15–20.

Stellin, S. (1997). Privacy in the digital age: Part 1: Who's watching you on-line? (on-line), *CNET;* **http://www.cnet.com/Content/Features/Dlife/Privacy/**

Stellin, S. (1997). Privacy in the digital age: Part 2: How private is your personal information? (on-line). *CNET;* **http://www.cnet.com/Content/Features/Dlife/Privacy2/index.html/**

Swaine, M. (1996). Surfin' safari: finding the perfect Internet search engine (on-line). *MacUser.* Ziff-Davis Publishing Co. **http://www.zdnet.com/macuser/mu_0696/net/traveler.html/**

Tomaiuolo, N. G. (1995, July–August). Accessing nursing resources on the Internet. *Computers in Nursing,* 13 (4), 159–164.

Tyler, J. M. (1995, June). The Internet: legal rights and responsibilities. *Medsurg Nursing,* 4 (3), 229–233.

Wright, K. B. (1996, June). The Internet and nursing: a vital link. *Medsurg Nursing,* 5 (3), 209–211, 203.

Yerks, A. M. (1996, January–February). The Internet and pediatric nursing: guide to the information superhighway. *Pediatric Nursing,* 22 (1), 11–15.

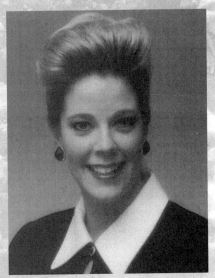

Sharon A. Brigner,

BSN, RN

Sharon A. Brigner, BSN, RN served as the National Student Nurses' Association (NSNA) President in 1996–1997, and is a recent graduate from Texas Woman's University-Houston (TWU) nursing school in Houston, Texas. During her first semester of school, Sharon was elected the Texas Nursing Students' Association President (TNSA), the following month was elected Chair of the Council of State Presidents (which is a liaison position to the NSNA Board), and the following year was elected NSNA President. Sharon credits her leadership experiences in NSNA with providing the "global picture" of nursing. In NSNA, she states she was able to learn about legislative issues, new emerging fields, and other topics that are not always discussed in the classroom.

During her education, Sharon worked part-time for a year as a student nurse professional at the Methodist Hospital Neurology and Otorhinolaryngology Intensive Care Unit in Houston, Texas. She volunteered frequently at an elderly Hispanic clinic, instructed cardiac pulmonary resuscitation (CPR) courses, and earned her certification in Advanced Cardiac Life Support (ACLS).

In her last semester of nursing school, Sharon attended the Nurse in Washington Internship where she interfaced with senators and legislators on Capitol Hill and learned how to become proactive concerning legislation that impacts nursing. This internship sparked her interest in policy making legislation.

During her senior year, she became a member of Sigma Theta Tau Honor Society (Beta Beta Chapter), Who's Who Among Students in American Universities and Colleges, and the Golden Key Honor Society.

Upon graduation in May of 1997 with a Bachelor of Science in Nursing, Sharon was hired by the National Institutes of Health Clinical Center, in Bethesda, Maryland. She will be working on the neurology unit and eventually pursue a Masters in Public Policy. Her career ambition and goal is to work in the legislative arena and public health policy process involving nursing. Sharon Brigner is now an active member of the Maryland State Nurses Association, the American Association of Neuroscience Nurses, and a sustaining member of NSNA..

CHAPTER 19

The Privilege
and Challenge
of Entering the
Profession
in Today's World

INTRODUCTION

This chapter will outline the working environment that nursing students are facing today and will provide tips and advice on preparing yourself to be a more marketable candidate. What makes this chapter unique is that it is written from my very recent perspective as a nursing student, as I graduated in the Spring of 1997. I am honored to have been approached to give my views on the profession in today's world. As the chapter continues, I will give you more information on my background, my experiences on job hunting, and many other things that I think you will find helpful as you, too, navigate the waters.

Entering the nursing profession in today's world brings us many challenges in this changing health care environment. But, along with those challenges comes a great privilege. As new nurses, we have a unique opportunity to impact the profession in many ways. The United States Department of Health and Human Services recently published a 1997 White House Briefing that stated—there are currently over two and one half million nurses in the United States, with 60 percent employed in hospitals. Thirty-two percent of the nurses are associate degree prepared, 31 percent are baccalaureate prepared, and 27 percent are diploma prepared registered nurses. It is interesting to note that in 1996, only nine percent of registered nurses were under 30 years of age. By the year 2000, it is likely that over half of the nursing workforce will be over 45 years of age, which implies that many of the new professionals are bringing varied experiences and backgrounds to the nursing arena. This diversity is a great benefit to the profession. The statistics also show that the majority of new graduates are beginning their careers in areas other than the traditional acute care centers. Community-based nursing opens up a whole new world of opportunities for the nurse in education, home care, and managed care. With the trend toward early hospital discharge, patients are now receiving highly skilled nursing care in their homes. Nurses have a whole new challenge to empower their patients with knowledge and confidence so they are capable of caring for their personal health and their loved one's health. It is the nurse's responsibility to give guidance in the delivery of that care.

With expanding work opportunities for the nurse, the new graduate is faced with more options at graduation. However, there is another challenge that the new graduate is facing. With the emphasis on cost cutting measures, hospitals are downsizing and nursing jobs are getting more competitive in the acute care centers. Many hospitals say they are not hiring new graduates because they have a large selection of experienced nurses from which to select. New graduates are now competing with experienced nurses, as well as foreign nurses, who are recruited to the hospitals from their native countries. This competitive environment forces the new graduate to be flexible and open to other work opportunities, such as the community-based home health care agencies. Many community-based health care agencies require a year of medical-surgical work experience before considering a nurse for employment. This experience is difficult for the new graduate to obtain when those jobs are limited in hospitals. However, home care agencies are exploring the development and implementation of internships for newly licensed graduates. In these internships graduates would precept with an experienced home care nurse for a few months, and then the new nurse would work independently in the role of registered nurse in the home health setting.

Employment for nurses has had distinct cycles over the years. However, in the light of managed care, many of these changes appear to be here to stay. Nurses must remain flexible and marketable as we adapt to the turbulent environment and create innovative and marketable ways to use our valuable skills. As a recent graduate from nursing school, I will share my perspective on how nursing students can maximize their potential and become competitive, cutting edge applicants for the jobs they desire.

BACKGROUND

To begin, I want to start with a bit of my history, and how I was able to be a "successful nursing student." When I was accepted into Texas Woman's University (TWU) in Houston, Texas, I was thrilled to be on my way to fulfilling my lifelong dream of being a nurse. For me, nursing is the most incredible profession because it allows the nurse to help people in a very holistic way . . . spiritually, physically, and emotionally. In my opinion, however, attending classes and clinicals did not complete the picture of nursing. I knew that there were many other places that I should and could learn different aspects of the profession on which I was embarking.

From the first day of orientation, the local nursing student organization, TWU's Texas Nursing Student's Association (TNSA), began introducing us to this world of student networking. Being a social person, I wanted to meet other students, especially ones who could shed some greatly appreciated advice on my upcoming journey through nursing school. I became involved in the local chapter, and one month later, I decided to run for TNSA President. Some students may think I was crazy for placing undue stress of a campaign on myself along with the new stresses of clinicals and class work. However, I realized that the board positions were being filled every year with nursing students who were in my exact position. I knew that this was an opportunity that would greatly enhance me as a student and future professional. After assessing my leadership qualities and realizing that I had the support and encouragement of my husband, my school, and faculty, and even my new nursing class, I vigorously prepared for my campaign.

The wonderful thing about the student nurses organization is that it is composed of many traditional and non-traditional students. As the Department of Health and Human Services verified, the definition of a traditional student now is very different from 10 years ago. So, as you can imagine, our organization was composed of men and women with a variety of ages ranging from 20 to 55 years of age. The candidates who ran for board positions were representative of this diversity.

My personal objective was to convey to the entire membership at this convention that I had many qualities to offer to the organization, driven by one definite force: A real love and enthusiasm for nursing and the desire to unite and help prepare my colleagues for our future employment. I believe that the membership saw that my motives were honest and sincere, and I was elected President of the Texas Nursing Students' Association.

This position required me to hold board meetings, assist in running conventions, represent Texas on the national level, and speak at various engagements representing nursing students. One month from the state election, I attended the National Student Nurses' Association (NSNA) convention where I ran for the office of Chair of the Council of State Presidents. The state presidents elected me to serve in this position as a liaison to the national board, while I also held the position of Texas' President. It did not take long for me to realize that my biggest challenge was the task of organization and prioritizing, which I think we can all agree is the essential component of being a nurse. Throughout that year, I learned more than I could have ever imagined. My attitude was marked by my effort to do my very best in my elected position. The membership had the confidence to place me there, and I had the duty to live up to that responsibility.

At the end of my term as state president and national board liaison, I decided to run for office again at the national level. This time, I ran for the office of president of the national organization and was elected to represent over 38,000 nursing students. Campaigning at the national level shared many similarities with the state level but was on a larger and more comprehensive scale. I had to have a national perspective, instead of only knowledge of state issues. This required extensive research on the Internet, reading journal and legislative material, attending conferences on legal and ethical issues, and studying issues with a mentor who was well informed on the current events in nursing. I had the privilege of serving as NSNA President in 1996–1997.

I encourage every student to attend a state or national convention at least once for the experience, networking, and learning opportunities. The experience of gaining that broader state or national perspective is so important. There are numerous opportunities to gain leadership experience that range from duties as a delegate, running for an elected office, or seeking an appointed office. It can also help you, as a student, begin to understand the importance of one unified voice in nursing.

All nurses must become united and share common goals, despite our differences. It was refreshing and encouraging to see this attitude displayed in the many arenas where I represented NSNA. After a year of traveling to national conferences, speaking at state conventions, and fulfilling other obligations, I ended my term without regrets and with many wonderful learning experiences that have opened many doors. Now that I have given you my organizational and educational history, I want to give you the benefits, both short- and long-term, that I reaped from my activities.

BENEFITS FROM ORGANIZATIONAL INVOLVEMENT

Today's nurse must be extremely skilled in many areas. It is not uncommon for the new graduate to be charge nurse on a nursing unit within six month's time. This job requires the nurse to have communication, leadership, and conflict management skills, all of which were essential during my terms in office. These skills are necessary on the unit and for life in general, whether you are a manager or a staff nurse. Unfortunately, school cannot provide us with multiple opportunities to learn and use these integral skills. This is where students must take responsibility for their own learning and their own career paths. We must actively seek opportunities that will provide us with those skills. The student nurses' association provided many avenues to practice the group dynamic skills of decision-making, conflict-resolution, and other leadership activities. Balancing the unique personalities and needs of a variety of individuals who comprise a board is a human relations workshop. I learned a great deal about people skills. Students need to seek these opportunities. We must not wait for someone to direct us or urge us to apply for positions. We need to take the initiative to find the right opportunity to challenge ourselves.

The second benefit of organizational involvement is knowledge of legislative issues. You may not think that politics have anything to do with you obtaining a job and advancing in your profession. This is a great misconception. Non-nursing people are making decisions about nursing daily. As the people who are being affected by *their* decisions, we should be actively involved and aware of this process. Again, the student nurses' organization educates the members on legislative issues that are influencing the profession, as well as employment trends and tips for success. This education is done on the national level through the NSNA publications titled, *Imprint* and *NSNA News,* and on the local and state level through newsletters, focus sessions held at conventions, and in many other ways that enhance our awareness of legislative issues.

Over the past two years, many students have asked me to name the single most important reason why they should spend the money for a membership fee and the precious time that they do not have to spare on a student organization. In addition to the reasons that I have already covered, there is one overriding benefit to belonging to and participating in the organization. That reason is . . . networking . . . networking . . . networking. My mentor, Dr. Lynn Wieck, always spoke to students and said that you never know when you might be sitting across the table interviewing with a person whom you have met at a convention or meeting. Her words rang true when I applied for a nursing student position in a Neurology Intensive Care Unit at a local hospital. When I entered the room for my interview with the head nurse and charge nurse, I happily recognized them both from a regional nursing organization meeting that I had attended as state president of Texas. Because we all had met a few weeks ago, they already had a preconceived notion that I was actively participating in learning about my profession and serving in a leadership position. As you can imagine, this previous encounter greatly assisted me in obtaining a position that I held for over a year.

The benefits of participating in these extracurricular activities and nursing organizations may not be realized immediately. The rewards may seem to be late in coming. You may not receive support or accolades from classmates, faculty, or family. You may not see how your energies will leave you with anything but less time to study for that crucial test. But I guarantee you that I have seen organizational involvement benefit *Every* student who has participated in it, one way or another, whether they were an officer or an active member in the association.

As you continue to develop as a leader, it is important that you learn to grow from constructive criticism. Part of becoming a better leader, nurse, spouse, and person is to be able to be open to other's advice and perceptions and turn it into something useful and beneficial. At the same time, it is important to take this guidance with a grain of salt in some instances, for criticism can also be nonconstructive. We must realize that not everyone will agree with us in life. However, you can use other's negative, as well as positive, words of advice to your advantage by choosing which battles to fight and giving your best effort when you believe the effort is worth it.

BENEFITS OF WORK EXPERIENCE

Another important component of my growth in nursing school was the opportunity to work part-time as a student nurse in the hospital setting. For me, this time was very valuable and rich in learning experiences. The difference in the quality of learning in the work setting versus the clinical school setting is that in the work setting you do not have the anxiety of having to complete care plans, review charts, or prepare for an instructor to come by to quiz you on the history of your patient. When I worked, it was strictly my time to learn what I wanted to cover. I believe that I am a self-directed, independent learner. I found that by setting weekly objectives, I was able to articulate to my preceptor exactly what I wanted to learn. One of my weak student clinical areas was the process of medication delivery. It would take me over 15 minutes to gather the drugs, research the medicine in the drug book, and prepare to deliver them to my patients. Because I worked on an eight bed intensive care unit, I was able to plan time into my daily work schedule and would pre-arrange with my preceptor for me to go through the motions of planning, looking up adverse reactions, and dosage information for the medications that her patients would receive that day. After a few months of this educational ritual, I found that I easily surpassed the required objectives that were outlined in my university's clinical syllabus. I also learned a tremendous amount of pharmacology that assisted me throughout the remainder of my education. It was a boost to my self-confidence to become accustomed and comfortable with the medication delivery process.

It is interesting to note that it became clearly evident to both students and instructors which of us were working part-time and which were not. I am not sure if it was the new sense of assurance they displayed, the decrease in their anxiety when performing new procedures, or a healthy invincible attitude that caught other's attention. But, I do know that working as a student nurse was a positive adjunct to my education process.

By working on the unit, I learned valuable communication skills with patients, co-workers, and managers. In clinical settings, students often miss out on the feeling of being part of a team. Due to time constraints and role expectations, our work with the unit nurses never seemed to feel like it resulted in a mutual, giving relationship to me. However, when I began working part-time, I experienced that rewarding feeling of team work from collectively working towards a goal. There were many patient situations that I would have missed if I had not been employed as a student nurse. It was difficult, with shorter hospital stays, to experience the full diversity of patient problems needed to get a "real world" picture of nursing. Professors agree that to a large extent, nursing cannot be taught to us solely in the classroom but must be learned and experienced with a hands-on approach. From the beginning of school,

I had heard from advanced level students and professors how important it is to work while you are in school. During the first year, I desperately wanted to excuse myself from working because I was spending so much time with association duties and activities. However, it is a fact that while organizational involvement builds self-confidence and leadership skills, it does not help build your clinical confidence on the unit with your patients. Because clinical exposure is necessarily limited during school, students must assume some responsibility for becoming competent professional nurses. Therefore, it is reassuring that students can actively take steps to enhance their clinical skills outside of the school realm.

In today's work environment, one of the most important benefits to working is gaining experience to cite on your résumé. That was clearly illustrated by my recent job hunting experiences. When I began calling human resource departments throughout the country to inquire about staff nurse positions for new graduates, over three-fourths of the institutions stated that they would only accept applications and interview experienced nurses. However, many quickly mentioned that they would be willing to consider new graduates who had a history of work experience throughout school. I encourage all nursing students to work, even if it is just one weekend a month, so that they can boost skills, clinical knowledge, and confidence.

One option currently being discussed on a national level is the development of nursing externship/internship programs. State boards of nursing, nursing colleges, and various health care and home care facilities are collaborating in the discussion. It is essential that nursing students are also granted a voice in the development of such programs.

ENHANCING MARKETABILITY

As I have mentioned, I just finished interviewing for my first nursing job. When people ask me when I started preparing for interviews and getting serious about my job hunt, I reply that I started during my first month of nursing school. The simple fact is that you must start preparing for that job as soon as possible, because you are competing for jobs with highly qualified nurses, as well as new graduates who bring a wealth of past professional experiences with them. Your résumé makes a much stronger statement about your commitment to nursing if all of your accomplishments, volunteer, and/or leadership activities have not taken place exclusively during your last semester of nursing school.

When we started nursing school, many of us were told that the academics of nursing school would be our greatest challenge, and that we should keep our activities and social life to a minimum. But, I believe that it is possible to volunteer, work, attend conventions, run for office, do well in school and grades, and maintain a family life. I did, however, have to release the obsession to make a 4.0 GPA. This ability to accept less than perfection is a great challenge to the high-achievement type people who accept the challenge of becoming a nurse. I went on my intuition and on guidance that by working on many aspects of my career preparation, I would benefit more in the long-run than if I solely concentrated on grades. That was the single most valuable piece of advice that I had received throughout school. I guarantee that the employers today do not think of a successful student as one who has achieved a 4.0 GPA. Instead they seek potential employees who have accomplished a holistic, well-rounded set of achievements that cannot be exclusively defined within a grade point average. Please do not think that employers do not value class achievement. They do. The employers with whom I have recently interviewed did want me to have at least a 3.0 GPA before they would even interview me. In addition, I personally realized that I needed to achieve above average grades so that I could learn the material for the National Council Licensure Examination for Registered Nurses (NCLEX), which is the national standardized test for licensure. In summary, it is absolutely essential for you to have well rounded achievements to add to your marketability.

The first step is to start analyzing your career path with the method that we all use, the nursing process. Assess your resources. I suggest finding those faculty members who are willing to provide guidance and direction. Observe, listen, and learn from them. So many students feel that there is a barrier between them and their teachers. I feel that we must overcome the "we-they" stigma and realize that after nursing school, we will be among them as colleagues. There are those faculty who perpetuate the separatist image and make it difficult to develop a rapport outside of the classroom. However, it has been my predominant experience that there are more faculty who are willing to help and motivate students in and outside of the classroom. To illustrate my point, I will relay my personal experience and explain how I used my resources to my advantage.

I feel that it is important to seek a mentor and a role model. I was blessed to have discovered my mentor, role model, and friend in a faculty member during the first month of school. Dr. Lynn Wieck is a precise nurse clinician, innovative thinker, eternal optimist, and admirable leader, serving as the Vice-President in the state organization, Texas Nurses Association. When I first met her, I realized that Dr. Wieck possessed qualities I desired and she had a wealth of information that she was willing to share. She inspires students to believe that they can do and be whatever they want if they put their minds to it. During my first semester, I went to Dr. Wieck and explained that I desired to be involved in the state student nurses' association. I asked for her input on whether she felt I would be able to handle school, clinicals, and this extra responsibility. She provided me with facts, and honesty, encouraging me with each of my goals. When I speak to student groups, I cannot stress enough how valuable it is to have a trusted faculty member to consult with during your student life. In my situation, my positions required a great deal of travel. There were times that she was able to intercede on my behalf to the other faculty members. Because of our relationship, I was able to apply for scholarships and extracurricular organizations and societies that required a recommendation from a faculty member who knew me well. In return, I volunteered for her elderly clinic that she had founded and assisted her in any way possible. When she needed help at meetings or events, I was there, attempting to return all of the benefits that I was gaining from her. Even at this early stage in my career, I was learning how to be collegial and how to network. Now that I have graduated, I continue to admire Dr. Wieck and her accomplishments. This personal story of mentorship was meant to convey the importance of fostering a relationship with a faculty member that can help you throughout your career, even after graduation.

I firmly believe that mentors are in each and every educational facility; however, it is up to us as students to seek out and utilize the many resources that we have available to us. Your friends might accuse you of trying to get close to a teacher, otherwise known as "brown-nosing." My philosophy is . . . what is wrong with finding a professional individual with whom you can relate, learn, grow, and receive valuable direction? You will have to make personal decisions when you apply for a job, ask for written recommendations, and plan your career. Why not make a personal decision to begin a collegial relationship with more experienced nurses early in your career. It is up to you to seize control of your destiny and future. I feel these tips can help you do just that.

Some additional steps assisted me with my development as a nursing student. I created a mission statement during nursing school. This statement includes your reasons for entering nursing, goals, personal philosophies, and overall vision for your nursing leadership. Examples of potential goals and objectives might include: (1) completion of nursing education with a masters or doctoral degree; (2) turning every problem into an opportunity to succeed; (3) refusing to quit in the face of diversity; or (4) getting that certain job you always wanted.

It is also important to make one, two, five, and ten year strategic plans. It is essential to develop goals because there are many things that we all want to accomplish, and it can be difficult to put them in perspective. You can list your short-term and long-term goals and mix them with your dreams and aspirations. Put it in a visible place and refer to it at regular times throughout the year to see if you are actively taking steps to accomplish your plan. If you find that you are not being successful at completing some of your goals, do something about it. If you are not constantly working and evaluating how you are making yourself a more marketable applicant for that job, you need to do something about it immediately. Obviously, you cannot always be successful in everything all of the time throughout nursing school, but you can find out what you can do better.

Finally, surround yourself with positive people. It is intriguing how people start talking and acting like those with whom they spend the most time. If you find yourself around people who act negatively and are bitter and disillusioned about the profession, you will find that you and your dreams will be smothered. Surround yourself with other dreamers, achievers, and optimists.

JOB-SEEKING EXPERIENCE

The highlight of serving as President of NSNA was having my eyes opened to the numerous, diverse opportunities for nurses today. By meeting and speaking with individuals who are making new paths in our profession, it inspired me to do just that. The one thing that they all had in common was that they coupled their strong attributes, their interests, and love for nursing with creating an innovative niche for themselves. Because I am fascinated with legislative issues, my long-term career aspiration is to obtain a master's degree in public policy and work in the political arena for nursing. Therefore, I decided it would be best to relocate to the Washington, DC area and begin my nursing career in the region in which I would like to eventually study and work. To make sure that I was exploring all options and gaining experience with the interview process, I decided to seriously interview in both my hometown, as well as the northeastern region of Baltimore, Bethesda, and Washington, DC.

About five months before I began contacting nurse recruiters, I worked diligently on refining and updating my résumé for distribution. Résumé writing may not be covered extensively in your nursing school, but you do have avenues to making it your most important asset. I would suggest visiting the library and using reference books and Internet information to find out what is expected and what is discouraged on today's résumé. Once I compiled a fairly complete and refined résumé, I gave it to a few of my professors for their opinions and constructive criticism. You will also want to speak to nurse recruiters and get their viewpoints on writing a résumé and what they feel should and should not be included. You will probably have several different versions of your résumé if you are applying for various positions that would require elaboration on certain components of your experience. Update your résumé continually, using the finest quality of paper and print on your final draft. Again, you should refer to your job placement division at your school to assist you with information on cover letters, résumé tips, and interview guidance.

MAKE A LIST

Before you start your job search, evaluate and make a list of the things that are important for you to have in your first job. I had definite views on the kind of institution in which I wanted to begin my career. Do not have the attitude that it is only for a year, so if you do not like it, you can leave. Before it gets to that point, do yourself a favor and research the facility, their mission statement, the workers and their views on their workplace, as well as the management philosophy. I personally attended seminars of various institutions, researched the Internet, visited with employees of different hospitals, and attended state nurse association meetings to meet those who were working in the institution. This information is valuable to know for your interview as well.

Orientation

First, I wanted my first job to have a sufficient orientation time, so that I could get acclimated to the environment as well as the patient workload. We all know how uneasy we feel the first few times on a new unit of our clinical rotation. It takes time and experience to feel competent and familiar. Until we reach that level, we are not performing at our maximum. Therefore, I felt that this was extremely important to have a few weeks of preceptorship and orientation before I accepted full patient assignments and all of the expectations that come with it.

Management Style and Philosophy

Second, I looked at the employer's management style and philosophy. During my educational period, I had grown accustomed and enjoyed the shared governance form of management. This style empowers staff nurses to give input, participate, and be involved in decision-making levels that affect the workplace. Upon graduation, I knew that I did not want to just put my time in on the nursing unit. Instead, I wanted to contribute to the institution and to my co-workers. Another important pre-requisite was for my nurse manager to support advanced education and obtaining of higher degrees. I also looked at the availability of tuition reimbursement from the employer.

Unit Climate

Finally, I wanted to observe the unit climate, including the interaction between the nurses and other interdisciplinary teams on the floor. On one of my interviews, part of the interview was a four hour "share day" that I (the interviewee) spent on the unit in scrubs. I was not able to work or assist in procedures but was assigned to a preceptor who oriented me to the unit and hospital protocols and answered my questions about the unit. This time was equally beneficial to the nurse manager who received a report of my knowledge and adaptability to the unit. If you do not have an opportunity to spend some time on the unit or floor for which you are interviewing, I suggest that you request such a time. To my surprise, I actually changed my opinion about the units at the end of my share day. I had finished the interviews and tour by the nurse manager and had distinctly preferred one unit over the other almost immediately. However, after four hours among the patients and staff and after collecting detailed information from the preceptor, I reversed my work-site preference.

THE NEXT STEP

To enhance my job search, I researched and compiled a list of all of the hospitals that were located in the vicinities in which I would consider relocation. I then called the human resource department in each hospital. This endeavor was one of the most challenging components of my search because it was extremely difficult to speak with a nurse recruiter. In many cases, even though I asked, the secretaries would not just mail an application or give their fax number so that I might fax my résumé . It takes a lot of persistence to kindly ask the secretary to have the recruiter return your call. Once you make contact with the nurse recruiter, the next hurdle is to convince him or her that you are not an average new nursing graduate. At this point, I had to sell myself and my experience to the recruiters so that they would at least consider my application and possibly offer an interview. This need to sell yourself is precisely why I would suggest doing all of the above in person, if at all possible.

An interesting event occurred in my job search. I was having difficulty getting a nurse recruiter from a particular hospital to return my calls. Ironically, I met her the following week at an exhibitor's booth at the student national convention where she was advertising for the hospital. After we had a moment to speak and make personal contact, she immediately set up an interview time for the following week. I interviewed and received a job offer. This incident is another perfect illustration of how networking in our pre-professional organizations proves beneficial.

The types of interviews you encounter may be distinctly different depending upon the region of the country. Upon speaking to many of my colleagues, I found that they also had distinct experiences. One clear difference was the line of questions that I was asked by the human resource personnel and the nurse managers. In one region, the questions were strictly the traditional topics of your past experience, attributes, and goals for the future. In other regions, the questions included the previously mentioned topics with additional, specific, technical questions. These technical questions were similar to sample N-CLEX questions that we would see. They ranged from explaining what a physician's orders would state for a particular patient, to effects of certain medications, to arranging a prioritized list of patients you would visit first on your rounds. I did not expect to have so many detailed technical questions. Therefore, when you are preparing for your interviews, scan the Internet for interview questions. I found that extremely helpful for my interviews. Your school or university will probably have a job placement center that offers advice, free videotaping, and other valuable tools to use in preparation.

Here are some of the questions that I received at some of my interviews:

1. Tell me about yourself.
2. What is an example of your worst failure in life, and how did you cope with it?
3. What is an example of a clinical situation where you had a conflict with a fellow worker, and how did you solve it?
4. What is an example of a conflict with a boss or superior, and how did you solve it?
5. What role do you expect a nurse manager to play on the unit?

6. Where do you see yourself in the next 5 years? 15 years?

7. How do you think starting nursing on this unit will help you achieve your goals?

8. What was your best clinical rotation during school and why? Your worst rotation and why?

9. How do you handle stress in your life? What are your coping mechanisms?

10. What was your most difficult course in school?

11. Do you feel that your grades are indicative of your performance or knowledge level?

12. Why did you choose nursing?

13. What do you plan to do this first year of work in your personal life? volunteer? (where) organizations?

14. What is cardiac output?

15. What are the six rights of medication administration?

16. What are some uses of Epinephrine, and what other drugs have you used in your clinical practice?

17. A 58-year-old small bowel obstructed male walks in the emergency room and is in great pain. What do the doctor's orders look like exactly? (They wanted to know that you would see an order for NG tube for distention relief, a KUB stat to visualize the obstruction, an antacid, an anti-anxiety medication, and probably much more.)

18. You are a nurse coming on shift, and you have four patients that need immediate attention. Tell me which ones you would see in an exact order, and why you selected that order. I will not repeat the case scenarios. You have a patient who needs pre-operative medications and is due for surgery in a half hour, a patient that is sputtering and having difficulty breathing, a head injury patient that is flailing around and very restless and unrestrained and not oriented, and a patient who is vomiting and in great GI distress. (After I gave the order of visits and why, she then asked me what physician orders I might see and how I would quickly assess and treat each of the four patients.)

19. Why would a patient be getting hemodynamically unstable and what would some signs and symptoms be? What would you do to treat it?

20. Why did you choose to get certified in Advanced Cardiac Life Support?

21. What are four qualities that you feel a nurse must possess? why?

22. What four qualities do you have that would make you a proficient nurse?

23. How do you feel about unlicensed personnel that serve as nurse technicians in the hospital?

24. How would you evaluate the competency of assistive personnel on tasks you are delegating?

25. Tell me about your organizational/prioritizing skills.

26. How do you prepare for your day once you have received report?

27. What area of your nursing skills do you feel most deficient in and feel will need the most work?

28. What area of your nursing skills do you feel will be your greatest strength?

29. How would your instructor describe you in a few words? your classmates? your patients?

30. What is your greatest challenge as you make the transition from nursing student to registered nurse?

31. What frightens you about the transition?

32. How would you deal with a physician who began publicly and loudly criticizing your performance, saying derogatory statements to your face?

33. What do you expect or what are you looking for in your first job?

34. What do you think about policy and procedure?

35. Do you think that you should have a different or greater scope of responsibilities if you have a bachelor's degree or specialty certification? How do you think your education has prepared you for a leadership role?

36. Do you believe in teamwork in an ICU setting?

37. Do you have any interest in participating in committee meetings or hospital projects or assignments?

38. What kind of scheduling do you prefer? (self-staff scheduling or manager scheduling)

39. What did you like most about your boss in your student professional nurse job? Least about your boss?

40. How would you approach your boss if you felt that she/he was ignoring an unethical or unprofessional activity on the unit and you disagreed with how it was being handled?

41. What type of management style do you like best?

42. When you are working in a group, what role do you take? (facilitator, peacemaker, . . .)

43. Who was your favorite nursing theorist and why?

44. What type of nursing do you like best? (team, primary)

45. Do you have a copy of the nurse practice act of this state?

46. Have you contacted the state board as to how you will receive reciprocity? If so, what did they say were the requirements?

47. What is your motto in life?

48. What is the motto or mission statement of this institution basically about?

49. And finally, (my favorite zinger of all) . . . "We have not hired a new graduate in the past four and a half years. We simply do not need to, because we have a great selection from experienced nurses out there. Why should we consider you and what could you offer?"

In summary, be as informed as possible as you prepare to interview. First impressions are your only impressions when applying for a job and you want to feel confident and prepared.

PREPARING FOR LICENSURE

Every nursing student throughout the country will take the national standardized exam for the registered nurse licensure. It will matter, however, how you prepare for the exam. There are a variety of review books, courses, computer disks, audio tapes, and more available for your preparation. Evaluate your self-discipline, finances, and the methods of studying that work best for you. I am an auditory and visual learner. I felt that I needed some encouragement and discipline to review over two year's worth of material. So, for me, I benefitted greatly from a four day review course, audio tapes to listen to in the car and computer disk simulated questions. Whatever your preference, you should remember that preparation will help decrease anxiety. It is only natural that everyone will have a certain degree of anxiety upon taking this exam that leads to nursing licensure. I intensely reviewed, on my own, for the entire week before the exam date that I had scheduled. After I took the exam, I felt that the process was convenient and quick to complete on the computer. My reviews gave me the assurance to take the test confidently. If you ask any nurse who has taken the exam over five years ago, you will feel greatly relieved that we do not go through a rigorous two-day, paper and pencil examination with results that took many months to receive.

I applied for state licensure in Texas before I had made the decision to move. Therefore, I immediately had to contact the state board of my new home to inquire about the requirements and the procedure for application in that state. Each state has certain rules and regulations on receiving licensure, as well as how to receive reciprocity. Reciprocity is the permission to receive a license and privilege to work in a state other than the state of your original license. So if you are planning to move, I suggest that you find the number of the state board in that particular state. Also important for you to know, some states will allow new graduates from nursing school to begin working immediately after graduation as a graduate nurse. Other states require a current license in hand before you can work. Most state boards of nursing phone numbers are listed in the government pages of the telephone directory.

SUMMARY

One of my goals for this chapter was to share with you my personal thoughts about the steps needed to be a successful nursing student and competitive applicant in the job market of today's world. It is my hope that you, the reader, might be able to adapt some of my philosophies in your own career path.

Remember, organizational involvement is a lifelong commitment for the registered nurse. Wherever you get your first job, seek out the state nurses association and get acquainted and involved. The challenge and the privilege of professional nursing are one and the same—the opportunity to provide quality nursing to the public as a health care provider. Together as nursing's future leaders, we move forward into the next century empowered to get involved and make a difference!

CRITICAL THINKING QUESTIONS

1. What are your positive attributes and talents? How can you communicate those on a job interview?
2. What are your one, five, and ten year goals? academically, personally, and professionally?
3. There are many leadership opportunities available to you as a nursing student. What are your short-term and long-term goals while in nursing school to capitalize on those opportunities?
4. What do the headlines in today's paper mean to nurses and health care consumers? Do they impact you as a nursing student? If so, how?
5. What employment opportunities are available to nursing students in your community? Are there any summer internships you can apply for? (See your faculty advisor for suggestions of where to go for information.)

ACTIVITIES

1. Subscribe to a nursing journal or go to a local library and read a journal every month to become familiar with the nursing issues and occurrences within the profession. I suggest the *American Journal of Nursing, Imprint* (NSNA Publication), and *Nursing '97.*
2. Join the National Student Nurses' Association and get involved at the school chapter, state level, and national level. Attend local, state, or national student nurses meetings or any career fairs available to you so that you can learn more about the endless opportunities in your profession.(Information on NSNA available at 212-581-2211.)

3. If you have a particular area of interest in a nursing specialty, join the nursing association at a student rate and enjoy benefits of the organization such as journals, conventions, and networking with those individuals within that specialty.

ADDITIONAL SUGGESTED READINGS

Kelly, L. Y., & Joel, L. A. (1995). *Dimensions of Professional Nursing* (7th ed.). New York: McGraw-Hill.

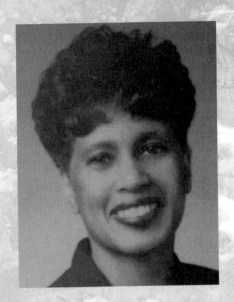

Beverly L. Malone,

PhD, RN, FAAN

Beverly Malone is currently serving a two-year-term as President of the American Nurses Association (ANA). ANA is the nation's leading professional organization representing the major health care, practice, and work place issues of the nation's two million registered nurses. Dr. Malone is on leave of absence from her role as professor at the School of Nursing at North Carolina Agricultural and Technical State University, in Greensboro.

In North Carolina, Dr. Malone has served on the Governor's Task Force on the Nursing Shortage; commissioner of the North Carolina Commission on Health Services; vice-chair of the Board of Trustees, Moses Cone Health System; Board of Directors of the Adolescent Pregnancy Prevention Program; and President of the North Carolina Council of Baccalaureate Deans and Directors.

In her clinical career, she has worked as a surgical staff nurse, clinical nurse specialist, director of nursing, and assistant administrator of nursing. Dr. Malone is also a licensed Clinical Psychologist. Since she began her presidency in 1996, Dr. Malone has been appointed to President Clinton's Advisory Commission on Consumer Protection and Quality in the Health Care Industry and its Quality Measurements Subcommittee. Dr. Malone is an exceptional, motivating speaker and long-time advocate of leadership development of nursing students.

Dr. Beverly Malone extends her gratitude to Jan Jones Schenk, MNA, RN, CNA for her valued assistance on the chapter.

CHAPTER 20

Career Mapping: Visioning Your Future

INTRODUCTION

"What we call the beginning is often the end. And to make an end is to make a beginning. The end is where we start from." T. S. Eliot

There is an abundance of talk around organizations these days about the importance of vision and values to organizational success. Personal success has the same formula. Recent research on why college-bound students choose nursing confirms some beliefs we have had and confirms nursing as a good path for fulfilling those stated needs: "those who chose nursing cited the desire to help people, to do important work, and to work with a variety of people" (Tomey, Shwier, Martiche, & May, 1996, p. 28). These are basic values that may direct a career in nursing. But, what are the personal values that are individually important in one's work, and how do they come together with competencies, trends, and networking to create a personal career vision? In this chapter, we will explore the components of successful career mapping. In this discussion, career mapping is a process of converging personal skills, knowledge, and values into an individual strategy.

As we evaluate information on trends in health care and market forces affecting nurses and nursing careers, we are challenged to look to career mapping as a plan for proactively managing not just careers but also personal fulfillment. This is not just about planning a career in nursing but about bringing who we are to what we do. If vision is the world we want to create and values are the beliefs we honor as we reach out to the world, then it is individual values that create the unique practice pattern of each nurse (Koerner, 1996). We must start with values to make the map.

VALUES

". . . follow your bliss." Joseph Campbell

We start by clarifying those core qualities that give meaning to life. What are those qualities or aspects of human life that have worth for us? It is sometimes helpful to start with a list of ideas and beliefs that describe what we believe and what we want to demonstrate to others through personal example. Values are truly "words to live by." They express our deepest beliefs about ourselves and our relationships with others. One way to begin is by asking why. Why did I choose nursing? You might answer, "I chose nursing because I want to work with people." Why do you want to work with people? "I want to work with people because I enjoy the learning I experience when I get to know someone else's situation." Why is the learning important? "The things I learn help me to be more effective with other people I work with." Why? The exercise can continue as long as new information surfaces. There are no right or wrong answers, only personal truths about why you do what you do. The why exercise helps to hone in on the meaning you are able to gain from your nursing life. There are many personal values inventories available to assist in self-assessment. You may wish to use the list of values printed at the end of this chapter as a starting point for your own journey to enhanced self-knowledge (Cavouras, & Eddy, 1996). Experiencing self-understanding is the first step toward clarifying personal work values to use in career mapping.

IMPORTANCE

"It is not critical that your values be fulfilled via your work environment. What is important to your happiness and well-being is that your work environment not be eliminating the fulfillment of any of those values which are truly important to you." Art Schwartz

At a recent retreat, our group leader had us identify 15 core values as a prelude to strategic planning (a process not unlike career planning). Each of us made our choices very carefully. We thoughtfully examined the list before us, generated some of our own "values words," and held each up for careful examination of how it fit or was reflected in our lives. After several grueling minutes, we each had our personal list of absolute values. Then the group leader said, "We're going on a trip and the airplane will only hold 10 values for each of you. You must now choose only 10 of your original 15 values." We were indignant! Surely she knew these were our absolute values. How could we possibly narrow such an important and inclusive list down to 10? We argued that it couldn't be done . . . . . and she gave us five minutes to do it. Another careful, deliberate but quicker process was undertaken by each member of the group as we each discarded five of the things that just minutes before made our lives "worth living." "Now," said the group leader, "we're on the plane and it's overloaded. We'll crash if we don't throw some things out. Each person choose your top five values and throw the rest out!"

Now this story serves to point out a few lessons about values. Obviously there isn't some magic number of absolute values for each person. But, when we prioritize our values, we clarify how they fit into our lives. That clarity can be a powerful step in planning. When pushed by other circumstances (like the pretend scenario of a plane crash), we can and must identify those values that we won't discard. This ability to prioritize is useful in all stages of career planning. It helps initially to choose directions, but it also serves well during times of change and chaos when roles and expectations change, sometimes quickly and arbitrarily. While a career choice may not fulfill all your values, it is important to know what aspects if any may violate or conflict with your values. This requires a willingness to reassess, maintain a personal connection with your values, and to know how to prioritize.

VISIONING

"All things are created twice. There's a mental or first creation, and a physical or second creation to all things." Stephen R. Covey

Once you know the why and the importance or order of magnitude of certain values in your professional life, you can begin the step of creating your own preferred future. Covey talks about the "mental creation" as the essential step toward achieving or enacting that vision (Covey, 1989). Creating the vision requires personal courage and commitment. If you can envision it, it can happen but only if you are willing to measure the differences between the realities of today and the requirements of the vision. For example, if you were to envision yourself as a nurse researcher but you had no research skills and made no place in your career map to obtain those skills, the vision is empty. In making a career vision, the first step is self-assessment. Self-assessment is difficult and time-consuming, but without it, achievement of your goals is unlikely.

What are the skills, abilities, and competencies you have developed thus far? Reflect on some of your personal achievements in other areas of your life. What were those achievements? What skills did you use to accomplish the goals?

Use this *List of Skills and Competencies* to help you identify your personal strengths:

Advocate	Design	Lead	Plan
Assess	Document	Listen	Prioritize
Analyze	Evaluate	Make Decisions	Reading Information
Articulate	Empathize	Maintain Records	Research
Budget	Expedite	Make Arrangements	Sell/Market
Communicate	Edit	Manage	Studying/Learning
Critical Thinking	Follow Through	Motivate	Supervise
Coordinate	Interview	Mediate	Teach
Coach	Implement	Monitor	Visualize
Delegate	Initiate Change	Organize	Write

(Adapted from *Developing Your Nursing Career: A Working Guide* by the Arizona Nurses Association)

Have the strengths you've identified from other experiences in your life also proven beneficial to you as a nursing student? Typically you will find that the strengths you have utilized in other aspects of your life are the same strengths that have brought you success as a nursing student. The skills assessment also may clarify areas that aren't well developed for future learning.

In 1995 as part of the *Pathway Evaluation Program for Nursing Professionals,* Glaxo, Inc., identified twenty important aspects of the practice of nursing. Prioritization of each of these critical factors offers yet another opportunity to assess how one might plan and choose a career path.

The twenty aspects are:

_____ Patient contact
_____ Continuity of relationships
_____ Colleague relationships
_____ Interacting with a team
_____ Status among colleagues
_____ Patient education
_____ Innovative thinking
_____ Autonomy
_____ Accountability
_____ Social responsibility

_____ Manual activities
_____ Technology
_____ Work schedule
_____ Pressure
_____ Diversity of activities
_____ Focus of expertise
_____ Sense of accomplishment
_____ Opportunity for advancement
_____ Job security
_____ Income/Benefits

When you rate each aspect on a scale of one to ten, it becomes more clear what aspects of a role may create personal satisfaction or dissatisfaction. For example, if you really enjoy manual activities and focus of expertise, a good match might be infusion therapy or a career in specialized procedures such as Cardiac Procedures Lab.

If patient education and patient contact are high on your list, perhaps a long-range plan for a career in diabetes or chronic disease management would be satisfying. For those that prefer autonomy and lots of accountability, advanced practice nursing would be a good choice.

TRENDS

Having identified personal values, a preferred vision, and a self-assessment, the next step is to consider industry trends and career options. Nursing is a highly diverse field with many options. The four traditional categories of nursing careers—clinical, education, research, and administration—have become even more rich as health care has become more complex. In 1996 the United States Bureau of Labor Statistics compiled a list of top nursing jobs:

1. Advanced practice nursing
2. Case management
3. Home health
4. Gerontological nursing
5. Traveling/temporary nursing

Each of these nursing careers has an obvious similarity, all require ongoing continuing education and a strong basic knowledge base. While only the APRN requires an advanced degree today, it is likely that both case management and gerontological nursing will require increased education in the future. Additionally, in this information age, the Department of Labor estimates that by the year 2000 the most highly prized of all workers' skills will be in competencies related to the gathering, processing, retrieving, or analyzing of information. Nurses who combine the expertise of one of the top demand job areas above with increased data competencies through the use of technology will greatly increase their employability (Cavouras, 1996).

CERTIFICATION

Achieving and maintaining certification is a public demonstration that a nurse has achieved mastery of his or her chosen area of practice. Professional certification is an important step in career mapping for both personal empowerment and public acknowledgment. Certification not only validates competence but demonstrates professional commitment, enhances career opportunities, and demonstrates a kind of self-regulation that is the hallmark of a profession (Styles, 1997). Certified nurses must meet certain criteria that include an educational requirement (these vary depending on the certifying agency and the type of certification being sought), practice requirement, evidence of continuing education, and clinical leadership. There are many voluntary credentialing organizations throughout the country, but the largest is the American Nurses Credentialing Center. ANCC offers 27 different exams from generalist to specialist in all areas of practice. As health care continues to transform itself, there is an ever greater need for ways for consumers to identify and evaluate competency, skill, and in quality in both providers and organizations. Nurses who are "Board Certified" by ANCC or any of the other accredited credentialing organizations will increasingly be seen as safe, high quality, highly competent providers.

NETWORKING

One frequently overlooked but highly effective career strategy is networking. Members of National Student Nurses' Association are already developing a professional network that will ensure personal exposure to new ideas and new opportunities. After graduation, participation in the American Nurses Association and pertinent specialty groups is an essential beginning to the development of a lifelong career network that provides personal support, information, and contacts—all necessary for a career to flourish. Such affiliations also provide opportunity for personal growth and the development of new skills that are useful and transferrable to the workplace. The American Nurses Association offers many volunteer leadership opportunities that serve the organization and also provide personal development for those who step forward to actively participate. The best place to begin this important affiliation is with your State Nurses Association. SNA committees and activities are focused on service to members but also help to create linkages between nurses from all settings within the community. These linkages, like all long-term relationships, need nurturance. But, there is no more powerful tool in times of need (whether the need is for advice, support, or information) than well-established and nourished professional relationships.

One often overlooked aspect of networking is the need to network with other professionals in other disciplines (Vicenzi, White, & Begun, 1997). The trend in patient-care management is toward interdisciplinary planning and care provision. Being able to effectively work with other types of professionals is an essential survival skill in todays' environment. This sort of networking requires some personal "stretching." As Vicenzi describes it, ". . . listening to others' interpretations and discussing issues amplifies your knowledge, because the diversity in the backgrounds of team members enhances the possibilities for 'frame breaking, innovative thinking, and discovery'" (Vicenzi, 1997, p. 29). Once again there are personal benefits to be gained from a career perspective in developing a broader base of relationships.

A final networking consideration is the value of building a personal, community-based network. Whether it is through a community service organization, community-based health organization, the public schools, or the city council, nurses have unique knowledge that is often overlooked in public dialogue at the community level. The relationships developed through working on community projects provide another source of information, knowledge, and support from neighbors who share a commitment to the community you share. From a larger perspective, nurses become more visible and our message is heard in places and in ways that can have a more significant local impact.

MENTORING

As stated in Unit 4, traditional mentoring involves a relationship between two individuals with different levels of power and authority. The more senior, powerful member of the organization becomes a coach or guide to the less powerful member moving up the nursing career ladder within the organization. Most nurses have had limited experience with mentoring. Yet recently, the concept of preceptoring has served as an example of an assigned mentor protégé relationship. However, mentoring relationships are usually intense and require great emotional investment by both the mentor and protégé.

The mentor sees something in the protégé that she or he likes and perhaps reminds the mentor of her or himself. It is the generativity of the best of one's life that the mentor frequently gains from a mentoring relationship. The protégé is moved to the fast-track of an organization and learns to lead with the safety net of her or his mentor. With the mentor's support, the student learns to risk. Without risk-taking, there is no creativity and no leadership.

Mentoring is an essential element of preparing nurse leaders. Every nursing student who wants to be a leader should have a mentor or be involved in a search process for a mentor. The following is recommended when searching for a mentor:

1. Be visible. Let prospective mentors know that you are looking for a mentor. Let them also know you bring creative skills, talents, and abilities.
2. Choose and approach your potential mentor.
3. Give in return.

Mentors are frequently in need of assistance, such as research assistants, a sounding board, or a general helper. Be ready to give back to the mentor.

FROM HERE TO THERE: A PRESIDENT'S PERSPECTIVE

My road to the Presidency of the American Nurses Association must have started with the beloved attention of my family. There were so many of us that any one of us who could hold everyone's attention was rewarded. This affinity for attention was displayed and nurtured in the Baptist Church as the congregation allowed a four-year-old to summarize the Sunday School lesson while they attentively listened. This experience provided my first external applause outside of my family.

My mentors were at every crossroad and decision-making point along the way. Miss Addie, my great grandmother, Ms. Eleanor Douglas, my sixth grade English teacher, Ms. Sadie Tate, fourth grade math and Ms. Martin, fifth grade English. They were all committed to my growth and development as a future leader.

After graduating from my undergraduate program at the University of Cincinnati, I attended Rutgers the State University in the graduate adult psychiatric nursing program chaired by Dr. Hildagard Peplau. This was a critical event. During that time, Dr. Peplau was President of the American Nurses Association. I had my first reality-based vision of being president. She exposed her graduate students to campaigning. The politics and power of nursing unfolded right before my eyes. At that point I realized my attraction to the idea of being President of ANA in the future.

The years following my graduate studies were filled with marriage, children, clinical practice, and various roles as a clinical nurse specialist, director of nursing, and assistant administrator. I also acquired a doctoral degree in clinical psychology. Even during these busy years, I was involved at my district and state level of ANA.

With the strong support of state nursing leaders, I progressed to the elected position of Vice-President of the Ohio Nurses Association. My career path seemed simple. The next step would be President of the Ohio Nurses Association and from there to the national level with the eventual outcome—President of ANA. Dorothy Cornelius, past president of both ANA and the International Council of Nursing had discussed with me these possibilities.

However, due to an academic career move, I relocated to Greensboro, North Carolina. Not surprisingly, my North Carolina colleagues were not anxious to re-order their line-up of committed nurses who had been prepared for state and national leadership positions. I had to move to the back of the line.

With a sense of urgency, I went back to work at the district level in North Carolina. Within a two-year-period, I ran for my first national office, the ANA Board of Directors. In a six-year-period, I ran for national office three times, twice as a Director-At-Large and once for Second Vice-President. Each win built a wider base of recognition and acceptance. These campaigns, which were eagerly anticipated by my children, became models for planning and implementation when working with large groups. My fourth successful national campaign was for President of ANA.

The winning ingredients seem to consist of excellent leadership for management of the campaign; personal interaction with nurses all over the country through speaking engagements not necessarily related to campaigning; and a disciplined understanding of the dynamics of small and large groups. Approximately six years before seeking election at the national ANA level, I had started a career of speaking to nursing and non-nursing groups. Being on the speaker's circuit greatly contributed to my success in campaigning.

My appreciation for group dynamics in organizational life was developed through an association with the A. K. Rice Institute. This institute focuses on experientially addressing issues of power and authority when working with organizations. A system's perspective provided me with a firm foundation for effectively functioning in my organizational leadership roles within ANA.

The road to the ANA presidency was neither simple nor direct. At times, I could not visualize that I would actually arrive at my destination. I was carried by a strong belief, even when my vision was foggy, that I was the right person, at the right place, at the right time on a mission with a higher purpose than my own personal goals. My mission was simply to make a difference in the lives and the care of patients. As President of ANA, this remains my mission.

SUMMARY

A consistent theme throughout this discussion of career mapping is a commitment to lifelong learning. But the learning is not limited to nursing skills and competence. The learning for successful career planning requires a continued pursuit of self-knowledge, an ability to accurately assess ones strengths and weaknesses at every stage and measure them against changing career goals, and the commitment to maintaining and achieving new competencies through leadership development opportunities, certification, and academic pursuits. Self-awareness is the cornerstone to effective career planning and choosing. Each of us must appreciate our inner workings as we appreciate the beating of our hearts. Being self-directed in your career means *you* plan the moves along the way. . . . it is not a linear one-time process (Henderson, & McGettigan, 1994). Each choice, each opportunity is measured against your personal inventory of skill and knowledge married with your personal career values and vision.

Thus career mapping is not even a step-by-step process. It requires *constant* reconsideration and adaptation. And today more than ever, the ability to adapt is elemental to a successful career. Your career map begins as you vision your future roles. As one of nursing's future leaders, you must be encouraged to imagine yourself in leadership roles. Then through development and use of your career map that vision will become a reality. I invite you to begin—imagine yourself as President of the American Nurses Association.

CRITICAL THINKING QUESTIONS

1. What personal values have you identified that are *elemental* to your personal and professional happiness and success in life? (For help describing your values, see Activity #1 on page 300.)

2. What top five aspects of nursing have you chosen as most important to you and most congruent with your values?

3. In thinking about the aspects of nursing in context with your values, what career roles would be most fulfilling of your chosen aspects of nursing? Identify two or three different roles.

4. In terms of the career roles identified in question 3, make a list of activities that you think should be completed to prepare for the role in each of the following categories. Make a separate list for each role identified:
   - basic nursing education
   - advanced nursing education
   - clinical experience
   - certification

- networking (include professional affiliations and organizations)
- mentoring (include relationships both within and outside of nursing)

5. If a new nursing student asked you to list at least five ways that having a career map will impact your career in nursing, what would you say?

ACTIVITIES

1. Use the following values list and/or add your own words to enhance this listing. Begin by choosing up to ten words that represent your most closely held values. As you make the choices, examine each value against the personal expression of that value in your work and personal life. This exercise will enable you to identify and clarify values that have great meaning to you and to measure if your stated values are honored through the work and personal choices that currently describe your life. You may also use this list and your personal list to do a prioritization exercise as mentioned in the chapter.

VALUES EXERCISE LIST

Accountabiltiy	Courage	Health	Recognition
Authenticity	Enlightenment	Honesty	Serenity
Beauty	Fairness	Independence	Spirituality
Balance	Family	Insight	Social Justice
Charity	Flexibility	Justice	Strength
Comfort	Friendship	Kindness	Success
Communication	Freedom	Liberty	Support
Compassion	Fun	Loyalty	Trust
Cooperation	Grace	Patience	Truthfulness
Competition	Growth	Peace	Understanding
Creativity	Happiness	Power	Wealth

Adapted from *Developing Your Nursing Career: A Working Guide*, Arizona Nurses Association

2. Attend your State Nurses Association Convention and introduce yourself to your State President. Ask to meet the nurse leaders from the District you live in. The Keynote Speaker's Session at the convention would be an inspirational session for you to attend. Also, sit in as a guest at the House of Delegates meeting to learn about issues affecting nurses in your state.

3. Start your career map today by writing down your four top goals for your nursing career. Keep this list and develop your map one step at a time. Remember it will require constant reconsideration and adaptation.

REFERENCES

Cavouras, C. A., & Eddy, L. D. (1996). *Developing your Nursing Career: A Working Guide.* Phoenix, AZ: Arizona Nurses Association.

Covey, S. R. (1989). *The Seven Habits of Highly Effective People.* New York: Simon & Schuster.

Glaxo, Inc. (1995). *Pathway Evaluation Program for Nursing Professionals.*

Henderson, F. C., & McGettigan, B. O. (1994). *Managing your Career in Nursing.* New York: NLN Nursing Press.

Koerner, J. G. (1996). Congruency between nurses' values and job requirements: A call for integrity. *Holist Nurs Pract, 10* (2), 69–77.

Styles, M. M. (1997, September). *Competence, Credentials, and Careers.* Paper presented at the Career Transitions Workshop, University of Utah College of Nursing in collaboration with the American Nurses Association, Salt Lake City, Utah.

Tomey, A. M., Schwier, B., Martiche, N., & May, F. (1996). Student perceptions of ideal and nursing career choices. *Nursing Outlook, 44,* 27–30.

Vicenzi, A. E., White, K. R., & Begun, J. W. (1997). Chaos in nursing: Make it work for you. *American Journal of Nursing, 97* (10), 26–31.

ADDITIONAL SUGGESTED READINGS

For more information on career strategies:

Chenevert, M. (1997). *The Pro-Nurse Handbook: Designed for the Nurse Who Wants to Thrive Professionally.* St. Louis, MO: Mosby.

For more information on career trends in nursing:

Aiken L., & Fagin, C. (1992). *Charting Nursings' Future: Agenda for the 1990s.* New York: J. B. Lippincott.

Fondiller, S. H., & Nerone, B. J. (1995). *Nursing: The Career of a Lifetime.* New York, NY: National League for Nursing, Nursing Press.

For more information on values:

Styles, M. M., & Moccia, P. (1993). *On Nursing: A Literary Anthology.* New York, NY: National League for Nursing, Nursing Press.

Conclusion:
The Stepping Stones—
From Nursing Student
to Nursing Leader
and Beyond

Throughout this text, the goal has been to illuminate the stepping stones that can move you from nursing student to nursing leader and empower you as you begin your own path to leadership development in nursing. Through sharing current leaders' biographies, thoughts, visions, and passion for nursing, you have been challenged to think critically. We have tried to change you, inspire you, and motivate you to join nursing's leadership as the profession moves into the twenty-first century. In the *Conclusion, Part One: This is Where the Change Begins,* you'll review the book and go on to take a first glance at the future stepping stones that can move you from nursing leader to nursing's vision. In the *Conclusion, Part Two:* you will discuss *Following Your Path to Leadership Development* by exploring the vision of a leader who served as President of the National League for Nursing (NLN) and Sigma Theta Tau. Our journey continues.

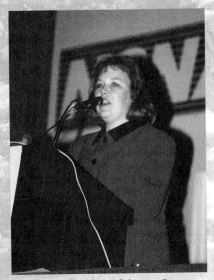

Photo © Todd Lengnick/Focus One

Carol A. Andersen,

BSN, RN

(Continued from page 2). She was appointed to the American Nurses Association HIV Resource Task Force, and was actively involved in the development of the ANA Position Statement on HIV and Student Nurses during her term as NSNA President. Carol was also an invited speaker/panelist at the National Conference on Gerontological Nursing Education during that time.

Carol has spoken at state nursing student meetings, as well as many national meetings about leadership roles and leadership development for nursing students. From 1995–Fall 1997, Carol served as a state consultant to the Iowa Association of Nursing Students (IANS). It has been rewarding for her to mentor new nursing leaders and see the growth of IANS, an association that she previously led in 1990 as IANS President. Her articles have been published in the *American Nurse* and the *Pharmacy Student* regarding the strong future for nursing.

Carol Andersen is an active member of District Seven of the Iowa Nurses Association (INA). She served as INA Third Vice-President in 1994, and Chair of the INA Policy Committee, served on the state membership committee, and was an Iowa delegate to the American Nurses Association House of Delegates Meetings in 1994 and 1995. Carol looks forward to future leadership roles in her state Nurses Association, the American Nurses Association, and active leadership roles as part of nursing's voice in the twenty-first century. She is a member of Sigma Theta Tau Honor Society, Phi Eta Sigma Honor Society, and serves on the Grand View College Alumni Board. Carol was named to *Who's Who Among Students in American Universities and Colleges.* She is an active member of Windsor Heights Lutheran Church, the Danish Brotherhood/Sisterhood in America, and is a supporting member of the arts in Iowa. She is also an individual sustaining member of NSNA.

More biographical information on Carol A. Fetters Andersen, BSN, RN, can be found on page 2.

CONCLUSION: PART 1

This Is Where the Change Begins

INTRODUCTION

As we conclude the book, let's consider some important areas that can impact your path to leadership development in nursing. The title of this chapter *This Is Where the Change Begins,* sets the direction for our efforts.

You should know that I'm a firm believer in each of us making a difference in nursing, so that the future "becomes what we make it." I look forward to observing these efforts and results from you, and you can expect no less from me. And so, the journey from *Nursing Student to Nursing Leader* begins.

THE FRAMEWORK FOR YOUR PATH

In the Introduction of this book, I proposed a framework for your path to leadership development that is built on stepping stones that will help support you along the way. There are also "key stones" that *you* must supply: courage, commitment, purpose, and unity, all strengthened by education and professionalism.

UNDERSTANDING THE IMPACT OF NURSING EDUCATION ON LEADERSHIP

In Unit One we:

1. Looked at the beginning development of nursing (Chapter 1—Tarbox, M.),

2. Discussed the important role that nursing education and research will play in your role as a future nurse leader (Chapter 2—Fitzpatrick, M. L.; Chapter 3—Felton, G.),

3. Learned about the valuable contribution your faculty makes when they mentor accountability and then instill it in you. Those seeds of accountability and ethics are planted there to take root and provide you with strength and vision in your role as a twenty-first century nurse leader—a leader who will be well grounded in the integrity of nursing, perhaps best demonstrated by nursing's commitment to patient advocacy (Chapter 4—Strachota, E.; Chapter 5—Weingarten, C.).

Also in Unit 1, we explored through nursing's history how various paradigm shifts occurred in nursing care. We looked at the example of nursing's focus moving from community-based care in the days of Lillian Wald to acute care/illness care after the discovery of the germ theory and now back towards community based care with an emphasis on wellness and prevention. *What have you learned from nursing's experiences of the past and from your own nursing curriculum?*

As I look back to evaluate the impact that my curriculum had on me, I find that my baccalaureate program in nursing at Grand View College in Des Moines, Iowa, provided me with a valued liberal arts education. One that has helped me to be:

1. Holistic in my care
2. Prepared for case management roles
3. A strong patient advocate
4. A leader who incorporates in her various roles both vision and professional involvement

What are the written outcome objectives for graduates of your nursing curriculum? Certainly, the challenge for nursing will continue to be the development of curriculum models that focus on the essence of nursing and yet remain dynamic enough to adjust to rapid changes in the health care environment. As changes in nursing programs continue, encourage students who come after you to remain an active part of curriculum committees. For it's through working together that faculty and students can best achieve positive outcomes.

Undoubtedly, many of you reading this will continue your education and will one day assume leadership roles in nursing education. You will be charged with the task of developing, evaluating, and redesigning the nursing curriculum models of the future. That task calls for your attention and critical thinking, beginning today. *Be sure you understand how your nursing curriculum was developed and also its mission and goals.* It may also prove valuable for you to explore new and innovative curriculum models in the country. One example that I have personally observed is the innovative *Caring Curriculum* now being utilized at Grand View College, where I serve on the college's Alumni Board of Directors. This is one example out of many new and innovative curriculums that you can explore. Even your own nursing program has most likely gone through many changes in the past 10 years. Begin today to observe, assess, and evaluate how nursing education programs are impacting nursing's future leaders.

SHARING EXPERIENCES—A WAY TO EXPAND YOUR VISION

Another way that this book has attempted to empower you to take steps towards leadership has been through sharing portraits of the paths taken by some current nurse leaders. Through the following chapters: Introduction: Part 2 (Joel, L.), Chapter 6 (Foley, M.), Chapter 15 (Mallison, M.), Chapter 16 (Anderson, C., & Bednash, G. P.), in the Conclusion: Part 2 (Donley, Sr. R.), and in parts of other chapters you have been given a personal glimpse into how and why each nurse's leadership evolved and what each one's path to leadership looked like.

Let me emphasize that our purpose is not to narrow your horizons by suggesting that your steps mirror those taken by the nurse leaders included in this book. But rather, our purpose is to expand your vision and empower you to glean the best of what you see here and apply it to the ever-changing environments you will face. You must factor in your own unique gifts of vision and talent, and then you can begin to solidify your own path.

UNDERSTANDING THE IMPACT OF PRACTICE AND EXPERIENCES ON LEADERSHIP DEVELOPMENT

Have you written down your nursing story—how you've gotten to this point in nursing, what you've learned, and where you'll go from here? This is a very valuable exercise for you to do. Just by writing it down, you will be focusing your thoughts and vision. It will also allow you to later look back at what you've written, "in hindsight."

It's an exercise that I did prior to writing an article that was published in the *American Nurse, Directions* (p. 2), October, 1991. Through the exercise, I realized that my energies and experiences in nursing up to that time had been directed in two main areas—professional involvement and leadership development in nursing. The resulting article addressed those areas.

An Experience Using Hindsight to Discover Change

In writing this book, I took the time to look back "in hindsight" at the article. I found that both my nursing story and my understanding of the impacts on nurses today have expanded and evolved.

Changes have occurred in my perception. I've learned that as nurses grow and gain experience in practice not only do their opportunities for leadership change, but also their perceptions of where to lead changes. This can have both positive and negative consequences on nursing's voice.

A positive consequence of growth and maturity in nursing is that as nurses gain experience within specific roles, they begin to see things from a more defined frame of reference. Then nurses begin to have an impact on patient care because of the experience focused leadership that develops as you move from *novice* to *expert* (Benner, 1984). In other words—experience talks and other nurses listen.

It is true that experienced nurses can see specific details in a specialty area that might be missed from a novice, or more generalist view. But, while this transformation of nurses to a more detailed specialty focus can have a positive impact on nursing's voice, let's look at what we lose in the process.

The potential negative consequences are that:

1. As a nurse develops expertise and focuses primarily or exclusively in one practice area, he or she risks losing the broader perspective of nursing and health care. This is especially dangerous in today's managed care markets where the movement is away from specialization towards generalist practice. And it also becomes a clear threat to the unity and strength of nursing's voice. A threat that I believe is magnified when nurses belong only to their specialty nursing organization and not ANA.

2. As nurses gain experience, participate, and react to unplanned changes in their roles, they move away from the idealism, creativity, and flexibility that they had as new nurses. In the extreme, this leads to cynicism, resistance to any change, and if left unaddressed to burn-out and nurses leaving the profession.

While experienced nurses have often been put in situations where they can only react to change, newer nurses have trained in today's world to be proactive and plan for change. As a result, newer nurses bring a fresh vision to nursing.

So, what is the answer for nursing? How can nurses find win/win solutions to what we've just discussed? I believe the answer lies in active professional involvement for **all** nurses from the early days as a student and first licensure continuing throughout one's lifetime. Nursing's voice must become stronger, unified, reflect nurses in all settings, and include both experienced and novice nurses. The expertise of experienced nurse leaders is valuable as they may see specific practice details to problems that newer nurses might miss. But, it is just as critical that newer nurses are given an active voice. The new nurse's global perspective, enthusiasm, commitment, fresh vision, and active change experience *must* also be part of nursing's voice for it to "be complete."

When I've served in the ANA House of Delegates as a delegate for Iowa, I was alarmed to see that over the years less than five percent, and often less than one percent, of the delegates in the House have been in practice less than five years. This will soon impact you—for often the nursing future that we vision and plan in the ANA House of Delegates is yours. But, how are current nurse leaders mentoring and encouraging your active part in nursing's voice? I authored and presented to our 1997 Iowa Nurses Association House of Delegates meeting a resolution to allow at least one of Iowa's (INA's) delegate seats in the ANA House to be held by a nurse that has been in practice five years or less and to continue to seek ways to actively involve those new nurses in active district and state level roles. The INA House endorsed the concept and referred the proposal to the INA Board for study and implementation. I encourage all states to follow Iowa and other state's mentoring example and to seek the same. Current nurse leaders have a responsibility to nursing's future to be sure that new nurses become and remain an active part of nursing's unified voice.

Just as crucial to nursing's twenty-first century voice will be our need to bring on board more nurses from all settings. Too many of our nursing colleagues in practice do not belong to either ANA or their specialty organization. We must not forget that every nurse's voice is important, and we are strongest when nursing speaks as one.

We touch on these concepts in Chapter 10 (Andersen, C.), Chapter 13 (Andersen, C.), and Chapter 14 (Vance, C.), by discussing the need for nursing's collective identity and the process of mentoring nursing students to become future nurse leaders.

Besides the impacts we've discussed so far, your path to leadership will also be impacted by external forces. Today, the most immediate and significant external impact appears to be in the area of managed care reforms.

UNDERSTANDING THE IMPACT OF MANAGED CARE: A LEADERSHIP OPPORTUNITY?

When we discuss managed care, we are really looking at health care reform and its political and practice impact on nursing. In Chapter 12 (Betts, V.), we discussed the need to strengthen nursing's voice through political action for nurses. We also explored the development of nursing's vision for political involvement, and assessed what nursing has accomplished so far. To provide you with examples, Chapter 16 (Anderson, C., & Bednash, G. P.), explored some paths to political roles taken by nurse leaders.

You are entering nursing during a time of dramatic changes to the environment of health care. The current changes in our country's health market structure impact nursing and quality patient care. Nursing *must* have politically active leaders if we want to be active participants in the changes. Earlier in the book we reviewed that health reform in these late 1990s is being driven by market place predictions and adaptations to real and perceived change. We see a movement through what insurance and medicine often call phases of managed health care markets.

It will be critical for you to remain aware of the changes that are occurring in this area. To help you begin, let me summarize what I've observed through attending speeches and presentations on managed care. When discussing managed care, speakers usually cite four market phases. The progressive movement flows from:

1. Phase 1 Markets, where health care is largely unstructured, through

2. Phase 2 Markets, that have loose frameworks, resulting in more control and less choices, then continuing through

3. Phase 3 Markets, where consolidation of large HMO's occurs and provider networks evolve. There is movement away from specialty roles towards general practice, discussions occur related to capitation of fees and services. We see declining hospital profit margins, and then with even more consolidation the move is towards

4. Phase 4 Markets, where managed competition occurs, and everything is consolidated and controlled by the managed care network, as they serve what are called "covered lives." This market type consists of consolidation of insurers, hospitals, clinics, physicians as employees, and employers as "the purchasers" of care plans for those "covered lives," all joined together into one entity.

This is only a thumb-nail sketch of what's being discussed and presented. The trends also include the increased use and sophistication of information systems—where as we learned in Chapter 17 (Delaney, C.) nursing is invisible in current health care databases. I wanted to share this brief sketch of managed care market phases with you as I have some significant concerns about these external market impacts on nursing.

My concern involves the movement away from more patient focused care systems, towards control of risk, expenses, and providers. Nurse leaders must have leadership roles in their state and nationally within each market phase to ensure that nursing care, advanced nursing care, and our patient's voice is represented in the discussions and decisions that are made. Nurses must also understand and be an active participant in developing information systems for health care, to ensure that nursing care is not invisible in health information systems of the future. Let me emphasize that *the time is now for your involvement to occur.* When managed care moves from Phase 1 Markets towards Phase 4 Markets, it becomes increasingly difficult to involve new ideas and new providers.

In Chapter 7 (Evans, M.), Chapter 8 (Cipriano, P.), Chapter 9 (Porter-O'Grady, T.), Chapter 17 (Delaney, C.), and Chapter 18 (Huey, F.) we have laid a solid foundation of knowledge to help you understand and prepare for the impact of these areas. Our goal is to empower you to be both proactive to change and to remain actively involved in health reform, whatever future path that reform takes.

HOW TO BEGIN YOUR LEADERSHIP DEVELOPMENT

You should begin today to develop as a nursing leader. The best way is to become an active member of the National Student Nurses' Association (NSNA). It is the one pre-professional association that includes membership for all nursing students preparing for RN licensure. Please don't be dissuaded into joining only a specialty nursing student group exclusively, rather than taking part in NSNA. For that moves you away from our bigger voice and fractions and divides us even at the student level. *Let our generation be the one that stands for unification of nursing's voice.*

Nursing needs your involvement and experience in the bigger picture of NSNA. As you gain that global perspective and vision as a nursing student leader, you can bring that, along with your idealism, creativity, commitment, and vision into nursing practice and professional involvement after graduation.

Chapter 11 (Mancino, D.) and Chapter 19 (Brigner, S.) discussed the importance of developing your nursing leadership skills now as a student and continuing to do so throughout your career. We also reviewed some helpful hints about interviewing and job placement. These hints for that stressful and exciting time we all face and other ideas that were shared will serve you well as you travel from nursing student to nursing leader.

NURSING LEADERSHIP'S FUTURE AND YOU

I want you to picture yourself graduated, and a licensed RN. This is probably your favorite picture right now as you long to be done with nursing school! You are almost to a point of merging theory with practice.

Whatever your chosen area of nursing practice becomes, you enter nursing at a unique time in history. In my parent's generation and the early part of my life, society's work ethic and goal was to find employment with a reputable facility, firm, or corporation. The employee would then work there gaining skills and seniority and often retire from the same employer. In fact, employees who changed jobs or career areas several times were looked at in disapproval by employers. Today's marketplace is vastly different. With moves to different cities and consolidation of companies and roles, it's not unusual for executives and employees to change employers, roles, and locations many times in their careers.

The word *career* has taken on a life-time perspective rather than a role perspective. This has called for nursing leaders to develop *career maps* to assist in their professional development throughout their lifetimes. In Chapter 20 (Malone, B.) we reviewed ways that you can do just that. This will prove extremely valuable to you as you try to keep on track with your goals.

The other way that you can organize your development in a specific nursing role and/or in professional involvement is through strategic planning. Strategic planning involves setting a three to five year plan of where you want to proceed, your goals, objectives, and implementation strategies of how you propose to get there. When matched to your career map, you will be well on your way to *creating* opportunities for yourself, rather than only reacting to those that happen your way. The concept of strategic planning may be foreign to some of you. Since I am a very visual learner, I know that if I can relate a concept to something I already know, I can understand and internalize it much better. I've included for you in Appendix D a strategic planning model that I've developed to help me and the students I work with complete strategic plans. I invite you to use it to assist you in developing your own strategic plan.

SUMMARY

In the Introduction: Part 1 (Andersen, C.) we looked at the model for *The Critical Path to Leadership Development in Nursing*. The model follows here to allow us to look at it again, for a final overview.

First, please note that there is a space between *nursing student* and the beginning of the center of the path to leadership in nursing, *patient centered care*. This is because entering the path to leadership development requires a conscious decision by you to begin. Second, you'll see that patient centered care flows from that first committed step through to nursing's vision. It is in fact central to the entire path, just as it is central to nursing.

Also, there are stepping stones that lay along side the center in close proximity, while there are those stepping stones that have to join patient centered care directly to be part of the path. Although patient centered care is essential to all areas of your path, those stepping stones that will be most effective with patient/patient's family involvement are:

1. Networking
2. Interdisciplinary collaboration
3. Patient advocacy
4. Fostering self-care and community involvement

In this book through our study of the *Critical Path to Leadership Development in Nursing,* we've explored the efforts that will be needed to move you from the first cross bar of *Nursing Student,* upward and onward on the stepping stones to the next cross bar of *Nursing Leader.* We've looked at related issues and impacts of *nursing education, practice, professional involvement, mentoring,* and *networking* on your path.

The model is missing one important element, **you.** It is my sincere hope that the discussions, visual examples, motivation, and challenges presented to you within this text have changed you, inspired you, and empowered your active involvement in nursing's voice.

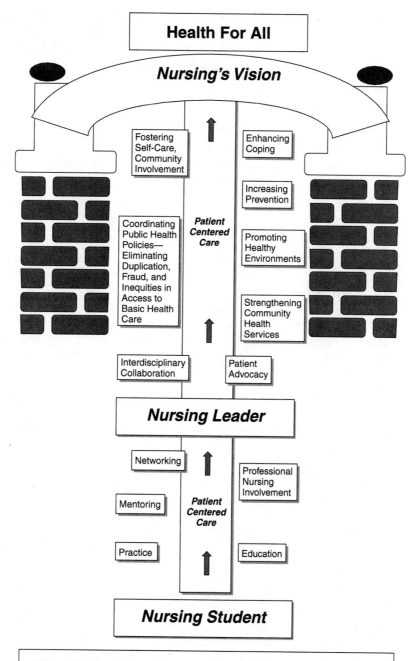

Health For All

Nursing's Vision

Fostering Self-Care, Community Involvement

Enhancing Coping

Increasing Prevention

Patient Centered Care

Coordinating Public Health Policies— Eliminating Duplication, Fraud, and Inequities in Access to Basic Health Care

Promoting Healthy Environments

Strengthening Community Health Services

Interdisciplinary Collaboration

Patient Advocacy

Nursing Leader

Networking

Professional Nursing Involvement

Mentoring

Patient Centered Care

Practice

Education

Nursing Student

The Critical Path To Leadership Development In Nursing

Together, you and I will move with other nurse leaders (both experienced and new) along the second half of the *Critical Path to Leadership Development*. There, as we move towards *nursing's vision of health for all,* we will encounter many new stepping stones to guide our way. The ones that I foresee involve:

- Patient advocacy
- Interdisciplinary collaboration
- Strengthening community health services
- Promoting healthy environments
- Coordinating public health policies and eliminating duplication, fraud, and inequities in access to basic health care
- Increasing prevention
- Enhancing coping
- Fostering self-care and community involvement

This second half of the model is offered as a guidepost for our future leadership development in nursing. But our paths will not lead to nursing's vision, nor be complete without each nurse leader's critical thinking, creative problem solving, visioning, and active participation. As we continue to grow in our leadership roles in nursing, I hope that someday we can revisit the second half of this model together and see how far we've come. Together, we will then explore our continued movement along the path to leadership development as we travel from *Nursing Leader to Nursing's Vision.*

For now, please know that it has been a gift and privilege for me, and all the contributing authors to define, discuss, and share with you about the important progression from *Nursing Student to Nursing Leader,* and *The Critical Path to Leadership Development in Nursing.*

In closing, those of you who know me, know how much I dislike goodbyes. We have a great deal of work ahead of us as we continue to develop as nurse leaders for the twenty-first century. And, if we are all actively involved—as we should be—our paths will cross many times. So, I will close with the same words that I used to close my NSNA Presidency. *"I do not say goodbye, but rather, that I will be waiting for you on the floor of the ANA House of Delegates."*

CRITICAL THINKING QUESTIONS

1. What do you think is the most effective way to learn? How has your nursing curriculum structured learning for students?

2. What is your nursing curriculum's mission and goals? Do you agree with them? If you were to design a nursing curriculum to prepare nursing students to meet the ever changing demands of our health care system in the United States, what areas would you have as required objectives and experiences?

3. Do you feel ready to enter nursing? If not, what can you do to be sure you become ready? If so, why do you believe you are ready? Do you think Boards of Nursing should require internships of nursing students?

4. Why should you become involved in professional nursing as well as practice? Have you begun today as a member of NSNA? If not, why not? If so, what have you gained so far from the experience, and how has it helped in your education?

5. Have you stepped onto *The Critical Path to Leadership Development* in nursing? What stepping stones have you included in your path to becoming a *nursing leader*? How can you become an active part of nursing's unified voice?

ACTIVITIES

1. Write down how you have gotten to this point in nursing, what you've learned, and where you go from here. This will help you focus your thoughts and vision. Take this exercise back out in a year, and after five years, and evaluate where you are then compared to where you are now.

2. Consider doing an independent study in nursing leadership as part of your remaining experiences in your nursing program. The National Student Nurses' Association (NSNA) has developed a sample independent study plan that includes objectives and ways that your NSNA involvement can help meet the proposed competencies of the independent study. A copy of NSNA's Independent Study Model can be obtained by contacting NSNA at (212) 581-2211. Discuss the independent study with your faculty advisor and Dean or Director of your nursing program. They will assist you on how and where to proceed.

REFERENCES

Benner, P. (1984). *From Novice to Expert: Excellence and Power in Clinical Nursing Practice.* Menlo Park, CA: Addison-Wesley.

Fetters, C. (1991, October). Message to nursing students: This is where the change begins. *The American Nurse, Directions,* 2.

ADDITIONAL SUGGESTED READINGS

Read the text of the brochures *Every Patient Deserves A Nurse* and *Nursing's Agenda for Health Care Reform,* that follow after the Conclusion chapters in Appendix A and Appendix B. Although *Nursing's Agenda* is no longer in print, the central tenets of the document still apply to nursing's overall efforts. The American Nurses Association is completing a document on managed care that will be valuable for you to review when it becomes available. Also, ANA has developed nursing report cards that talk about evaluation and outcomes of nursing care. You can contact ANA directly about publications at 1-800-274-4ANA.

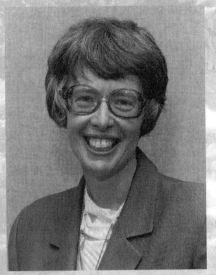

Sister Rosemary Donley,

RN, PHD, FAAN

Sister Rosemary Donley, RN, PhD, FAAN, an Ordinary Professor of Nursing at The Catholic University of America, Washington, DC. Sr. Rosemary Donley received a diploma from the Pittsburgh Hospital School of Nursing, holds a BSN summa cum laude from St. Louis University, and a MNEd. and PhD. from the University of Pittsburgh. Her major interests are health policy and decision-making.

Prior to assuming her current position Sr. Rosemary served as Executive Vice-President and Dean of Nursing at The Catholic University of America. In 1977, Sr. Rosemary was elected to be a Robert Wood Johnson Health Policy Fellow under a grant from the Robert Wood Johnson Foundation and the Institute of Medicine, National Academy of Science. Sr. Rosemary is a Fellow in the American Academy of Nursing and a member of the Institute of Medicine. She is past President of the National League for Nursing and Sigma Theta Tau International Honor Society of Nursing, and past Senior Editor of *Image: The Journal of Nursing Scholarship*. She serves on civic, college, and health system boards in addition to the editorial boards of five journals. She served as a member of the Secretary of Health and Human Service's Commission on Nursing; has been a consultant to the United States Army and Navy Medical Commands; and is recipient of six honorary degrees.

Sr. Rosemary has over 80 publications in professional journals and has contributed chapters in five recent publications. Her research is in clinical decision-making and health policy. Sr. Rosemary has presented papers throughout the United States, Kenya, Spain, The Peoples Republic of China, the Philippines, Guam, Okinawa, Japan, Korea, Taiwan, Hong Kong, Brazil, Argentina, Germany, Israel, Canada, and The Union of Soviet Socialist Republics. She has also participated in numerous seminars, panel discussions, and workshops in the United States. In the summer of 1997 Sr. Donley was elected to be a member of the leadership group of her religious community, the Sisters of Charity of Seton Hill.

CONCLUSION: PART **2**

Following Your Path to Leadership Development— The Vision of a Leader

INTRODUCTION

L eadership is identified as a desirable trait. Most people study leaders or leadership behaviors as part of their professional development. Nurses are no different. If nurses look for models of leadership within their profession, they find leaders within their ranks. These are the men and women who made the practice of nursing different and better. People know leaders because they see evidence of their presence in the world about them. Leaders change how people think and what they do. For many students, the search for leaders brings them to libraries and usually to the writings of Florence Nightengale, Isabel Hamptom Robb, or Lavinia Dock. Others seek leaders closer to home, a great teacher, an admired nurse in the community, or someone who is emulated because of what he or she has spoken or written. This text traces and defines the pathways forged by modern nurse leaders. It is hoped that by walking the journey with contemporary nursing leaders, students and all members of the profession will be inspired to improve the world of nursing practice and education.

I have been asked to contribute to this anthology by describing my career as a nursing leader. This is not easy for me to do, because I do not think of myself as a nursing leader. However, this essay is not about self-perception. It is an effort to lay out the forces and factors that helped shape my professional and personal life. Unlike many of my colleagues, I did not grow up with the idea that I would be a nurse. I wanted to do something important with my life, and I wanted to help others. The idea of entering a convent and being a sister appealed to me. I was fascinated with the talent and the professionalism of the sisters who had taught me in high school. The idea of being a Catholic sister was so engaging that it distracted me from thinking about any other professions or careers. At some level, I wanted to be a teacher of English or a librarian. It was my religious superiors that decided that I should study nursing. I began to do this as a novice. Because my work in nursing is inspired and motivated by religious values, I have looked to religion for some foundation for my life. During my first year in nursing school when the course work was in the basic sciences, I read the histories of nursing. I was particularly drawn to the accounts of nursing in the early Christian period and at the time of the Crusades. I also liked the history of nursing during the Second World War. I was not influenced by any particular person in my study of the history of nursing. I wanted to know about nursing practice and needed some images of nurses to inspire me in the anatomy and chemistry labs. I found wonderful stories of nursing in this literature, accounts of what the nurses did and the heroism and compassion that their actions expressed. My notions about the type of nurse I wanted to be were also influenced by the nurses whom I met during my formative days of clinical education. I looked for nurses to whom I would entrust the care of my family. I was not trying to intuit the qualities of a leader in a healing profession. I was seeking some constellation of qualities to which I could aspire. I was searching for an answer to an important question. . . .

WHAT IS A GOOD NURSE?

It seemed then that the good nurse should be knowledgeable, honest in her dealings with others, responsible, and compassionate. Knowing the discipline and the sciences that undergird it has always been significant for me. I was conscious, even as a beginning student, of how much there was to know about nursing. I also took responsibility for learning more than was required to pass the course. I did not want any patient to suffer because I failed to offer him the best insights that were available. Many of my classmates liked the clinical work and put up with the classes. I liked to study and learn more about the pathophysiology of disease. For me, the clinical experience was an opportunity to see a disease process in a particular person. How was it manifested? How did the person live with it? I was also impressed with the need for personal and professional integrity. In the early days of my studies, many of my patients were not able to represent themselves. They depended on their nurses for food, support, medicine, positioning—their very lives. They could not say what had happened to them on any shift. Not only did I need to be responsible for my behavior, I had to be honest and forthright in describing the nursing encounters. One of my teachers told me that the word of a professional is all that is needed, and that all professionals were judged by their reputations in the community. I also learned that the only account of what had happened the day or the night before was that written by my colleagues. I came to rely on the nursing and medical documentation as a guide to my own practice. It was also very important to me that the patient be treated with respect. Nurses of my era were taught to address patients by their titles, not their first names or their nicknames. We were schooled in confidentiality and in enhancing the patient's personhood. In the world in which I first studied nursing, the patient was sacred. At the beginning of my studies, I could not quote Virginia Henderson's definition of nursing. I knew, however, because of the environment in which I was being educated that the nurse often became the alter ego of the patient. Not only did the nurse do what the patient was not able to do, she acted in the patient's interests. I was impressed with the responsibility that nurses assumed. Even in the years when physicians had control over many decisional paradigms, nurses were responsible for the care of the patients. Some observers of hospital nursing practice in the '60s and '70s have complained that nurses had responsibility, but not authority over patient care. This responsibility covered 24 hours a day, seven days a week, fifty-two weeks a year. It required the total assessment and complex management of the physical, emotional, intellectual, social, and spiritual well being of the patient. As a student, I was imbued with my responsibility for my practice and patient care. I felt responsible not only for the patient, but also for the environment of his or her care. I was in charge. It was important that I and my classmates could be counted on to be there and to be on time. One of my early learnings as a student was the devastating effect of illness on the person and his or her family. Anxiety, fear, pain, toxicity, fever, and suffering are only a few of the experiences common to those who are ill.

In the hospital schools of nursing in the '60s, there were 40 hour weeks. There were classes during this period, but students were with patients more than 30 hours each week. The average length of stay was longer for patients. It was not uncommon for women to stay in the hospital five days after childbirth, or for patients to spend 10 to 14 days in the hospital after a myocardial infarction. Students were with patients on the evening and night shifts. It was possible to learn about the effects of disease and treatment on the patient and the family. Because nursing is a relationship, it was important to learn how the nurse responded to the patient's disease and its manifestations. I brought more than knowledge and a responsible presence to the patient's bedside, I brought myself.

What then should be the attitude of persons charged with alleviating the symptoms of illness? It seemed that nurses and all health care workers should understand the suffering of their patients and seek to enter into their experiences. I call this effort to participate in the experience of the patient—compassion. As a student of nursing, I was attracted by the nurses who were kind and compassionate to the patients. These nurses listened to the patients and understood their symptoms and behaviors.

MY EDUCATIONAL PATH

My initial study of nursing took place at a diploma school of nursing operated by the Sisters of Charity of Seton Hill. The school, the Pittsburgh Hospital School of Nursing, was located in a section of the city that had known better times. While much has been written about the positive and negative values of hospital-based education, my memories of my education and the depth of the clinical knowledge that I gleaned in that small school on Finley Street are deep and sustaining. While a student, I was fortunate enough to realize that nursing was very complex. I also knew that I had more to learn. Successfully writing the State Board of Nursing examination, what the NCLEX was called in the sixties, was not enough. If I were to be a good nurse, I needed to learn more. I was very pleased when my religious community told me that I was to continue my studies at St. Louis University. In the mid-'60s, St. Louis was a very different world than Pittsburgh. The school of nursing that I was to attend was part of an academic health center. There were many students from the health professions on campus and in the hospitals. There were also other people on the campus who were concerned about philosophy, history, and aeronautical engineering. I had entered a world of ideas. In the clinical part of the program, we studied in five hospitals, each designed to offer specialized care to a defined group of patients. We also studied public health in a community-based clinic in a poor section of the city. Among the clinical insights I gained in St. Louis was the idea that there are many right ways to deliver nursing care. I also learned new ways of thinking about patient care and my responsibilities. In the city where I first went to school, patients did not leave the unit to go to the cafeteria or to take a walk. They stayed in their beds, in their rooms, or perhaps walked to a solarium at the end of the hall. I remember one frantic, hot evening in St. Louis searching for a patient, a man who was being treated for diabetes. When he returned at dusk, he told me of his dinner in the hospital cafeteria and his walk around the lovely garden area surrounding the hospital. I can't remember whether I revealed my anxiety. I still recall how happy I was that he came back. That evening I reflected that I had become overly protective of the patients. They were not my prisoners or my children. What better way to test diabetic management than to have a real life. Now when I recall my days at St. Louis University, it is the courses in English and Philosophy that shine forth. I learned to think at the university. I learned to discuss ideas and to expand my awareness. While my search for competence began in the diploma school of nursing, my search for meaning in nursing began at St. Louis University. If I would describe myself as a nurse, I would say that I have spent my professional life struggling to give meaning to nursing. After graduate studies in nursing at the University of Pittsburgh, I would borrow a phrase from Peter Drucker to describe me and what I wanted nurses to be—"knowledge workers." I mean to convey that nursing is work built on knowledge. Part of what has shaped me as a nursing leader is the opportunity to have studied nursing in good schools. I believe that a leader must value and express knowledge.

THE INFLUENCE OF PROFESSIONAL NURSING INVOLVEMENT

The next major influence on my life was the nursing organizations. This force developed as I was finishing the diploma program. In those days, the faculty of the diploma schools in Pittsburgh literally signed their new graduates up! I joined the American Nurses Association and the National League for Nursing as a new graduate. I attended district meetings and was a faithful member. When I finished my master's work at the University of Pittsburgh, one of my teachers was elected President of the Pennsylvania Nurses Association. Lucie Kelly appointed me to the State Nurses Association's Committee on Nursing Education. I was very pleased and very scared. The other members of the Committee were seasoned professionals. They had careers. Some of them had written in the journals. They led the influential nurses in the state. As time went on, I realized I had something to contribute at the meetings. I had ideas and an incredible optimism for nursing. I continued to be involved with the Pennsylvania Nurses Association and later the American Nurses Association in their efforts to raise the educational standards and enhance the continuing education of the nursing community. My introduction to Sigma Theta Tau International occurred shortly after I was inducted into the Eta Chapter at the University of Pittsburgh.

SIGMA THETA TAU A MORAL DECISION FOR EXCELLENCE

My classmates explained that being a member of Sigma Theta Tau looked good on the curriculum vitae. For me, the decision to join Sigma Theta Tau (we were not then an international society), was a moral decision. I was invited to membership in the society when schools were adopting a pass/fail system of grading and everyone was to be thought of as the same. How then could I join an elite society? Accepting membership in Sigma Theta Tau was more than signing a card, paying dues, or making an entry on a curriculum vitae. I had to face who I was and what I aspired to be. I had graduated summa cum laude from St. Louis University and was first in my class in my diploma and master's program. Did I want to identify with the best educated and most academically able of my colleagues? Did I want to foster professional standards and encourage creativity in patient care? Did I want to be a leader? When I said yes to the invitation to join Eta Chapter, I was saying yes to the gifts I had been given. It was a fortunate choice. I found the chapter meetings at Eta Chapter to be delightful. The lines among faculty, young graduates, students, and nurses in practice disappeared in dialogue. We talked about practice and ways to improve care. As a young clinical teacher, I was enriched by these meetings. I could get advice and strategic suggestions from experienced practitioners. My questions and observations were not heard as iconoclastic efforts to undermine nursing or its modes of practice. Networking, social support, and mentoring became "things to do" in the '70s.

I learned what colleagueship meant at the meetings of Eta Chapter. One evening, the chair of the nominating committee asked me to run for office. She said they needed another name for the president's slot. Assuming I was too young in the society to be elected, I said yes. Several weeks later, I learned I was not as young as I thought!

Many of my ideas about leadership and its importance in nursing developed because of my work in Sigma Theta Tau. I was privileged to be President of Eta Chapter and later Vice-President and eventually President of Sigma Theta Tau International. Over the years, because of this, I worked closely with many important leaders in nursing. When I became associated with Sigma Theta Tau International, the organization was small. I and my colleagues built an organization that could be a force for excellence in many communities. The officers of Sigma Theta Tau were very engaged then in expanding the boundaries of the organization and in using programs as a way of advancing scholarship and research. Nell Watts, the Executive Officer of Sigma Theta Tau International, has written a history of her years in the organization. It is an account of the leadership experience of a group of nurses who believe that nurses are scholars and who used a nursing organization to express this vision.

My years in Sigma Theta Tau International were devoted to strengthening and enriching the members of the society. At one level, we were extending the network of nurse scholars by chartering chapters in schools of nursing around the world. At another, we were disseminating information about the best practices in nursing via conferences, publications, monographs and on-line access to a nursing data base. Recognizing achievement and building the scientific base for nursing practice became the task of the society's leaders. It was fun to work with such talented and dedicated nurses. I will always be indebted to Nell Watts and Rebecca Markel for their wisdom and leadership in the organization.

From them and from my other colleagues, I learned that a group can do more than an individual. Later when management gurus said that the leader of the future will be a small group, I knew exactly what they meant.

ROBERT WOOD JOHNSON HEALTH POLICY FELLOW

Another leadership experience that influenced my life occurred in the late-70s when I was nominated by the University of Pittsburgh to be a Robert Wood Johnson Health Policy Fellow. In the spring of 1977, I and five gentlemen were selected as the Robert Wood Johnson Class of 1977–1978. My year "on the Hill" was an experience in political leadership and policy development. I had the opportunity to work with members of Congress in the Senate and in the House and to attend agency briefings and legislative and policy development sessions. We also traveled to Ottawa, Canada for a comparative experience in budget building. When I returned to the University of Pittsburgh at the end of the year, leadership included policy development.

THE CATHOLIC UNIVERSITY OF AMERICA

In the fall of 1979, I became Dean of Nursing at The Catholic University of America. Although I have been President of Sigma Theta Tau International, I had never held a formal leadership position in an organization. In 1986, I became the University's Executive Vice-President. My colleagues were faculty from 10 schools, three presidents and a talented group of academic administrators. Academic leadership involved articulating the vision of the University and its mission so that it could be understood by a constituency that was diverse and frequently distant from the campus. These positions gave me a "hands-on" experience with budgeting, the fiscal and managerial direction of a school and then a university, and experience in fundraising.

LEADERSHIP ROLES IN THE NATIONAL LEAGUE FOR NURSING

During my deanship, I was elected to be the President of the National League for Nursing (NLN). I had the good experience of working with members of the very talented staff of the NLN and also with the Tri-Council—comprised of the Presidents and Executive Officers of the American Nurses Association (ANA), the National League for Nursing (NLN), The American Association of Colleges of Nursing (AAON) and the American Organization of Nurse Executives (AONE). Our challenge was the defeat of the proposal of the American Medical Association for registered care technicians (RCTs). This event gave me and my colleagues the opportunity to use individual and collective leadership skills.

While unlicensed multipurpose workers are employed in the contemporary health care environment, their presence and practice is not institutionalized because of this effort.

In the summer of 1997, I was elected to be a member of the leadership group of my religious community, the Sisters of Charity of Seton Hill. While I do not yet feel the completeness of coming full circle, the new work has reconnected me to my spiritual and cultural roots.

SUMMARY

As I write this essay, I am searching for what gives meaning to nursing in this profit oriented age of managed care. The new practice paradigms require leaders who have a vision of nursing that is grounded on a reality that is more complex than what is offered by economic and management theories. I am seeking to ground nursing in its heritage and traditions because I believe that getting in touch with these values will enable nurses to provide spiritual leadership and direction to a very troubled health care industry that has lost its purpose and identity. It is our hope that through this book we've connected the nursing leaders of the past, their vision and you. There is much work to be done, and I seek your help.

CRITICAL THINKING QUESTIONS

1. What is a good nurse?
2. Do you see yourself as a leader? If so, what qualities do you possess that define your leadership style?
3. My notions about the type of nurse I wanted to be were influenced by the nurses I met while in nursing school. Which nurse leader/leaders featured in this book exemplify the kind of nurse leader you want to be?
4. Peter Drucker used the phrase "knowledge worker." What does this mean to nursing?
5. What is your leadership story?
   Start living it and writing it today.

ACTIVITIES

1. Examine your career trajectory and select activities that are appropriate for where you are.
2. Examine and describe the values that you espouse and that give meaning to your practice. In your efforts to practice holistic nursing, nurture and support your own spirituality, and advocate for the unique spiritual and cultural needs of your patients.
3. Study the life and/or the writings of one nursing leader.
   Create your ideal curriculum vitae.
4. Identify concrete strategies to meet one or two life objectives each year.
5. Join a nursing organization and work toward achieving a leadership goal.
6. Become active in a civic or business group.
7. Encourage your colleagues to be nursing leaders.

ADDITIONAL SUGGESTED READINGS

Aiken, L, & Fagin, C. (1992). *Charting Nursing's Future: Agenda for the 1990's*. New York: J. B. Lippencott.

Fondiller, S. H. & Nerone, B. J. (1995). *Nursing: The Career of a Lifetime*. New York: National League for Nursing, Nursing Press.

Henderson, F. C. & McGettigan, B. O. (1994). *Managing Your Career in Nursing*. New York: National League for Nursing, Nursing Press.

Kelly, L., & Joel, L. (1995). *Dimensions of Professional Nursing* (7th ed.). New York: McGraw-Hill.

Styles, M. M., & Moccia, P. (1993). *On Nursing: A Literary Anthology*. New Yrok: National League for Nursing, Nursing Press.

Appendix A: Nursing's Agenda for Health Care Reform

This document is reprinted with the permission of the American Nurses Association. Although *Nursing's Agenda* is no longer in print, the central tenets of the document still apply to nursing's overall health advocacy and health reform efforts. It is a significant historical document for nursing in the twentieth century. It serves as published documentation of how organized nursing united with one voice to advocate equal access to affordable, quality health care for Americans. While our country debated national health care reform, nurses were there testifying to Congress, talking to community groups, and insisting that patients and their families were allowed to be part of the discussion. This reprint is provided for your review as you prepare to become one of nursing's leaders in the twenty-first century.

EXECUTIVE SUMMARY

America's nurses have long supported our nation's efforts to create a health care system that assures access, quality, and services at affordable costs. This document presents nursing's agenda for immediate health care reform. We call for a basic "core" of essential health care services to be available to everyone. We call for a restructured health care system that will focus on the consumers and their health, with services to be delivered in familiar, convenient sites, such as schools, workplaces, and homes. We call for a shift from the predominant focus on illness and cure to an orientation toward wellness and care.

The basic components of nursing's "core of care" include:

- A restructured health care system which:
  - Enhances consumer access to services by delivering primary health care in community-based settings.
  - Fosters consumer responsibility for personal health, self care, and informed decision-making in selecting health care services.
  - Facilitates utilization of the most cost-effective providers and therapeutic options in the most appropriate settings.
- A federally-defined standard package of essential health care services available to all citizens and residents of the United States, provided and financed through an integration of public and private plans and sources:
  - A public plan, based on federal guidelines and eligibility requirements, will provide coverage for the poor and create the opportunity for small businesses

and individuals, particularly those at risk because of preexisting conditions and those potentially medically indigent, to buy into the plan.

— A private plan will offer, at a minimum, the nationally standardized package of essential services. This standard package could be enriched as a benefit of employment or individuals could purchase additional services if they so choose. If employers do not offer private coverage, they must pay into the public plan for their employees.

- A phase-in of essential services, in order to be fiscally responsible:
  — Coverage of pregnant women and children is critical. This first step represents a cost-effective investment in the future health and prosperity of the nation.
  — One early step will be to design services specifically to assist vulnerable populations who have had limited access to our nation's health care system. A "Healthstart Plan" is proposed to improve the health status of these individuals.
- Planned change to anticipate health service needs that correlate with changing national demographics.
- Steps that reduce health care costs include:
  — Required usage of managed care in the public plan and encouraged in private plans.
  — Incentives for consumers and providers to utilize manage care arrangements.
  — Controlled growth of the health care system through planning and prudent resource allocation.
  — Incentives for consumers and providers to be more cost efficient in exercising health care options.
  — Development of health care policies based on effectiveness and outcomes research.
  — Assurance of direct access to a full range of qualified providers.
  — Elimination of unnecessary bureaucratic controls and administrative procedures.
- Case management will be required for those with continuing health care needs. Case management will reduce the fragmentation of the present system, promote consumers' active participation in decisions about their health, and create an advocate on their behalf.
- Provisions for long-term care, which include:
  — Public and private funding for services of short duration to prevent personal impoverishment.
  — Public funding for extended care if consumer resources are exhausted.
  — Emphasis on the consumers' responsibility to financially plan for their long-term care needs, including new personal financial alternatives and strengthened private insurance arrangements.

- Insurance reforms to assure improved access to coverage, including affordable premiums, reinsurance pools for catastrophic coverage, and other steps to protect both insurers and individuals against excessive costs.
- Access to services assured by no payment at the point of service and elimination of balance billing in both public and private plans.
- Establishment of public/private sector review—operating under federal guidelines and including payers, providers, and consumers—to determine resource allocation, cost reduction approaches, allowable insurance premiums, and fair and consistent reimbursement levels for providers. This review would progress in a climate sensitive to ethical issues.

Additional resources will be required to accomplish this plan. While significant dollars can be obtained through restructuring and other strategies, responsibility for any new funds must be shared by individuals, employers, and government, phased in over several years to minimize the impact.

NURSING'S AGENDA FOR HEALTH CARE REFORM

Nurses provide a unique perspective on the health care system. Our constant presence in a variety of settings places us in contact with individuals who reap the benefits of the system's most sophisticated services, as well as those individuals seriously compromised by the system's inefficiencies.

More and more, nurses observe the effects of inadequate services and of the declining quality of care on the nation's health. Firsthand experience tells us that the time has come for change. Patchwork approaches to health care reform have not worked. While preserving the best elements of the existing system, we must build a new foundation for health care in America. It is this realization that drives *Nursing's Agenda For Health Care Reform*.

Nursing's plan for reform converts a system that focuses on the costly treatment of illness to a system that emphasizes primary health care services and the promotion, restoration, and maintenance of health. It increases the consumer's responsibility and role in health care decision making and focuses on partnerships between consumers and providers. It sets forth new delivery arrangements that make health care a more vital part of individual and community life. And it ensures that health services are appropriate, effective, cost efficient, and focused on consumer needs.

A HEALTH CARE SYSTEM IN CRISIS

The strengths and weaknesses of our nation's health care system are well documented. Every day, many Americans profit from the system's technological excellence, extensive medical research, well-educated health professionals, diverse range of providers, and myriad of facilities. Millions of people live longer lives because of the care they receive.

But America's health care system is also very costly, its quality inconsistent, and its benefits unequally distributed. Although the system provides highly sophisticated care to many, millions of Americans must overcome enormous obstacles to get even the most elementary services. In short, health care is neither fairly nor equitably delivered to all segments of the population.

As caregivers in a diversity of settings, responsible for providing care and coordinating health care services 24 hours-a-day, nurses clearly understand the implications of the system's failings. The more than two million nurses in American are at the front lines—in hospitals, nursing homes, schools, home health agencies, workplaces, community clinics, and managed care programs. And what nurses see are the alarming effects of a system that has lost touch with the communities it is supposed to serve:

- More and more people must overcome major barriers to gain access to even the most elementary services.
- Too many Americans receive treatment too late because they live in inner cities or in urban or rural areas where service levels are inadequate.
- People enter hospitals daily in advanced stages of illness, suffering from problems that could have been treated in less costly settings or avoided altogether with adequate disease prevention and health promotion services.
- The lack of access to prenatal care contributes to an alarming number of infant deaths and low birth weights each year.
- Obstacles to obtaining fundamental services, such as childhood immunizations, are largely responsible for a resurgence in preventable diseases.
- Disproportionate amounts of resources are used for expensive medical interventions, which all too often provide neither comfort nor cure.
- Every year, expensive nursing home care impoverishes an alarming number of residents and their families.

Major changes in the health care system can no longer be put on hold. Further analysis and investigation will neither change the facts nor diminish the problems.

Today, more than 60 million Americans are either uninsured or underinsured. This fact alone cries out for health care reform. Now, the system's inability to contain costs is placing more and more Americans with "adequate" insurance coverage at risk of hardship when major illnesses do occur. Employers and employees alike are desperately seeking solutions to the dual problems of rising health care costs and increased premium rates that threaten basic coverage for most American workers and their dependents.

Americans cannot afford to sit idly and do nothing. Health care costs are approaching 12 percent of the gross national product (GNP). Health care is expected to cost over $756 billion in 1991.[1] If nothing is done to control expenditures, health care spending is expected to reach $1.2 to $1.3 trillion by 1995—an increase of some $500 billion in less than five years. At this rate, if the system remains unchanged, spending will reach between $2.1 and $2.7 trillion by the year 2000.[2]

THE FRAMEWORK FOR CHANGE

Nurses strongly believe that the health care system must be restructured, reoriented, and decentralized in order to guarantee access to services, contain costs, and ensure quality care. Our plan—the product of consensus building within organized nursing—is designed to achieve this goal. It provides central control in the form of federal minimum standards for essential services and federally defined eligibility requirements. At the same time, it makes allowances for decentralized decision making which will permit local areas to develop specific programs and arrangements best suited to consumer needs.

Nursing's plan is built around several basic premises, including the following:

- All citizens and residents of the United States must have equitable access to essential health care services (a core of care).
- Primary health care services must play a very basic and prominent role in service delivery.
- Consumers must be the central focus of the health care system. Assessment of health care needs must be the determining factor in the ultimate structuring and delivery of programs and services.
- Consumers must be guaranteed direct access to a full range of qualified health care providers who offer their services in a variety of delivery arrangements at sites which are accessible, convenient, and familiar to the consumer.
- Consumers must assume more responsibility for their own care and become better informed about the range of providers and the potential options for services. Working in partnership with providers, consumers must actively participate in choices that best meet their needs.
- Health care services must be restructured to create a better balance between the prevailing orientation toward illness and cure and a new commitment to wellness and care.
- The health care system must assure that appropriate, effective care is delivered through the efficient use of resources.
- A standardized package of essential health care services must be provided and financed through an integration of public and private plans and sources.
- Mechanisms must be implemented to protect against catastrophic costs and impoverishment.

The cornerstone of nursing's plan for reform is the delivery of primary health care services to households and individuals in convenient, familiar places. If health is to be a true national priority, it is logical to provide services in the places where people work and live. Maximizing the use of these sites can help eliminate the fragmentation and lack of coordination which have come to characterize the existing health care system. It can also promote a more "consumer friendly" system where services such as health education, screening, immunizations, well-child care, and prenatal care would be readily accessible.

At the same time, consumers must be the focus of the health care system. Individuals must be given incentives to assume more responsibility for their health. They must develop both the motivation and capability to be more prudent buyers of health services. Promotion of healthy lifestyles and better informed consumer decisions can contribute to effective and economical health care delivery.

Finally, in implementing reforms, attention must be directed to the unique needs of special population groups whose health care needs have been neglected. These individuals include children, pregnant women, and vulnerable groups such as the poor, minorities, AIDS victims, and those who have difficulty securing insurance because of preexisting conditions. Lack of preventive and primary care for this sector has cost the nation enormously—both in terms of lives lost or impaired and dollars spent to treat problems that could have been avoided or treated less expensively through appropriate intervention.

Access to care alone may not be sufficient to resolve the problems of these vulnerable groups. For those individuals whose health has been seriously compromised, a "catch up" program characterized by enriched services is justified. Coverage of pregnant women and children is critical. This first step represents a cost effective investment in the future health and prosperity of the nation.

It is this set of values that distinguishes nursing's plan from other proposals and offers a realistic approach to health care reform.

A PLAN FOR REFORM

Nursing's plan for health care reform builds a new foundation for health care in America. It shifts the emphasis of the health care system from illness and cure to wellness and care. While preserving key components of the existing system, it sets forth new strategies for guaranteeing universal coverage; making health care a more vital part of community life; and ensuring that the health care services provided are appropriate, effective, and cost-efficient.

The following pages provide a general overview of nursing's vision for a better health care system.

Universal Access to a Standard Package of Essential Services

Nursing's plan envisions a new and bold approach to universal access to a standard package of essential health care services and the manner in which these services are delivered.

The federal government will delineate the essential services (core of care) which must be provided to all United States citizens and residents. This standard package will include defined levels of:

- Primary health care services, hospital care, emergency treatment, inpatient and outpatient professional services, and home care services.
- Prevention services, including prenatal and perinatal care; infant and well-child care; school-based disease prevention programs; speech therapy, hearing, dental, and eye care for children up to age 18; screening procedures; and other preventive services with proven effectiveness.
- Prescription drugs, medical supplies and equipment, and laboratory and radiology services.
- Mental health services and substance abuse treatment and rehabilitation.
- Hospice care.
- Long-term care services of relatively short duration.
- Restorative services determined to be essential to the prevention of long-term institutionalization.

By taking this approach, traditional illness services are balanced with provisions for health maintenance services which prevent illness, reduce cost, and avoid institutionalization. Thus, hospital coverage and emergency care are covered, as are such services as immunizations, physical examinations, and prenatal and perinatal care.

The creation of federal minimum standards for essential services will necessitate modifications in existing public programs. The ultimate goal will be, over time, to merge all government-sponsored health programs into a single public program.

Coverage Options. Universal coverage for the federally defined package of essential services will be provided through an integration of public and private plans and resources.

- A public plan, administered by the states, will provide coverage for the poor (those below 200% of the federal poverty level), high-risk populations, and the potentially medically indigent. Any employer or individual will also have the option of buying into this plan as their source of coverage.
- Private plans (employment-based health benefit programs and commercial health insurance) will be required to offer, at a minimum, the nationally standardized package of essential services. This package could be enriched as a benefit of employment or individuals could purchase additional services from commercial insurers if they so choose.

All citizens and residents will be required to be covered by one of these options. Under both the public plan and private plans, no one will be denied insurance because of preexisting conditions. If employers do not offer private coverage, they will be required to pay into the public plan for their employees. Employer payments will be actuarially equivalent to the costs of employee and dependent coverage. Financial relief will be made available to small businesses (25 employees or less) for whom this provision would not be feasible. Individuals with no source of private coverage could also buy into the public plan. To assure universal coverage for essential services, systems will be developed to identify the insurance option through which each individual's needs are met.

Premiums and Payment Rates. Access to health care services will be enhanced by offering insurance premiums that the public can afford and payment rates to providers that are equitable and inclusive.

Both the public and private plans will utilize deductibles and copayments to ensure that beneficiaries continue to pay for a portion of their own care and, therefore, have financial incentives to be economical in their use of services. Deductible amounts and copayment rates, however, will never serve as barriers to care. Provisions will be made to waive or subsidize deductions and copayments for households with incomes below 200% of the federal poverty level. Deductibles for certain types of programs and services (e.g., health promotion, such as well-child care, immunizations, and mammograms; and managed care plans) will be held to a minimum to encourage wider use of cost-efficient, wellness-oriented options.

Public and private players will be required to offer fair and consistent rates of payment to providers. To protect access to care, providers will not seek payment at the point of service; nor will they be permitted to engage in balance billing. Because providers will be reimbursed fairly through insurance and the problems of uncompensated care will be largely eliminated, there will be no need for providers to charge consumers amounts above the established rate. Consequently, the consumer's financial responsibility for health care services will be more predictable.

To make insurance more affordable to individuals and to reduce costs to insurers and employers, nursing's plan calls for reforms in the private insurance market. These reforms may encompass a variety of strategies, including:

- Community rating for all insurers.
- A cap on the out-of-pocket expenses individuals must pay for catastrophic care, including nursing home and other long-term care.
- State reinsurance pools to protect insurers and consumers against high costs of insuring a broader range of patients.

Special Programs for Vulnerable Groups. Countless individuals suffer from long-term health problems associated with inadequate access to basic health services over time. Often, the poor and many members of minority groups are in this category. Special programs will provide services and outreach to vulnerable populations in order to compensate for formerly inadequate care and its consequences.

For infants and children (e.g., low birthweight babies, battered and neglected children, pregnant teenagers, children who abuse drugs, and young victims of violence and homelessness), such programming could be viewed as a health service ("Health-start") equivalent to the Headstart Program for those who are educationally disadvantaged. An expanded version of the Women's, Infants and Children (WIC) Program may be needed to produce quality outcomes in maternal-child health for poor and minority populations. Other special population groups also may warrant compensatory health programs beyond the scope of essential health benefits and services.

It is important to note that the ultimate goal of improved health is not achievable exclusively within the confines of the health sector. Social failures also have serious health consequences. Improvements in the broader environment have a major impact on health status and health care costs. While the focus of this plan is on the health care system, nursing's long-term policy agenda for the nation is much broader. National health reform must also consider the interrelationships between health and such factors as education, behavior, income, housing and sanitation, social support networks, and attitudes about health. Better health cannot be the nation's only goal when hunger, crime, drugs, and other social problems remain. Consequently, nursing is committed to pursuing reform in other areas affecting health. Discussion of such reform, however, is beyond the scope of this paper.

Long-Term Care. The high costs of long-term care often threaten to impoverish patients and their families. Nursing's plan seeks to prevent impoverishment and the potential loss of dignity by recognizing both public responsibility for long-term care and continued personal commitment to planning for such care. Financing arrangements will provide "front-end" coverage for chronic care and long-term care services of short duration through a variety of public and private options.

Beyond addressing short-term needs, individuals will be expected to assume personal responsibility for long-term care through strengthened private insurance programs and a variety of innovative financing arrangements. Such strategies will include privately purchased long-term care insurance, new savings and tax incentives, and home equity conversion opportunities. Such steps are essential to prevent individuals and their families from becoming impoverished by necessary care that can be anticipated and planned for. Emphasis on personal responsibility, however, does not ignore the fact that there will always be some individuals who will be left without resources and who must reach out for public assistance.

Catastrophic Expenses. Length and/or intensity of illness may generate catastrophic costs. Given this fact, limits will be placed on individuals' out-of-pocket payments for catastrophic health care expenses. Costs to insurers or individuals that exceed preset limits will be covered through a state reinsurance pool, to which all insurers must contribute. Under nursing's plan, insurers will tap into the pool when the cost of the insured exceeds preset limits. When costs decline, they will resume normal financing.

Decentralized Delivery System. Although standards for essential health services and eligibility requirements are to be mandated at the federal level, delivery mechanisms for health services will be decentralized in terms of planning and administration to foster greater consumer orientation. Because local needs differ, states will have the authority to modify implementation in order to reflect geographical diversity.

To promote greater use of disease prevention and primary health care, services will be delivered, whenever possible, in convenient, familiar sites readily accessible to households and individuals. Maximizing the use of local settings, including schools, homes, places of work, and other community facilities, will help reduce the fragmentation of primary health care delivery and promote a more consumer-friendly system.

Cost Effective, Quality Care

By properly balancing individual health needs and self care responsibilities with provider capabilities, care can be provided in a more efficient and coordinated manner. It can be more effectively directed at health promotion activities that will ultimately improve outcomes and reduce costs. Nursing's plan for reform is designed to achieve such a balance.

Provider Availability. Financial and regulatory obstacles, as well as institutional barriers, that deny consumer access to all qualified health professionals will be removed. The wider use of a range of qualified health professionals will increase access to care, particularly in understaffed specialties, such as primary health care, and in underserved urban and rural geographical areas. It will also facilitate selection of the most cost-effective option for care.

Under this arrangement, health providers must be reasonably and fairly compensated for their services. Where fee-for-service payment arrangements continue, payments for patient services must be made directly to providers.

Consumer Involvement. Consumers will be encouraged to assume more responsibility for their own health. Health professionals will work in partnership with consumers to evaluate the full range of their needs and available services. Together, the consumer and the health professional will determine a course of action that is based on an understanding of the effectiveness of treatment.

Outcome and Effectiveness Measures. Development of multidisciplinary clinical practice guidelines is essential to the proper functioning of the health care system. These guidelines will be used to sensitize providers and others to the proven effectiveness of practices and technologies. With clear-cut information on the value of various procedures, payers, providers, and consumers can work together to eliminate wasteful and unnecessary services. Moreover, increased dissemination of research findings regarding health care outcomes will enhance provider and consumer involvement in making the most effective choices about care and treatment. By taking this approach, the likelihood of serious disputes or litigation over appropriateness of care will be minimized. Likewise, the need for defensive practices designed to protect providers against malpractice suits will be greatly reduced.

Practice guidelines and directives derived from research, while providing an element of control, will be supportive of innovation. Coverage will be extended to procedures shown to be significantly more effective and less costly than existing approaches, and/or useful in improving patient outcomes and quality of life. At the same time, an effort will be made to carefully weigh new therapeutic approaches with high start-up costs that may ultimately be less expensive than present methods.

Use of advancements in clinical practice and technology will be conditioned on satisfying criteria related to cost efficiency and therapeutic effectiveness. Such an approach will not deny people essential services. It will, however, carefully assess the appropriateness of providing high-tech curative medical care to those who simply require comfort, relief from pain, supportive care, or a peaceful death.

Review Mechanisms. State and local review bodies—representative of the public and private sectors and composed of payers, providers, and consumers—will be established. These groups, operating under federal guidelines, will determine resource allocation, cost reduction approaches, allowable insurance premiums, and fair and consistent reimbursement levels for providers. Such review will be sensitive to ethical issues.

Managed Care. Managed care will be instituted both to reduce costs and to assure consumer access to the most effective treatments. Nursing's plan envisions managed care as organized delivery systems which link the financing of health care to the delivery of services—serving to maximize the quality of care while minimizing costs. To promote the use of managed care, enrollment in approved provider networks will be a requirement for those covered by the public plan. Managed care will also be encouraged for recipients of private coverage through reductions in deductibles and copayments.

In the past, managed care has been used, in many instances, to protect the pocketbooks of insurers rather than the rights of consumers. Managed care must be restructured to retain the maximum possible consumer choice and to place a premium on services that address the health of consumers.

Case Management. In contrast to managed care systems, case management is rooted in the client-provider relationship. Case management services will be used to integrate, coordinate, and advocate for people requiring extensive services. The aim of case management is to make health care less fragmented and more holistic for those individuals with complex health care needs. A variety of health care professionals are qualified to provide this service. The first allegiance of these providers will be to their clients. Acting as advocates, they will provide both direct care and negotiate with systems on behalf of their clients. They will be authorized to access services for a given client.

Both case management (provider) and managed care (delivery systems) models are important to the smooth functioning of the health care system.

A Realistic Plan of Action

Under nursing's plan, universal coverage will be achieved through implementation of both the public and private plan options. Employers will be motivated to collaborate with employees in shaping private plans which best satisfy their needs. At the same time, as larger numbers of more diverse groups participate in the public plan, the attractiveness of this option in terms of cost, quality, and image will be enhanced.

While the public and private sector plans can move forward simultaneously, it may be necessary to expand coverage to segments of the population in sequential steps. These steps would be introduced at an acceptable and financially reasonable rate until the ultimate goal of universal coverage is achieved. This approach would avoid excessive shocks to the health care system and allow the public to adjust to changing patterns of service.

Given this perspective, the first targeted population would include all pregnant women, children under age six, and those individuals who demonstrate a health status seriously compromised by a history of inadequate care. Improvements in coverage and benefits for these groups will have the greatest impact on the nation's future health and productivity.

As expeditiously as possible, other segments of the population would be covered. These groups might be targeted as outlined below; this sequence, however, is not necessarily intended as a rigid order:

- All children and young people, ages 6–18.
- All those above age 18 with incomes below 100% of the federal poverty level.
- All employees and dependents.
- All those with incomes below 200% of the federal poverty level.

The process will culminate with the merger of all entitlement plans into a single public program to provide coverage to all citizens and residents who do not have or cannot obtain coverage through a private plan.

The Fiscal Implications of Reform

It is impossible to predict the dollar amount which will be associated with the expansion of services or the efficiencies in nursing's plan. It is predictable that additional funding will be necessary to support start-up costs and transition. It is also possible that such expenditures will be recaptured over time.

A number of proposals for reform have been introduced. Among those proposals with cost estimates, additional health care costs range from $60–$90 billion.[3, 4] While nursing's plan for expanded coverage is similar in a number of ways to some of these proposals, offsetting proposed efficiencies integral to the plan will create significant dollars for reallocation. These resources will be directed to areas currently underfunded or excluded, including long-term care and primary care services.

While precise financial estimates are not possible at this time, several general observations can be made.

Cost Impact. Extension of coverage for essential services to the uninsured and underinsured will result in the dedication of more dollars. One source estimated that such coverage, if provided in 1990, would have added approximately $12 billion to health spending.[5]

It will also be necessary to dedicate more dollars to the expansion of long-term care services. Cost estimates for improved long-term care coverage vary. One 1990 study suggests that provision of comprehensive long-term care services, if implemented in 1990, would have cost $45 billion—$34 billion of which would have been new costs.[6] Nursing's plan, however, calls for more limited coverage supported through a combination of public dollars and enhanced personal responsibility.

In the initial phases of nursing's health care reform, the emphasis on preventive services will require dollars. Over time, however, improved health resulting from the availability of comprehensive primary health care services will produce a cost-reducing "health dividend." By placing greater emphasis on health promotion and disease prevention in community-based settings, the system will reach out aggressively to individuals and households to foster an increased commitment to healthy lifestyles, prevention of disease, periodic screening for early detection of illness and earlier treatment, and promote informed decision making by the consumer. All of this will contribute to cost-effective, early interventions which, over time, will reduce the need for more costly care.

Cost Savings. New costs associated with nursing's plan will be offset to a considerable degree by the following cost-saving initiatives:

- Required usage of managed care in the public plan and encouraged use in private plans.
- Incentives for consumers and providers to utilize managed care arrangements.
- Controlled growth of the health care system through planning and prudent resource allocation.
- Assurance of direct access to a full range of qualified providers.
- Development of health care policies based on effectiveness and outcomes research.
- Incentives for consumers and providers to be more cost efficient in selecting health care options.
- Elimination of unnecessary bureaucratic controls and administrative procedures, through such measures as standardized billing, simplified utilization review, streamlined administrative procedures, regulatory reforms, and consolidation of plans.

Sources of Revenue. To the extent that any additional dollars are needed, sources can be found. Responsibility for financing health care reform must be distributed equitably among individuals, employers, and government.

Individual will continue to pay a portion of health costs through copayments by households and individuals with incomes above 200% of the poverty level, and through reduced copayments for those whose incomes are 100–200% of the poverty level.

Employers will provide private health insurance that meets or exceeds minimum federal standards for their employees and dependents, or will provide coverage through the public plan. Accommodations will be made to provide small businesses with the necessary financial relief to meet this obligation.

State governments currently pay a portion of health care expenses for the poor and fund certain other health programs. Nursing's health care reform plan calls for consolidation of existing government health plans into a single public program. When this occurs, all states will contribute revenues to the program through maintenance-of-effort arrangements.

Revenues to pay for any increased costs could be derived from some combination of higher tobacco and alcohol taxes, additional payroll taxes, higher marginal income tax rates, and the increase or elimination of other income tax rates, and the increase or elimination of the income ceiling for FICA tax collection. A value-added tax (similar to a national sales tax) could also be considered.

A LOOK TOWARD THE FUTURE

The existing health care system stands as evidence of the futility of patchwork approaches to health care reform. America's nurses say it is time to frame a new vision for reform—time for a bold departure from the present. Reform of any single component of the system will not do the job. Insurance reform alone will not guarantee access to care if the health care delivery system is not restructured. Conversely, many people will remain unserved or underserved if health care services are so costly that millions of Americans cannot afford to purchase care.

To be most effective, a health care system must do more than provide equipment, supplies, facilities, and manpower. It must guarantee universal access to an assured standard of care. It must use health resources effectively and efficiently—balancing efforts to promote health with the capacity to cure disease. It must provide care in convenient, familiar locations. And it must make full use of the range of qualified health professionals and diverse settings for care. It is this insight that underlies nursing's plan for reform—making it the most viable solution to the nation's health care crisis.

SOURCES

1. U.S. Department of Commerce, 1991, *U.S. Industrial Outlook 1991*, Chapter 44, "Health and Medical Services," pp. 1–6.
2. National Leadership Coalition for Health Care Reform, 1991, "A Comprehensive Reform Plan for the Health Care System," p. 2.

3. *The Pepper Commission, A Call For Action: Final Report,* September 1990, p. 137.

4. Mark G. Battle, January 8, 1991, National Association of Social Workers, remarks during NASW's National Health Care Press Conference.

5. Lewin/ICF estimates, November 1990, *To The Rescue: Toward Solving America's Health Care Crisis,* Families USA Foundation, p. 13.

6. *Pepper Commission,* p. 151.

Nursing Organizations That Support *Nursing's Agenda for Health Care Reform* Are:

- Advocates for Child Psychiatric Nursing, Inc.
- American Academy of Nursing
- American Academy of Ambulatory Nursing Administration
- American Association of Colleges of Nursing
- American Association of Critical-Care Nurses
- American Association of Neuroscience Nurses
- American Association of Nurse Anesthetists
- American Association of Occupational Health Nurses
- American Association of Spinal Cord Injury Nurses
- American Holistic Nurses Association
- American Nephrology Nurses' Association
- American Nurses Association
- American Psychiatric Nurses' Association
- American Radiological Nurses Association
- American Society of Ophthalmic Registered Nurses, Inc.
- American Society of Plastic and Reconstructive Surgical Nurses
- American Society of Post Anesthesia Nurses
- American Urological Association Allied
- Association of Black Nursing Faculty in Higher Education, Inc.
- Association of Community Health Nursing Educators
- Association of Operating Room Nurses, Inc.
- Association of Pediatric Oncology Nurses
- Association of Rehabilitation Nurses
- Association of State and Territorial Directors of Nursing
- Chi Eta Sorority, Inc.
- Coalition for Psychiatric Nursing Organizations
- Commission on Graduates of Foreign Nursing Schools
- Dermatology Nurses' Association
- Emergency Nurses Association
- Florida Organization of Nurse Executives
- International Association for Enterostomal Therapy, Inc.
- Intravenous Nurses Society, Inc.
- Midwest Alliance in Nursing
- NAACOG, The Organization of Obstetric, Gynecologic, & Neonatal Nurses
- National Association of Hispanic Nurses
- National Association of Neonatal Nurses
- National Association of Nurse Practitioners in Reproductive Health

- National Association of Orthopaedic Nurses
- National Association of School Nurses, Inc.
- National Black Nurses' Association, Inc.
- National Conference of Gerontological Nurse-Practitioners
- National Federation for Specialty Nursing Organizations
- National Flight Nurses Association
- National League for Nursing
- National Nurses Society on Addictions
- National Nursing Staff Development Organization
- National Organization for Associate Degree Nursing
- National Organization of Nurse Practitioner Faculties
- National Student Nurses' Association
- New Jersey Association of Directors of Nursing Administrators/Long Term Care Facilities, Inc.

- North American Nursing Diagnosis Association
- Northeast Organization for Nursing
- Nurse Consultants Association
- Nurses House Incorporated
- Oncology Nursing Society
- Philippine Nurses Association of America, Inc.
- Society for Education and Research in Psychiatric-Mental Health Nursing
- Society of Gastroenterology Nurses and Associates
- Society of Otorhinolaryngology and Head-Neck Nurses, Inc.
- Society for Peripheral Vascular Nursing
- Southern Council on Collegiate Education for Nursing
- Western Institute of Nursing

Non-Nursing Organizations That Support *Nursing's Agenda for Health Care Reform* Include:

- American College Health Association
- Leukemia Society of America
- National Association for Health Care Recruitment

- New Jersey College Health Association

Reprinted with permission of the American Nurses Association.

Appendix B: Every Patient Deserves a Nurse

This brochure is reprinted for you with the permission of the American Nurses Association. It demonstrates organized nursing's efforts to inform the public of outcomes from quality care provided by *registered nurses,* and to protect public safety. This document was developed in the 1990s when hospitals in America were downsizing and replacing registered nurses with less qualified assistive personnel. After research based studies showed that care provided by registered nurses resulted in better outcomes for patients, and ultimately less cost for care because of fewer complications and more effective recoveries, this document was developed. In the future nurse leaders must continue to clearly define what it is that registered nurses do and the impact that care provided by registered nurses has on patient outcomes, and the valued role that experienced assistive nursing personnel can provide.

CONSUMER FACTS FROM THE AMERICAN NURSES ASSOCIATION

Every Patient Deserves a Nurse

In the fast-paced,
high-tech world
of modern health care,
it's hard to know what to ask
or whom to turn to.
The kind of nursing care
you receive while in the hospital
is extremely important,
and this brochure
will let you know what
to expect from the nurses
who care for you.

WHILE AT THE HOSPITAL, INSIST ON A REGISTERED NURSE

Did You Know?

Nurses are concerned about the quality of care you receive in hospitals. To save money, many hospitals are replacing registered nurses (RNs) with less trained and unlicensed workers, often called unlicensed assistive personnel, nurses aides, or patient care assistants. Nurses want to be sure that when you are sick you get safe care. When you are in the hospital, you expect and need a registered nurse to care for you.

The assistance that unlicensed personnel provide to nurses can be invaluable. The problems occur when these workers, who may have as little as four to six weeks of on-the-job training, substitute for nurses and provide direct care when you are seriously or critically ill—a job that they are not prepared to do safely. The few nurses who remain on the floor or unit are caring for many patients like yourself. An RN with responsibility for fewer patients will be able to provide you with higher quality care.

Quality Care

Research shows that you will recover better and faster when you receive care from registered nurses. After all, you have been hospitalized because you need around-the-clock nursing care.

Research studies have found that patients in hospitals with a higher number of registered nurses on staff have a shorter length of stay in the hospital, lower readmission rates, and fewer complications. In other words, your chances for a positive, healthy, and productive hospital visit increase when registered nurses take care of you.

Hospital Safety

A hospital is safely staffed when there are enough RNs on duty to provide direct clinical patient care activities. For example, RNs must be available to: monitor and assess your condition; respond and act quickly; and spend adequate time with you to answer questions and alleviate your concerns.

RNs are educated to provide patient care such as administering and monitoring the effects of medications; monitoring heart rate, blood pressure, and respirations; wound care; counseling; teaching; and any other activities that require specialized nursing skill and knowledge. Unlicensed aides can safely assist in providing a patient's basic hygiene and daily living needs by working closely with a registered nurse.

Every Patient Deserves a Nurse

After surgery, an RN monitoring your vital signs can check for bleeding, infections, and breathing problems. These are the most common concerns within the first 24 hours.

When an RN is monitoring your vital signs, he or she is combining these and other observations with his or her other education, skills, and professional judgment to develop a specific plan of care for you. An RN has the education and experience to make these judgments and to develop a plan of care that is essential to your recovery.

An RN can answer your questions so you can learn about your illness and recovery. If you are discharged on medications, you nurse will inform you about them. If you need assistance at home, your nurse will have suggestions and be able to teach you and your family members about your care. Time with your RN is essential to your recovery. As a consumer, you owe it to yourself to learn as much as you can about the care you will receive.

RNs in Action

- An elderly patient complains of shortness of breath. An RN assesses his condition and notes that he also has a rapid heart rate, a sudden unexplained weight gain, and is retaining fluid in legs and feet. By fully evaluating the patient's condition, the nurse recognizes the early signs and symptoms of heart failure.
- A teenager with a broken leg is hospitalized and placed in traction to stabilize the bone. On day five of her hospitalization, an RN notices a change in the oxygen level in her blood and a sudden rise in her temperature. By assessing her fully, the nurse can detect if the patient is at risk for a blood clot or fat embolism and take the appropriate action. If either were to go undetected, the result could be fatal.
- A diabetic patient who was in surgery 24 hours ago is given his morning insulin injection. During her rounds at the end of the day, an RN notices that the patient is unresponsive and is taking shallow breaths. The nurse checks the patient's chart and notes the patient vomited breakfast and lunch. By checking the patient's blood sugar level, the nurse determines that the patient may go into insulin shock, and works quickly to prevent the problem.

Remember . . . A Registered Nurse at the Bedside Is Your Best Safety Net

CHECKLIST FOR CONSUMERS TO ASSESS THE QUALITY OF NURSING CARE IN HOSPITALS

To make sure your hospital stay is as safe and productive as possible, call the hospital administrator's office and find out more. What follows is a list of suggested questions that will help you evaluate the care you can expect to receive in your hospital. If you are not satisfied with the nursing care in your hospital, ask your physician or other health care provider if you can be admitted to another hospital.

If you believe the care you are receiving is unsafe or of poor quality, you can contact the government agency that licenses hospitals in your state to register a complaint.

Pre-Hospitalization

- Will I have an RN caring for me?
- Will a plan of care be developed? How will I learn about the plan of care and how will staff caring for me learn about the plan?
- How many patients are assigned to each RN on the unit where I will most likely stay?
- Compare the number of RNs on the weekday, night, and weekend shifts.
- How does the hospital provide for RN staffing when there is an unexpected shortage in the unit?
- Will I be assessed by an RN at least once per shift?
- Will an RN provide education about what to expect before, during, and after medical procedures and treatments?

Hospitalization

- Will I have an RN assigned to me and will the RN be coordinating my care throughout my stay? What hours will my RN be there and assigned to me?
- What other health care personnel will be working with my RN? What are their qualifications? What tasks will they be doing?
- Will an RN review my plan of care with me? Will I understand who will be providing different aspects of my care?

Post-Hospitalization

- Will an RN discuss plans for discharge and follow-up with me?
- Will an RN teach me about medications, diet, activity, wound care, and what to expect when I get home?
- Will I need nursing care at home? If so, who will provide it? Has it been arranged?
- Whom can I call for answers to questions once I am at home?

Permission is granted to reproduce this document from American Nurses Foundation, Inc., Washington, DC. Copies of this brochure can be obtained by contacting ANF's Customer Service Center.

Appendix C: Nursing Bookmarks for the Internet

This summary of nursing bookmarks is an extension of Chapter 18 by Florence Huey, RN, MA. It is included for your use as you explore the Internet. Although the list is not exhaustive, it is intended to provide a good start for the nursing student who wants to investigate what nursing information is available as he or she surfs the web and explores Internet sites. Keep in mind that sites and addresses change from time to time. This list intends to give you enough information to have direction to explore for any of these bookmarks that may change over time.

Here is a small sample of the Web sites that may be useful or interesting to nurses. Nearly every site offers links to information on other sites. Some sites are only gateways to other sites, providing little or no original content themselves.

NURSING ORGANIZATIONS

Sites that contain .org in the URL clearly are Web sites maintained by organizations and usually feature information on membership activities and services, as well as links to affiliates with Web sites. Sometimes, an association's "site" is actually a section on an education site as an indicates.

- National Student Nurses' Association (NSNA) **<http://www.nsna.org>** This site includes information on the association's services and activities, plus links to sites maintained by the association's chapters and by other nursing associations.
- NursingWorld: The American Nurses Association **<http://www.ana.org>** or **<http://www.nursingworld.org>** It includes content on the history and structure of the association, background and full-text on nursing and health care policy and advocacy activities, plus links to Web sites of state nurses, the American Nurses Credentialing Center, and the National Student Nurses' Association.
- Sigma Theta Tau International Honor Society of Nursing **<http://sttiweb.inpui.edu>** It includes information on the history and activities of the association, such as research conferences, grants, and scholarships; membership information; and links to information on the history of nursing.

NURSING INFORMATION

- Academic Journal Directory **<http://www.son.utmb.edu/catalog/catalog.htm>** Published by the University of Texas School of Nursing, this site profiles 400 professional journals in clinical nursing, nursing education, research, and related health field where nurses can publish their work.

- NursingNet **<http://www.nursingnet.org>** It links to other sites rather than original content and includes links to National Library of Medicine, print publications, nursing schools, nursing associations, employment opportunities, and chat rooms/forums to talk with other nurses.

- Nursing.Net **<http://www.nursing.net>** This site (not to be confused with NursingNet above) contains forums for different interest areas, chat rooms, a book store, job search, and résumé writing assistance.

- Nurse Practitioner Support Services **<http://www.nurse.net>** This site primarily provides links to other Web sites such as Boards of Nursing, sites maintained by recruitment firms interested in working with advanced practice nurses, and educational offerings, but when the site was visited in August, 1997, it had not been updated since November, 1996. A more current visit to the site may show more recent updating.

- Nurses' Call **<http://www.nurses-call.org>** It features links to nurses' Web sites.

- NurseWire **<http://www.callamer.com/itc/nursewire>** This site features home pages of nurse entrepreneurs promoting their services.

- Virtual Nursing Center **<http://www-sci.lib.uci.edu/~martindale/Nursing.html>** A large, well organized resource center with links to a variety of information sources including: medical dictionaries, anatomy browsers, nursing case studies, pharmacology resources, and CEU courses. For students, there is a "Clinical Examination" section with tutorials on a variety of skills.

- Virtual Nursing College **<http://www.langara.bc.ca/vnc>** A site offering many resources for doing on-line searches, getting information on labs, diagnostic tests, and pharmacology. It also has links to job search sites.

- The WEBster **<http://www.cyberspy.com/~webster/index.html>** This is an eclectic site created by computer-nerd, pediatric nurse to provide patient and family support during illness; includes links to such health care resources as sites offering information on domestic violence, death and dying, hospices, funerals and burials, bioethics, transplants and organ donations.

- Whole Nurse **<http://www.wholenurse.com>** This features links to other nursing sites.

- World Wide Nurse **<http://www.wwnurse.com>** A site that contains hundreds of links to resources related to: nursing, developing a web page, web searches, and more. It will soon offer software reviews.

JOURNAL SITES

While some journal sites offer full-text articles, most offer only the article abstracts and perhaps the full-text of letters and editorials, but some may permit on-line ordering of articles.

- JAMA **<http://www.ama-assn.org>** This site of the American Medical Association offers information about the organization and its publications, such as JAMA. The publications feature abstracts of articles, letters to the editor, and medical news.

- New England Journal of Medicine **<http://www.nejm.org>** This site includes abstracts of original and special articles plus full-text of the case records, editorials, correspondence, and book reviews contained in each weekly edition of the New England Journal of Medicine.

- NursingCenter **<http://www.nursingcenter.com>** This expanded version of the AJN On-line, features abstracts from the American Journal of Nursing, MCN, Nursing Case Management, and Home Health Care Nurse. This site also includes nursing peer consultation forums, full-text CE articles, and career center; site plans to add a career-related feature, tentatively called *Build Your Own Home Page* that will allow nurses to create their own home pages on the site.

- SpringNet **<http://www.springnet.com>** This is the site of Springhouse, the publisher of *Nursing 1997, 1998, etc., Nursing Management,* and *The Nurse Practitioner.* It includes CareerDirectory, on-line CE tests, catalog for ordering books, videos, and copies of articles, plus nursing conference listings.

EDUCATIONAL SITES FOR HEALTHCARE PROFESSIONALS

- HealthAtoZ **<http://www.HealthAtoZ.com>** This is a self-described search engine for health and medicine. It is sort of a YAHOO-like site with a directory of more than 20 categories of health care topics such as "Nursing," "Medicine," "Diseases and Conditions," and "Diabilitites."

- MedConnect **<http://www.medconnect.com>** This site features continuing medical education, links to physicians' job placement, and to chapters of medical associations.

- Medscape **<http://www.medscape.com>** It features full-length, graphic-rich, and interactive articles that contain links to other pages within the site as well as to other sites. Access is free and unrestricted but registration on the first visit and logging in with a password for subsequent visits is required.

- Medical Matrix **<http://www.slackin.com/matrix>** This site features links to sites with full-text health care information by searching a term.

- Internet Mental Health **<http://www.mentalhealth.com>** This fist features full-text public domain articles and links to sites with full-text information on mental health for patients.

- International Network for Interfaith Health Practices: IHP Net **<http:///www. omteraccess.com/ihpnet/health.html#mgr>** This site features links to

CancerNet, to sites that provide parenting information, and to nursing and medicine-related search engines.

- OncoLink **<http://cancer.med.upenn.edu>** This site features disease and medical specialty menus for browsing and linking to information on the causes, prevention, and treatment of cancer. It includes links to government information sites like the National Cancer Institute and other Institutes within the NIH.

- University of Iowa Virtual Hospital **<http://vh.radiology.uiowa.edu>** This site provides patient care support and distance learning to practicing physicians and other health care professionals.

HEALTH INFORMATION SITES FOR CONSUMERS

- American Academy of Allergy, Asthma, and Immunology **<http://www.aaaai.org>** This site is an on-line physician referral database that provides information on the association.

- Disease Management Forums on Geenstone's Healthcare Solutions Site **<http://www.sapien.net/dm>** This site features live chat sessions on the 4th Wednesday of the month at 7 PM EDT.

GOVERNMENT SITES

- Agency for Health Care Policy and Research [AHCPR] **<http://www.ahcpr.gov>** This site provides full-text English- and Spanish-language clinical practice guidelines, quick reference guides for health care professionals, and consumer guides on such topics as pain management, depression, unstable angina, etc.

- Centers for Disease Control and Prevention **<http://www.cdc.gov>** This site includes full-text of the MMWR, treatment guidelines and recommendations, vaccine schedule.

- National Institutes of Health **<http://www.nih.gov>** This site includes clinical alerts, which are early findings from clinical trials, NIH Consensus Development Program statements on agreed-on treatment protocols, National Library of Medicine's Health Services/Technology Assessment Text (HSTAT), on-line resource of clinical practice guidelines, consumer brochures, and a search engine for locating NIH documents.

- Occupational Safety and Health Administration **<http://www.osha.gov>** This site contains text of worker health safety regulations and enforcement procedures.

- United States Department of Health and Human Services **<http://www.dhhs.gov>** This site provides links to the various agencies within DHHS, such as the Centers for Disease Control and Prevention (CDC), the National Institutes of Health (NIH), the Food and Drug Administration (FDA), and others.

JOB HUNTING ON-LINE

Several job sites have emerged on the Web. Some invite people to post their résumés by filling out on-line résumés. Some provide job search help, such as tips on résumé writing or interviewing. Some automatically notify job seekers when a job in their field becomes available. On-line job hunting makes it easy for a job applicant to check out a prospective employer if the company has a Web site. Below is a sample of the job banks that include positions and job placement services for professional nurses:

- Career Mosaic <**http://www.careermosaic.com**>
- Career Path <**http://www.career path.com**>
- Job Span <**http://www.jobspan.com**>
- Medsearch America <**http://www.medsearch.com**>
- Monster Board Career Center <**http://www.monster.com**>
- Online Career Center <**http://www.occ.com**>
- U.S. Labor Department's America's Job Bank <**http://www.ajb.dni.us**>

Appendix D:
Strategic Planning

This appendix is an extension of the Conclusion: Part 1 by Carol A. Andersen, BSN, RN. The Strategic Planning Model that follows is intended to be used to assist nursing students as they develop strategic plans for themselves and for the professional nursing groups that they will help lead.

A strategic plan is a three to five year plan that outlines where you or your group want to proceed. It may help to think of it as a combination of a road map, an itinerary, and a checklist for your journey. The *Strategic Planning Model* that follows is based on the concept of an umbrella. For those who have not been involved in strategic planning, it is offered as a simple first step to understanding the process.

The tip of the umbrella represents your *mission statement*. This will be a short statement of one or two sentences that share your "reason for being" as a nurse leader or as a group. If you apply the nursing process to your planning effort, this step involves broad *assessment*. Brainstorm words to describe what you do, or would like to do and your mission will emerge.

The *goals* of your strategic plan will be found as you move from your mission to the *diagnosis* of your areas of concern. It helps me to think of goals as the fabric on the umbrella. I would suggest that you develop six goals (approximately) for your strategic plan, with each one described by one or two words. Because these goals are not very functional at this point, you will want to further support them with objectives.

Your *objectives* will be the spines or supports of your umbrella that provide structure and a broad *plan* to your goals. Objectives make your goals time specific in a broad sense, as in "over the next three years" or "at the end of five years." The strategic plan is stronger, but still can't adapt easily to environmental changes.

The *implementation strategies* (represented by the center post of the umbrella) become the functional part of your plan that can support your objectives, goals, and mission statement. Through implementation strategies, you develop *interventions* that are more time specific and measurable than your objectives were.

The *evaluation* part of your strategic plan is the mechanism that most effectively makes the plan work. On the model, it is represented by the mechanical button on the center post that makes the umbrella quickly go up or down. The umbrella will work manually without the button, but it is slow, clumsy, and not as effective. In that same way your plan may, by chance, work without evaluation. But, you will be less assured of its timely success.

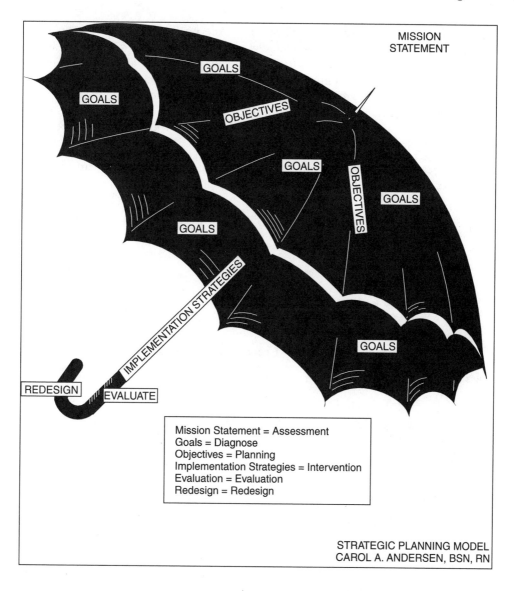

MISSION
STATEMENT

GOALS

GOALS

OBJECTIVES

GOALS

OBJECTIVES

GOALS

GOALS

IMPLEMENTATION STRATEGIES

REDESIGN

EVALUATE

GOALS

Mission Statement = Assessment
Goals = Diagnose
Objectives = Planning
Implementation Strategies = Intervention
Evaluation = Evaluation
Redesign = Redesign

STRATEGIC PLANNING MODEL
CAROL A. ANDERSEN, BSN, RN

Finally, and in my opinion most important, a step for *redesign* is added to your strategic plan. On the model, redesign is the handle of the umbrella that curves back up towards the objectives, goals, and mission statement. After recycling back up to your mission statement and back downward, the previous ideas and outcomes are applied as redesigned implementation strategies.

The secret to any successful strategic plan is to keep it dynamic by evaluating and redesigning frequently. In fact, when strategic plans are used by groups or organizations, responsibility for the implementation strategies, objectives, and goals should be assigned to one person or committee. Then at frequent planned intervals they should report back to the whole group in terms of progress, evaluation, and redesign that is needed. Of course for individual strategic plans the evaluation and redesign is done independently, or with a mentor. I hope that this model will assist you to become more comfortable in using strategic plans.

Although these suggested forms are formatted for use by a group, they can easily be adapted for individual use for personal strategic plan development.

STRATEGIC PLAN

Mission Statement:

1. Goal: (Use a page for each goal—I recommend 6 pages.)

Objective:

Implementation Strategies:

Assigned to:

STRATEGIC PLAN EVALUATION:

Assigned to:

Goal: (# and description of goal)

Objectives:

Implementation Strategies:

Evaluation:

Cost/Benefit Analysis (What were benefits/negative impacts of implementation strategies)

Detailed Summary

STRATEGIC PLAN EVALUATION (CONTINUED):

Recommendation:

Check One:

_____ **Redesign**   **Detailed**

                            Summary: _____

                            _____

_____ **Continue**

                            _____

_____ **Discontinue**

_____ **Completed**

Date_____

Signed_____ **, Chair** _____

Appendix E: Nursing Facts: RN Numbers and Demographics

This reprint of *Nursing Facts: RN Numbers and Demographics,* done with the permission of the American Nurses Association, is included to assist you in your assessment of the picture of nursing today. This data can also prove helpful to you in your own career choices as well as any future recruitment efforts of others into nursing.

NURSING FACTS FROM THE AMERICAN NURSES ASSOCIATION

Today's Registered Nurse—Numbers and Demographics

Registered nurses (RNs) are the largest segment of the health care work force. 2,239,816 people living in the United States are educated and licensed to practice as RNs, and 1,853,024 are employed RNs. RNs come from every socio-economic class, every state, and every neighborhood in America. This diversity grants them a special understanding of the people for whom they care. What follows is a statistical portrait of today's RN, compiled from *The Registered Nurse Population, Findings from the National Sample Survey of Registered Nurses, March 1992,* U.S. Department of Health & Human Services, Public Health Service, Health Resources and Services Administration.

Gender

Historically, more women than men have chosen nursing as a profession. That remains true today, but the trend may be changing. In 1992, only 4.3 percent of RNs employed in nursing were men. However, that number reflects a 97 percent increase from 1980 to 1992, in the number of men entering the profession. In the same period, the number of RNs grew by 35 percent.

Ethnic/Racial Background

White/caucasian RNs represent 90 percent of the population. Roughly 10 percent of the employed RN population come from non-Caucasian backgrounds. African-American RNs make up 4 percent of the population. Asian/Pacific Islanders account for 3.4 percent. Hispanics are 1.4 percent, and American Indian/Alaskan Natives are 0.4 percent of the RN population. RNs of non-Caucasian background most often practice in the Middle and South Atlantic states, as well as the East South Central and Pacific states. (See Geographic Distribution.)

Age

RNs reflect all demographics of this country, including age. As the typical American citizen ages, so does the typical RN. In 1992, only 11 percent of all RNs were under 30. More than 60 percent of RNs were 30–49 years old, with the average age being 43 years. These statistics are not so surprising when the average age at nursing school graduation is considered. For RNs who graduated in 1987 or later, the average age at graduation was 30 years. Now, RNs enter the work force later, with more life experiences to bring to the profession.

The Second-Career RN

The older RN brings not only general life experiences to the workplace, but usually specialized training as well. Almost 30 percent of RNs had worked in a health care occupation just before they entered nursing school. About two-thirds of these RNs had worked as nursing aides, and another 29 percent were licensed practical nurses or licensed vocational nurses. Another 8 percent had post-high school academic degrees—more than half had baccalaureates, and almost 27 percent of these had majored in liberal arts, followed by health-related majors (24 percent).

Family Status

A majority—72 percent—of registered nurses are married. Less than 17 percent are widowed, divorced or separated. The remainder have never married. More than half—55 percent—have children living at home, and 21 percent of all RNs have children under the age of 6. Almost a third of the RNs who are employed full-time in nursing have children.

Basic Nursing Education

To become an RN, candidates first must graduate from a state-approved school of nursing. The program may be a two-year associate degree program (usually based in community colleges), a three-year diploma program (usually hospital-based) or a four-year university program. Over the past 20 years, RNs have changed dramatically in the mode they have chosen for their basic nursing education.

In 1977, three-quarters of RNs graduated from diploma programs. Diploma programs were the first form of organized education for nurses. Usually associated with a hospital, the Diploma in Nursing combines classroom and clinical instruction. As nursing education has shifted from hospitals to academic institutions, fewer nurses are choosing this route. By 1992, the percentage of nurses who receive their basic nursing preparation in a diploma program dropped to 34 percent. Associated degree nurses accounted for 28 percent; nurses with bachelor's degrees made up 27 percent of the group. There was an obvious trend toward associate degree graduation—with 59 percent of all RNs who had graduated within the past five years getting an associate's degree. During that same period, 31 percent were baccalaureate graduates. Overall, 3 percent of the RNs in 1992 received their basic nursing education in a foreign country.

After earning their basic nursing preparation, about 21 percent of the RNs had completed additional education. Aside from RNs who sought graduate and post-graduate degrees, associate degree RNs and diploma nurses also returned for baccalaureate degrees. More then 60 percent of the RNs returning to school were enrolled in baccalaureate programs. Typically, the returning RNs attend class part-time while working full-time as nurses (65 percent).

Advanced Nursing Education

In 1992, 7.5 percent of the RNs had a Master's degree in nursing or a related field. The percentage of doctorally-prepared nurses was 0.5 percent. Of those with a Master's degree, 43 percent focused their graduate work on clinical practice. The doctorally-prepared RNs concentrated more often on education (36.8 percent) or on research (33.5 percent).

Financing Nursing Education

To pay for their education, 72 percent of RNs use personal resources. Employer reimbursement plans were used by 56 percent of RNs in 1992. Scholarships, grants, loans, and fellowships were listed by less than 15 percent of the nurses as the means they employed to finance their basic or graduate nursing education.

RNs ON THE JOB

Hospitals

In 1992, about two-thirds of employed RNs worked in hospitals, with almost 70 percent employed full-time. In the hospital, full-time RNs worked an average 41.6 hours during a survey week as opposed to the scheduled 39.4 hours. Younger RNs worked in hospitals—84 percent of all employed RNs under 30 worked in hospitals. Only half of those 50 and over did so. The vast majority of RNs in 1992 were employees of their facility. Only 2 percent relied on temporary agencies for their primary source of employment, and 2 percent were self-employed, a decline from 1988.

Within the hospital, 40 percent of RNs worked on general medical or surgical units. More than 18 percent worked in intensive care units. Just over 8 percent worked in operating rooms, and almost 7 percent staffed emergency rooms.

The types of patients that these RNs cared for at least 50 percent of the time included: coronary care, 16.7 percent; newborn infants and psychiatric patients, 7.5 percent each; pediatrics, 7 percent; obstetrics/gynecology, 5 percent; multiple units, 4 percent; chronic care, 3.3 percent; rehabilitation, 2.8 percent; and neurology, 2.4 percent. Just over 34 percent of RNs in hospitals had associate's degrees as their highest nursing education.

National average annual earnings for a hospital staff nurse: $36,618.

Community/Public Health

Almost 10 percent of RNs worked in community or public health settings in 1992, including health departments, visiting nurse services, non-hospital home health agencies, and substance abuse outpatient facilities, among others. More than 35 percent of those RNs held baccalaureate degrees.

National average annual earnings for a staff nurse in community/public health: $32,621.

Ambulatory Care

Almost 8 percent of RNs worked in ambulatory care settings, most of them physicians' offices. Other settings include nurse-based practices, freestanding clinics, health maintenance organizations and mixed professional practice groups. Just over 40 percent of these RNs had diplomas as their highest nursing educational preparation.

National average annual earnings for a staff nurse in ambulatory care: $27,949.

Nursing Home/Extended Care

Seven percent of RNs worked in nursing homes in 1992, which included those based in and out of hospitals, facilities for the mentally retarded and retired home residences. More than 45 percent of these RNs held diplomas as their highest nursing educational preparation.

National average earnings for a staff nurse in a nursing home: $31,298.

Other Areas

The remainder of nurses worked in: nursing education, 2 percent; student health, 2.7 percent; occupational health, 1 percent; and in miscellaneous areas, such as for state boards of nursing, health planning strategies and correctional facilities, 3 percent.

JOB DUTIES

In 1992, 69 percent of RNs spent at least half of their working time in direct patient care activities. A majority—52 percent—spent at least 75 percent of their time doing so. In general, RNs with diplomas and associate degrees spent more time (67 percent of their work time) in direct patient care. RNs with Master's degrees spent less than a third of their time in patient care. RNs with doctorates spent less than 7 percent of their time in hands-on patient care.

POSITION TITLES & AVERAGE ANNUAL EARNINGS

Of the registered nurses surveyed in 1992, 66 percent listed their position title as staff nurse. The average staff nurse working in all settings earned $35,212. (Hospital staff nurses reported $36,618.) Smaller proportions listed other position titles. Administrators (6.2 percent) earned $45,071. Instructors (3,.5 percent) earned $36,896. Supervisors (5 percent) earned $38,979.

Advanced Practice Nurses

Almost 140,000 RNs in 1992 reported having the education and credentials to work as advanced practice nurses. There are four categories of advanced practice nurses: clinical nurse specialists, nurse practitioners, nurse anesthetists, and nurse-midwives.

Clinical Nurse Specialist

To be a clinical nurse specialist, an RN must have earned a Master's degree in nursing that confers specialized knowledge, skills and training to the RN. Usually, the clinical nurse specialist works in a hospital, teaching patients and staff as well as consulting on complex patient cases. The RNs who fit this description numbered 58,185.

Average annual earnings of clinical nurse specialists: $41,226.

Nurse Practitioner

The 48,237 nurses who fit the description of nurse practitioner had received advanced education that culminated in a certificate or Master's degree. The practice area is an evolving one in which many states are allowing nurse practitioners the privilege of writing prescriptions and providing primary care to people. Almost 90 percent of this RN group practices in nursing, including 2,000 who had formal preparation as clinical nurse specialist as well as nurse practitioner.

Average annual earnings of nurse practitioners: $43,636.

Nurse Anesthetists

The oldest advanced nursing specialty is that of nurse anesthetist. Approximately 25,238 nurses in 1992 were nurse anesthetists. These RNs complete formal preparation beyond their basic nursing education, usually a two-year program. They administer anesthesia in a variety of settings from operating rooms to dentists' offices.

Average annual earnings of nurse anesthetists: $76,053.

Nurse-Midwives

The smallest group of advanced practice nurses is that of nurse-midwife. Slightly more than 7,400 RNs were nurse-midwives in 1992. They had completed formal education of at least 9 months in length after their basic nursing preparation. Nurse-midwives attend to or assist in childbirth in various settings, including hospitals, birthing centers and homes. They are also involved in well-woman care.

Average annual earnings of nurse-midwives: $43,636 (same as nurse practitioner).

CERTIFICATIONS

Certification is the process by which RNs establish that they have specialized knowledge of particular practice areas—for instance, critical care, medical/surgical care, pediatrics, geriatrics, etc. The 1992 survey found that certification made a difference in the employment status of advanced practice nurses. No information was given for RNs other than those in advanced practice positions.

- For clinical nurse specialists, 7,877 were certified by a national organization. The certified clinical nurse specialists were more likely to be employed than their noncertified peers, and also they were more likely to have a position title of clinical nurse specialist.
- About 58 percent of nurse practitioners were certified by national organizations. Of those who were certified, 95 percent were employed in nursing and were more likely to have the title of nurse practitioner.
- For nurse anesthetists, most had national certification. Of the certified registered nurse anesthetists (CRNAs), 93 percent were employed in nursing.
- Two-thirds of the nurse-midwives were certified by national organizations. At least half of these practiced nursing with the title of certified nurse-midwife.

GEOGRAPHIC DISTRIBUTION

The geographic distribution of RNs reflected the general population spread of the United States. Accordingly, more RNs practice on the East Coast (approx. 42 percent) and in cities than anywhere else (approx. 69 percent). The concentration of nurses was densest in New England with 991 employed nurses per 100,000 population, and it was sparsest in the West South Central states with 537 employed nurses per 100,000 population.

New England: Connecticut, Maine, Massachusetts, New Hampshire, Rhode Island, Vermont

This region represented 7 percent of the employed RN population. Fewer RNs were employed in hospitals in this region (62 percent), and more RNs worked in nursing homes (11 percent). It had the largest percentage of nurses with a diploma as the highest nursing preparation (41.9 percent), and the largest percentage of its population had a Master's degree in nursing (6.4 percent). Almost 3 percent of this region's RN population was from a non-Caucasian background.

Regional average annual salary for full-time RNs in staff positions: $37,785.

Middle Atlantic: New Jersey, New York, Pennsylvania

This region represented 18 percent of the employed RN population. A larger portion (4.5 percent) of this RN group worked in student health service than any other region. About 12.5 percent of this region's RN population was from a non-Caucasian background.

Regional average annual salary for full-time RNs in staff positions: $37,225.

East North Central: Illinois, Indiana, Michigan, Ohio, Wisconsin

This region represented 18 percent of the employed RN population. Approximately 5.4 percent of this region's RN population was from a non-Caucasian background.

Regional average annual salary for full-time RNs in staff positions: $33,453.

West North Central: Iowa, Kansas, Minnesota, Missouri, Nebraska, North Dakota, South Dakota

This region represented 8 percent of the employed RN population. Slightly more than 3 percent of this region's RN population was from a non-Caucasian background.

Regional average annual salary for full-time RNs in staff positions: $33,641.

South Atlantic: Delaware, District of Columbia, Florida, Georgia, Maryland, North Carolina, South Carolina, Virginia, West Virginia

This region represented 17 percent of the employed RN population. A tenth of this region's RN population was from a non-Caucasian background.

Regional average annual salary for full-time RNs in staff positions: $34,058.

East South Central: Alabama, Kentucky, Mississippi, Tennessee

This region represented 5.5 percent of the employed RN population. A larger portion (11.8 percent) of the RN workforce practiced in community/public health than any other region, and the smallest percentage (1.6 percent) worked in student health. Almost 38 percent of the RN population has an associate's degree as the highest nursing preparation. It had the highest proportion of RNs who were 29 years old and younger (14.9 percent). About 8 percent of this region's nurses was from a non-Caucasian background, including the largest proportion (6.7 percent) of RNs who were identified as African-American.

Regional average annual salary for full-time RNs in staff positions: $32,227, the lowest of all the regions.

West South Central: Arkansas, Louisiana, Oklahoma, Texas

This region represented 8 percent of the employed RN population. It had the highest proportion of RNs in the age group of 30–49 years old (65.6 percent) and the lowest proportion of RNs who were 50–64 years old (15.7 percent). About 11.2 percent of the RN population in this region was from a non-Caucasian background.

Regional average annual salary for full-time RNs in staff positions: $33,641.

Mountain: Arizona, Colorado, Idaho, Montana, Nevada, New Mexico, Utah, Wyoming

This region represented the smallest proportion of RNs nationally—5 percent of the employed RN population. Almost 6 percent of this region's RN population was from a non-Caucasian background. It includes the largest proportion (0.9 percent) of American Indian/Alaskan Native RNs.

Regional average annual salary for full-time RNs in staff positions: $32,551.

Pacific: Alaska, California, Hawaii, Oregon, Washington

This region represented 8 percent of the employed RN population. Of all the regions, it had both the highest percentage of RNs in the 50–64 age group (24.1 percent) and the lowest percentage of RNs in the category of 29 years and younger (6.1 percent). This region had the largest portion (16 percent) of RNs from a non-Caucasian background, with the most represented group being Asian/Pacific Islander (9.5 percent). Also, the Pacific region included the largest portion (2.7 percent) of Hispanic RNs.

Regional average annual salary for full-time RNs in staff positions: $41,315, the highest of all the regions.

SOURCE

Moses, E. B. (1992, March). *The Registered Nurse Population, Findings from the National Sample Survey of Registered Nurses, March 1992*, U.S. Department of Health & Human Services, Public Health Service, Division of Nursing, Health Resources and Services Administration.